THE FLUORIDE WARS

THE FLUORIDE WARS

How a Modest Public
Health Measure Became
America's Longest-Running
Political Melodrama

R. ALLAN FREEZE
JAY H. LEHR

WILEY

A JOHN WILEY & SONS, INC., PUBLICATION

Library of Congress Cataloging-in-Publication Data:

Freeze, R. Allan.
    The fluoride wars : how a modest public health measure became America's longest-running political melodrama / by R. Allan Freeze.
       p.   cm.
    Includes index.
    ISBN 978-0-470-44833-5 (cloth)
    1. Water–Fluoridation–United States–History.   2. Pressure groups–United States–History.   I. Title.
    RA591.7.F74 2009
    362.19'76010973–dc22

                                                        2008045482

Printed in United States of America

10 9 8 7 6 5 4 3 2 1

CONTENTS

ACKNOWLEDGMENTS

We wish to thank Rick Freeze and Lorna Richardson for their helpful comments on an early draft of the book. Gary Derksen reviewed much of the technical presentation from a dental research perspective and made many useful suggestions. Warren Wood and Frank Schwartz provided supportive reviews of the final manuscript.

We appreciate the efforts made on behalf of this book by our original agent, Janet Rosen of Sheree Bykofsky and Associates in New York.

The book would never have seen the light of day without the support and encouragement of Bob Esposito of John Wiley & Sons. We thank him for taking a chance on this offbeat slice of Americana.

Michael Leventhal and Rosalyn Farkas carried this book through the publication process at wiley with efficiency and goodwill.

A. R. F.

CHAPTER 1

A STORY OF OUR TIMES

The first purposeful fluoridation of a public drinking water supply took place in Grand Rapids, Michigan, in the late afternoon of Thursday, January 25, 1945. A technician working under the direction of W. L. Harris, chief chemist of the city waterworks, donned a face mask to protect against inhalation of fluoride dust, and working barehanded, dumped a barrel of powdered sodium fluoride into the hopper of the city's newly designed fluoridation system. A few minutes later, the first artificially fluoridated water in the world coursed through the pipes of the Grand Rapids water distribution system.

It seemed such a simple act at the time. A tap was turned, and water that had been chlorinated for many years without much fuss now carried a second chemical supplement to help keep us healthy. Soon, the taps would be turned in city after city across the nation. For most, it was another blessing bestowed on us by modern medical science. But for some, it was one chemical too many.

This book traces the history of how that simple act came to pass and what has happened since. It is a tangled tale of intrigue that starts as a medical mystery story and ends in political farce. It involves the use and misuse of science. It features persons of goodwill and bad, engaged in a bitter struggle for the public high ground. There are personality conflicts, unfair accusations, and ruined reputations. Political machinations and ethical conundrums abound. In short, it is a story of our times.

GRAND RAPIDS, MICHIGAN, FOUR O'CLOCK EASTERN WARTIME

The activities at the city waterworks in Grand Rapids on January 25, 1945, heralded the beginning of an experimental trial of water fluoridation that had been under consideration for several years. The trial was designed,

The Fluoride Wars: How a Modest Public Health Measure Became America's Longest-Running Political Melodrama By R. Allan Freeze and Jay H. Lehr
Copyright © 2009 John Wiley & Sons, Inc.

promoted, and carried out by the U.S. Public Health Service. The organizers hoped that the results would confirm the emerging consensus of the dental research community that regular ingestion of fluoridated drinking water would reduce the incidence of childhood tooth decay and improve the dental health of the nation. The children of Grand Rapids were the experimental subjects who would help confirm or refute this hypothesis.

If we could take ourselves back to Grand Rapids in early 1945, we would find a blue-collar city manning the homefront in the waning days of World War II. The city's thriving furniture trade was largely converted to wartime production. With the men off fighting for freedom in faraway lands, the women of Grand Rapids pulled double duty, staffing the production lines at the plants while shepherding their families through the daily crises of everyday life.

Like most Americans, the citizens of Grand Rapids were caught up in the optimism that the war would soon be over. Every evening they gathered around the radio cabinet in the living room and listened carefully as it crackled with the latest news of the world. Franklin Delano Roosevelt had just recently been inaugurated for his third term as president. The Allies had liberated Paris and were setting up shop for the final capitulation of the Third Reich. In the Pacific, American forces were leading the assault on a small island named Guadalcanal. After six years of bitter fighting on two fronts, peace was on the horizon. The men would soon be home.

Those who stayed on to listen to the local news that evening would learn that an event of some significance had taken place right in their own city, and it had nothing to do with homefront efforts to win the war. In the news item, the citizens of Grand Rapids were reminded that their city had been selected by the Public Health Service to be the flagship city in a historic experiment, and that this important study was now under way. For those close to the situation, the launching of the fluoridation trial was the culmination of many years of medical sleuthing, scientific study, and intense strategic planning. The fact that it reached fruition in the waning days of the war, with hopes running high and optimism for the future in ready supply, was largely serendipitous. In due course, the result of their experiment would have its own impact on the affairs of the nation.

On that wintery January morning in Grand Rapids, the trees were bare of leaves, the air brisk. That morning, a long-awaited shipment had arrived at the waterworks: a carload lot of 107 barrels, each containing 375 pounds of sodium fluoride. It was planned to introduce this chemical into the city water supply barrel by barrel over the next several months, and then, all going well, for several more years, in such a way as to produce a dissolved fluoride concentration in the water of exactly 1.0 part per million (ppm). Scientists at the Public Health Service deemed this to be the optimal concentration for the enhancement of dental health.

On that cold winter morning, the barrels were unloaded and trundled across the works yard to a building that housed the primary pumping station for the city. In that building, a small team of engineers and technicians had just completed one last check on the basins, hoppers, filters, and tanks that would be used to blend the sodium fluoride into the Grand Rapids water distribution network. The system was designed carefully to keep the fluoride content of the water within a hair of the desired 1.0 ppm concentration. Careful checks and balances were built into the system to ensure against any mechanical failure that could lead to an overfeed.[1] At exactly 4:00 P.M. Eastern Wartime, the first hopper of fluoride was released into the pipes. The fluoridation era had begun.

THE LONGEST-RUNNING CIRCUS IN TOWN

The events in Grand Rapids took place with little fanfare and almost no opposition. There were a few letters to the editor from local cranks, but by and large the citizens of Grand Rapids were solidly behind the enterprise. The *Grand Rapids Herald* crowed about how the city had been selected to confirm this historic medical breakthrough. Even those folks who didn't read the paper knew all about it, because for the previous year, all the children, from those in the first grade to those in the higher grades, had undergone an examination of their teeth by a team of dental examiners brought in especially for this purpose by the Public Health Service. Remarkable pictures exist in the Public Health Service archives of little girls lined up in school hallways, and young boys bravely undergoing their examinations in the primitive dental facilities set up in the back of Grand Rapids classrooms.

None of the participants knew then what they had unleashed: that this modest public health measure would become one of the most contentious issues of our lifetime. Certainly, the student subjects did not see the coming conflict, nor I suspect did Mr. Harris and his team of engineers at the waterworks. It was probably not even high on the list of concerns of the dental research community in the Public Health Service in Washington who had put the process in motion. Sixty years later, all is clear. But it wasn't then.

In retrospect, we can see the fluoridation issue in all its complexity. In many ways, it offers a mirror on late twentieth-century America. Fluoridation belongs on the long list of social developments that swept into the public conscience on the wings of scientific achievment. There are many parallels with the development of nuclear power, for example, or with the development of genetically altered food production, or with the chemical revolution that put thousands of new organic chemicals into widespread industrial production. All of these developments brought great benefits, but they also brought risks to human health: some real, some perceived. All required strong public funding and legislative support for their development. Ultimately, they all required regulatory legislation to protect society against the risks. Like the pasteurization of milk and the iodization of salt, fluoridation was delivered publicly rather than privately. Those that wished to avoid the governmental benevolence had to work to do so. In all these cases, the greater good of the many was given precedence over the fears of a few. In all these cases, a vibrant opposition eventually arose that instigated adversary litigation, influenced public policy, and affected political life.

In the years following the Grand Rapids trial, as fluoridation began to spread through the cities and towns of the nation, the voices of opposition began to be heard. Whispers of dissent rose to the surface in public discussions of the issue. Questions were raised about the wisdom of a community-based approach to dental health, the effectiveness of the scheme in reducing dental caries, the costs of the effort, and the safety of the delivery systems. Whispers turned into audible static. Some people bridled at what they saw as involuntary mass medication or an unacceptable government intrusion into their private lives. Intemperate voices shouted loudest. They shouted about health problems, and odd diseases, and secret government plots.

Some of you may remember when the fluoridation circus first came to your town. Perhaps you were a young suburbanite with two small kids, ensconced in your first new house, which was mortgaged to the hilt. When the civic election came along you mulled over the mayoral choices, paying scant attention to the fluoridation referendum that was also on the ballot. Given the almost universal support for fluoridation that was coming from every medical and dental quarter, you assumed that this measure was sure to pass. You viewed the proposition as a formality: a motherhood issue, like saving the whales or supporting the troops at war. But then, much to your surprise, the hubbub began. Suddenly, full-page ads began to appear in the paper screaming "poison" and "cancer." Self-proclaimed experts on both sides of the question descended on the city and filled the local halls with cheering devotees and hostile antagonists. Local lobby groups sprang up like weeds. Pro- and anti-fluoride signs popped up on the lawns of neighbors you had taken for apolitical. You may remember the pro-fluoride ads with the kindly white-haired dentist in his pressed lab coat peering out from your TV set, asking you if you loved your children. You may also remember a pleasant older lady who looked like your grandmother handing out pamphlets at the mall that featured a tap dripping little skulls and crossbones into a sink.

"Do you favor the addition of fluoride to the city drinking water supply for the purpose of childhood cavity prevention?" the ballot read. "Vote *yes* if you love your children," said the kindly white-haired dentist. "Vote *no* if you don't want to poison your children," screamed the pamphlet. You didn't really have time to look into it. In the end, you identified more with the kindly dentist than the wild-eyed pamphlet. You voted *yes*. To your surprise, you were in the minority. The measure was defeated, and the city returned to normal.

So is this all that fluoridation means to us after all the hue and cry: an excuse for dredging up memories of our youth? To be sure, the entire subject of fluoridation has a ring of the past about it. Surely, you are thinking, this is a tale of the 1950s, not of the new millenium. Elvis Presley wiggling his bum on TV. Hula hoops and bomb shelters. Beach blanket bingo.

Devotees of classic movies will remember the famous scene in Stanley Kubrick's film *Doctor Strangelove, or How I Learned to Stop Worrying and Love the Bomb*. Colonel Jack Ripper, commander-in-chief of Burpelson Air Force Base, played over the top by character actor Sterling Hayden, finally confirms what the viewer has suspected all along: that he is as mad as the March Hare. The man who has his finger on the red button that could blow up the world is certifiably unhinged. And how does he clarify this critical point in the story line? He does so by declaring that the fluoridation of our public water supplies is a communist plot, designed to lower America's guard through postcoital exhaustion. "Fluoridation," he says, is sapping Americans of their "precious bodily fluids."

But *Doctor Strangelove* is old news. Surely by now, satirizing kooky anti-fluoridationists wouldn't get much of a rise. Surely by now, fluoridation is a done deal, a genuine medical breakthrough that has saved our children from those dreaded trips to the dentist and the jackhammer whine of his evil drill. "Look, Ma. No cavities," say the smiling children in the old Crest ads, as they run toward their mother's outstretched arms. Who could argue against no cavities and a mother's love? Certainly not the American Dental Association, or the Surgeon General, or anybody else that matters, all of whom say that fluoride is good for you. That ought to be enough for most of us.

And so it is for most of us, but not for all of us. Even today, many citizens remain wary. Fluoridation of public water supplies has been practised widely now for over 60 years, but the issue just won't go away. The dental community continues to sing its praises, but local grassroots anti-fluoridation groups spring up like topsy every time the question surfaces. Concern over fluoridation is not just a thing of the past. It is an ongoing, never-ending American obsession. In the past decade, the citizens of more than 50 U.S. cities have faced the fluoridation issue yet again. In many cases it was the second time, or the third time, or in one case the fifth time that the battle had been fought in the same city. Most were local referendums. Some were statewide initiatives. Some were administrative decisions by city council. Some of the measures set out to fluoridate water supplies for the first time. Others tried to put a stop to existing fluoridation programs. Yet others tried to reinstitute past programs that had once been approved, then later repealed. There were measures to revoke city charters, and measures that would have broken state law if the voters had approved them. All took place in an environment of heated debate. Most votes ended up within a point or two of 50:50.

It seems that times haven't changed that much after all. Back in the 1950s, at one famous anti-fluoridation rally, a large vat of fluoridated water stood at one side of of the lectern labeled "rat poison," while speakers drank copiously from a pitcher on the other side marked "pure water."[2] Scroll forward to October 2000 in Mesa, Arizona, where Republican state representative Karen Johnson announced that she would move out of the city to avoid "the poison" if a fluoridation initiative passed in that city.[3]

At a public meeting during a fluoridation referendum in Connersville, Indiana, Rusty Ammerman, a fluoride supporter and traveling magician, consumed an entire tube of fluoride toothpaste just to prove that it wouldn't kill him. The anti-fluoride faction claimed that he had used sleight of hand to switch to a tube of nonfluoridated paste.[4]

In Gilbert, Arizona, the town's plan to add fluoride to its water supply won council approval despite heated opposition from the wife of the man who would have to oversee the change. Shelley Frost, wife of public works director Lonnie Frost, called fluoride "a toxic waste product" that could be harmful to children. "Thank goodness we're living in a world where Lonnie's wife feels she can say that," commented one councilman before voting in favor of the initiative.[5]

Referendums turn into armed combat. Public voices rise to a fever pitch. Personal animosities emerge, the information highway lurches into gridlock, and the politicians run for cover, hurling their best double-speak platitudes into the wind, sensing another no-win issue.

PRO OR CON?

You must be wondering by now where this book fits in. Is it going to be a pro-fluoridation hymnary, patting the medical establishment firmly on the back? Or is it going to be an anti-fluoridation diatribe, full of secret tales and dark conspiracies? Well, believe it or not, it is neither. Or perhaps, it is both.

The objective of this book is to present a social history of the fluoridation debate in the United States. There are wonderful stories to be told of the pioneering dentists and the research that led to their early public health victories. There are equally colorful tales of the lonely crusaders; the unfashionable Don Quixotes who fought fluoridation as if it were the work of Satan himself. Larger-than-life characters abound on both sides of the political fence, people of high principles and unbendable opinions. Their views, like those that swirl around the question of abortion, present a clash of absolutes.[6] The members of each group see only their own side of the argument. The views put forth by those on the other side produce incredulous frustration, even rage. Each group sees its members as honest and compassionate and at work on behalf of the public interest. Each group is suspicious of the motives of their opponents. They see nothing there but selfishness, thickheadedness, money, and greed.

In this book you will meet many of these protagonists. We trace the lifelong odysseys of Darlene Sherrell, the crusty *grande dame* of the Stop Fluoridation movement, and of John Yiamouyiannis, who believed that he had proof of a link between fluoridation and cancer. On the other side of the fence, we will meet Michael Easley, the founder of the National Center for Fluoridation Policy and Research and one of the chief pro-fluoridation spokesman for the American Dental Association; and Stephen Barrett, whose "Quackwatch" website disparages all those who do not recognize the miracle of fluoridation.

What will these two antagonistic groups think about this book? Both will probably be suspicious of our attempts to find middle ground. The antifluoridationists will assume that we are two more parrots of the American Dental Association and the U.S. Public Health Service, soft-pedaling a further cover-up of the poisoning of our water supplies. The pro-fluoridationists will worry about our establishment credentials, nervously flipping through to later chapters to see if we are toeing the establishment line. Or are we another pair of kooks that they will have to waste time debating? Or worse yet, a couple of reputable scientists to add to the list of those who have fallen off the wagon?

Well, we are none of these things. In this book we lead you through the story not as protagonists, but as questers. We trace the history and search out the facts. If you already have a strong opinion, I suggest that you try to park it in a corner for awhile. This is far too good a yarn to rush to judgment. It will come as a surprise to those of firm views, but there is some truth on both sides of the fence. Things are not black and white. We hope that rather than solidifying your position, the book will give you more sympathy for those of alternative viewpoints, more compassion for their concerns, and more curiosity about how things have come to such a pass.

Ultimately, we will find some reasoned positions to defend. We are sorry to say that they will probably not please the antis. We're pretty sure that they won't please the pros either. In the clash of absolutes, it isn't possible to gain the love of those on either pole unless you are willing to join their organization and use their secret handshakes. As we make our way through the historical record, the scientific evidence, the personal enmities, the complexities of motive, the legal challenges, and the political battles, we hope it will become clear that neither polar position is entirely tenable.

But remember! It is the trip that matters, not the finish line. All we promise is good company on the trek through the maze. Feel free to find your own destination.

REFERENCES

1. This brief description of the fluoridation of the Grand Rapids water supply is taken from R. R. Harris, *Dental Science in a New Age: A History of the National Institute of Dental Research*, Montrose Press, Rockville, MD, 1989; and F. J. McLure, *Water Fluoridation: The Search and the Victory*, National Institute of Dental Research, Bethesda, MD, 1970. A more complete description is included in Chapter 5.

2. J. M. Burns, The crazy politics of fluoride, *New Republic*, July 13, 1953, pp. 14–15.

3. *The Arizona Republic*, August 20, 1999.

4. http://www.CNN.com, November 1, 1999.

5. *The Arizona Republic*, April 27, 2000.

6. This term, which also forms the title of the next chapter, is taken from Laurence H. Tribe, *Abortion: The Clash of Absolutes*, W.W. Norton, New York, 1990.

CHAPTER 2

A CLASH OF ABSOLUTES

There was a time not so long ago when a writer embarking on research for a new book began in the library, combing the dusty shelves to clarify the historical record and perusing current periodicals to learn of the latest breakthroughs. Luckily for those of us who love rooting around library stacks, this step is still necessary. But it is no longer the first step. In the new millennium, the first step is to crank up your PC and start surfing the Internet.

The first time either of us brought up Google and typed in the keyword *fluoridation*, it was pure curiosity. We had no idea that we were about to encounter the massive fluoridation subculture, let alone join it. With alarming speed that is totally outside anyone's ability to comprehend, Google somehow assessed the relevance of 1,346,966,000 websites from all around the world in 0.08 second and produced a list of 47,300 sites having something to do with fluoridation. Well, actually it didn't produce the entire list, only the first 20 sites, ranked in order of relevance, with a promise that we could look at the other 47,280 if and when we desired to do so.

Forty-seven thousand three hundred sites! That's more hits than for Brigitte Bardot (1160); more even than for Raquel Welch (34,700); although it must be admitted that it doesn't quite match Pamela Anderson (538,000). Nevertheless, forty-seven thousand three hundred hits for a seemingly innocuous public health measure with no life or death implications. What is it about the promise of cavity-free teeth that can possibly be that controversial? What is it about this topic that makes the blood pressure rise for so many people?

DUELING WEBSITES

In 2002, when we first Googled up, the two most relevant fluoridation websites on the Internet, those at the top of the Google search list, were the

9

pro-fluoridation site of the National Center for Fluoridation Policy and Research and the anti-fluoridation site of the Stop Fluoridation USA movement. It would be hard to imagine a greater disparity in style and content than was exhibited between these two sites.

The National Center for Fluoridation Policy and Research was originally based at the School of Dental Medicine of the University of Buffalo, one of the many campuses of the State University of New York (SUNY). The center opened in 1996, and the website came online in 1998. Both the center and the website were the brainchild of Michael W. Easley, then a professor of oral biology at SUNY Buffalo. In subsequent years, Easley has made himself the voice of the fluoridation movement, involving himself in local referendums, lobbying state and local governments, organizing pro-fluoridation conferences such as the National Fluoridation Summit in Sacramento, California in September 2000, and writing articles with such titles as "Fluoridation: A Triumph of Science over Propaganda."[1] He perceived the need for a non-governmental organization that could counter anti-fluoridation propaganda by providing "reliable, timely, and scientifically based information" to public officials, educators, organizations, and concerned citizens. His organization is administered by a five-member executive advisory committee and a 23-member board of science, technology, and policy advisors. It boasts 167 collaborative partners from 16 countries and 30 states. The advisors and partners include many of the leading dental researchers in the world.

In 2003, the center shortened its name to the simpler National Center for Fluoridation (NCF) and moved its headquarters to Chicago, where it is now an arm of Oral Health America, an advocacy group "dedicated to improving oral health for all Americans." Michael Easley is still the director, although he is now based in Florida as the dental coordinator of the Florida Health Department.

The NCF is traditional and mainstream; it is the recognized voice of the medical–dental establishment in the United States. The NCF website is an exaltation of the benefits of community water fluoridation. C. Everett Koop, perhaps the most respected former Surgeon General of the United States (1981–1989), is quoted as saying that "fluoridation is the single most important commitment a community can make to the oral health of its children and to future generations." We learn that at the National Fluoridation Summit in 2000, then Surgeon General David Satcher announced the first-ever Surgeon General's Report on Oral Health, and that it includes the statement that "community water fluoridation is an effective, safe, and ideal public-health measure that benefits individuals of all ages and economic strata." Another former Surgeon General, Luther Terry, is cited for calling fluoridation "one of the four great mass preventive health measures of history" along with pasteurization of milk, purification of water, and immunization against disease.

We also learn on the NCF website that the Centers for Disease Control and Prevention, an arm of the U.S. Public Health Service (USPHS), have listed fluoridation of drinking water as one of the 10 greatest public health achievements of the twentieth century.[2] (The others: the eradication of small-pox and polio through vaccination; the saving of lives through improvements in motor vehicle safety; the control of work-related health problems such as black lung and silicosis; the control of infectious diseases through improved sanitation; the decline in deaths from coronary heart disease and stroke; the development of safer and healthier foods; the decrease in infant mortality through better hygiene and nutrition; the health benefits provided by better access to family planning and contraceptive services; and the recognition of tobacco use as a health hazard.)

If this is all starting to sound too doctrinaire, it is probably time to change the channel. In 2002, a flick of the wrist allowed us to enter the alarming, yet strangely alluring world of Stop Fluoridation USA. The original founder of this seminal anti-fluoridation website, Philip Heggen, died in 1999, and the webmaster in 2002 was a former frequent contributor named Darlene Sherrell. As this book goes to press, the Stop Fluoridation site is in temporary hibernation due to Sherrell's ill-health, but its 2002 content is mirrored in the literally hundreds of currently operating anti-fluoride websites.

It didn't take us long to realize that we had gone through a serious para-digm shift in moving to the Stop Fluoridation site from Michael Easley's NCF site. A big red stop sign welcomed us to the website. There were no more smooth assurances about the safety of fluoridation. In fact, one of Darlene Sherrell's longer contributions turned out to be a personal memoir of her own experiences of unwanted fluoride exposure. It was entitled "A Near-Death Experience." We also found links to book reviews for "The Fluoride Question: Panacea or Poison," "The Greatest Fraud: Fluoridation," and our favorite title on either side of the chasm, "Fluoridation and Truth Decay."[3]

Another article on the website pointed out that the nerve gas sarin, which was used in the Tokyo terrorist attacks of 1995, is 13.56% fluoride. We were told that the same chemical was also implicated in a military spill disaster in Utah in 1968 that was the basis of the George C. Scott movie *Rage*. It was stated elsewhere on the site that children have died in the dentist's chair after treatment with topical fluoride, and that adults have died during kidney dialysis due to fluoride overdoses. Excessive fluoride consump-tion was also blamed for cases of a rare disease known as crippling skeletal fluorosis. Links were provided to more aggressive anti-fluoridation websites that feature pictures of horribly disfigured third-world children said to be suffering from crippling skeletal fluorosis. There was also a link to the website of an organization called Parents of Fluoride Poisoned Children, which tells us sad tales of childhood cancer.

The anti-fluoride websites are proudly grassroots. There are no endorsements from famous doctors or scientists. In fact, membership in the medical establishment is clearly viewed with disdain. Anything that is endorsed by the American Dental Association (ADA), the American Medical Association, the U.S. Public Health Service, or any other mainstream health organization is seen as suspect. One organization that is seen as a particular bogeyman is the American Council on Science and Health (ACSH). On its own website the ACSH describes itself as "a nonprofit consumer-education organization dedicated to providing the public with mainstream scientific information on issues related to food, nutrition, chemicals, pharmaceuticals, lifestyle, the environment, and health." The president of ACSH is Elizabeth M. Whelan, the author of a book entitled *Toxic Terror*,[4] which strongly criticizes the scare tactics used by environmentalists in trying to ban chemicals that Whelan considers useful and safe. ACSH is also the publisher of the book *Facts Versus Fears: A Review of the Greatest Unfounded Health Scares of Recent Times*.[5] The ACSH is unabashedly pro-fluoridation. Michael Easley is on the editorial staff of their journal *Priorities*, and it was in this journal that he published his article on the triumph of science over propaganda.

Like the NCF, the ACSH also features a large advisory panel of scientists, doctors, and policy advisors. This list includes many of the most honored medical and dental researchers in the country, but it also includes scientists from several industrial laboratories, a fact that allows the Stop Fluoridation movement to identify the ACSH as an industry front. They see the fluoridation of public water supplies as a conspiracy by government and industry to help certain industries dispose of their fluoride wastes. In their eyes, government-sponsored fluoridation programs are a kind of kickback to industry for their political support. Pro-fluoridationists regard this type of thinking as paranoid. On the NCF site, they refer to it as *fluorophobia*, which is defined as an irrational fear of the element *fluorine* and its compounds.

Table 2.1 identifies a selection of representative websites on the Internet that support and oppose fluoridation. One can spend an interesting day flitting back and forth between them. The biggest and best of the pro-fluoridation sites favor carefully worded, heavily documented endorsements from unassailable sources. We learn that "the American Dental Association and the United States Public Health Service have continuously and unreservedly endorsed the optimal fluoridation of community water supplies as a safe and effective public health measure for the prevention of dental decay."[6] We learn that "fluoridation effectively, safely, and inexpensively helps prevent

TABLE 2.1 Some Representative Websites on the Internet That Support and Oppose Fluoridation

Internet Address	Sponsoring Organization
Pro-fluoridation	
www.ada.org	American Dental Association
www.cdc.gov	Center for Disease Control and Prevention, U.S. Public Health Service
www.nidr.nih.gov	National Institute of Dental and Craniofacial Research, U.S. National Institutes of Health
www.fda.gov	U.S. Food and Drug Administration
www.who.int	World Health Organization
www.derweb.ac.uk/bfs/	British Fluoridation Society
www.fluoridationcenter.org	National Center for Fluoridation
www.oralhealthamerica.org	Oral Health America
www.acsh.org	American Council on Science and Health
www.quackwatch.com	Independent site
Anti-fluoridation	
www.rvi.net/~fluoride[a]	Stop Fluoridation USA
www.nofluoride.com	Citizens for Safe Drinking Water
www.fluoridealert.org	Fluoride Action Network
www.fluoridation.com	Health Action Network
www.penweb.org/issues/fluoride	Pennsylvania Fluoride Leadership Team
www.orgsites.com/ny/nyscof	New York State Coalition Opposed to Fluoridation
www.trufax.org	Leading Edge International Research Group
www.citizens.org	Citizens for Health
www.thenhf.com	National Health Federation
www.all-natural.com	Natural Health and Longevity Resource Center
www.saveteeth.org	A consortium of sponsors, including Chapter 280, National Treasury Employees Union

[a]Temporarily in hibernation, 2008.

tooth decay in adults and children, regardless of socioeconomic status or access to care."[7] A bit bland, perhaps, but very authoritative.

The anti-fluoridation sites prefer a more colorful, anecdotal style. Robert Carton, a toxic risk specialist formerly with the Environmental Protection Agency, is quoted on several sites as describing fluoridation as "the greatest case of scientific fraud of this century." If you download the "action pack" from the Citizens for Health website, you can get a supply of postcards that feature a picture of belching smokestacks and a question-and-answer tagline. *Question*: "Since when is industry's toxic waste good enough to drink?" *Answer*: "When they call it fluoridation."

Some of the anti-fluoridation sites look a bit amateur compared with the pro-fluoridation sites of the ADA and the USPHS, but many are very professional. The California Citizens for Safe Drinking Water have a very classy website that features messages that move across the screen, multicolored U.S. flags waving in the breeze, and pictures of pre-teen kids holding signs at a fluoridation protest that read "Fluoride is More Toxic Than Lead." They offer pre-drafted anti-fluoridation letters to the editor, promotional items for use in referendum battles, and suggested wordings for anti-fluoridation ballot measures to be forwarded to your local elected officials.

The Preventive Dental Health Association offers a site that is limited to two topics: fluoridation and mercury fillings. In both cases the association lists the dangers associated with their use and suggests more holistic alternatives. Among the cavity-fighting alternatives to fluoridation that are touted are a salt-and-baking-soda mouthwash and tincture of prickly ash bark. Despite the official-sounding organizational name, the site is essentially the personal homepage of David C. Kennedy, an anti-fluoridation dentist who was one of the prime authors of a petition to ban fluoridation in California. His book *Fluoridation: A Fifty-Year-Old Blunder and Cover-up* concludes that scientific fraud has been employed to support the disposal of a toxic substance in public water supplies.

These anti-fluoridation sites are completely and unfairly one-sided. There is no chance of getting fair and balanced information from these sources. Perhaps this is not a big surprise, coming from organizations that are so avowedly single-minded. But what about the pro-fluoridation sites? Most of the bigger ones are maintained by government agencies, and rightly or wrongly, we might expect less biased and more complete coverage when the site is paid for with our own tax dollars. No such luck. The pro-fluoridation websites seem less strident, but in their own way they are just as partisan as the anti-fluoridation websites. They provide coverage of all the scientific studies that support the efficiency and safety of fluoridation, but not those that raise provocative scientific questions. They list all the organizations that support fluoridation, but not those that are opposed. They provide coverage of all the referendums that endorsed fluoridation, but not those where the issue was defeated. The anti-fluoridation forces use a hard-sell approach, the pro-fluoridation forces tend toward soft-sell, but the political nature of the endeavor is pretty clear on both sides.

QUACK, QUACK

There is probably no more loaded word in the medical lexicon than the word *quack*. A doctor who is called a quack has received the ultimate insult.

Webster's New Collegiate Dictionary defines a quack as "a pretender to medical skill, a charlatan." The word conjures up images of deceitful credentials, worthless treatments, botched operations, and hoodwinked grandmothers. Yet this is the word that Stephen Barrett boldly highlights in the title of his website, Quackwatch, a consumer health site that is designed "to combat health-related frauds, myths, fads, and fallacies."[8] Quackwatch gets upward of 1000 visitors per day, and it has won several national and international awards. On the site, Barrett pulls no punches. He identifies many health products, services, and theories as having no therapeutic value whatsoever. Included on his list of worthless remedies are aromatherapy, cellulite removal, chelation therapy, colon therapy, faith healing, hair analysis, magnet therapy, therapeutic touch, and many herbal practices. He is disdainful of most types of chiropractic medicine and describes certain aspects of acupuncture as "complete insanity." Homeopathy is described as an ineffective pseudoscience. "How long does it take to become a homeopath?" he asks. "Two seconds. You just call yourself a homeopath, and you are one." He gives no credibility to *Dr. Atkins New Diet Revolution* and calls the bestseller *Fit for Life* one of the "nuttiest books of all-time." The seven spiritual laws of Deepak Chopra are dismissed as "mumbo jumbo."

Stephen Barrett is a retired psychiatrist from Allentown, Pennsylvania. He is a medical doctor who practiced his profession for 35 years before setting his sights on what he sees as fraudulent health practices. Quackwatch is not his only website; he is also the webmaster for the National Council Against Health Fraud, a private nonprofit health agency that focuses on health misinformation, quackery, and fraud. The NCHF site is part of the "Skeptic Ring," an alliance of 147 websites that examine claims about paranormal phenomena and fringe science from a skeptical point of view. Barrett is also the editor of a weekly electronic newsletter called *Consumer Health Digest*. He has authored 47 books, including *The Vitamin Pushers: How the Health Food Industry Is Selling America a Bill of Goods* and *Health Schemes, Scams, and Frauds*. His best-known book is *The Health Robbers: A Close Look at Quackery in America*. In 1984 he received a Commissioner's Special Citation Award from the FDA for fighting nutrition quackery, and in 1986 he was awarded honorary membership in the American Dietetic Association. In his books, newsletters, and websites, Stephen Barrett rails against the shameful influence of quack science, and unhesitantly recommends that consumers get their health information from traditional establishment sources such as the American Medical Association, the American Dental Association, and the Food and Drug Administration.

Stephen Barrett is adamantly pro-fluoridation. He is a coeditor of a widely used strategy manual entitled *The Tooth Robbers: A Pro-Fluoridation Handbook*.[9] On the Quackwatch homepage he decries the scare tactics of misguided "poisonmongers" who have deprived many communities of the benefits of fluoridation. He claims that anti-fluoridationists create the illusion of scientific controversy where none exists. He accuses them of quoting statements that are out of date or out of context, and of playing on public fears by using scare words such as *cancer, leukemia,* and *Mongoloid births.* He notes that many of the "experts" who are quoted have no medical or scientific credentials. He condemns the use of innuendo and half-truth that might lead readers of anti-fluoridation propaganda to believe that fluoride is a synthetic chemical when it is actually a naturally occurring element of the Earth's crust that is commonly found in many rocks and minerals. In fact, he argues, water fluoridation simply "copies a naturally occurring phenomenon." (The NCF also emphasizes this point through its motto: "Fluoridation: Nature Thought of It First.") The Quackwatch statement on fluoridation ends with a statement of confident reassurance: "If you live in a community with fluoridated water, consider yourself lucky. Fluoridation is a modern health miracle."

The charge of quackery makes Darlene Sherrell furious. "What is quackery?" she asks on the Stop Fluoridation website, "and who decides?"[10] She quotes Barrett himself: "Most people think that quackery is easy to spot. Often it is not. Its promoters wear the cloak of science. They use scientific terms and quote (or misquote) scientific references."[11] This is exactly what her adversaries do, Sherrell argues. She charges that Stephen Barrett, Michael Easley, and former Surgeon General C. Everett Koop have all misrepresented the scientific literature on fluoride. "These men talk about hundreds of safety studies, but when asked to name one that didn't exclude everyone with symptoms, or use inappropriate methods, there is no response. ... No one can name a study because none exist. There have been no legitimate long-term controlled studies; and no attempt to identify, verify, or gather reports of suspected or confirmed cases of chronic fluoride poisoning in U.S. cities." She decries this selective silence and quotes a federal judge as follows: "Silence can be equated with fraud when there is a legal or moral duty to speak, or when an inquiry left unanswered would be intentionally misleading."

It may not be clear at this point who is misleading whom. In later chapters we will have a chance to examine carefully both sides of the argument about fluoride and health. Here, let it simply be said that quackery is plainly in the eye of the beholder.

THE $100,000 CASH OFFER

One of the past gambits of the anti-fluoridation forces featured a $100,000 reward for anyone who could prove that fluoridation is safe. The offer was first posted on a forerunner of the Stop Fluoridation website in the 1970s by

Philip Heggen. Darlene Sherrell, the longtime guardian of the website, regularly reported with great glee that the reward was never claimed. The offer promised to deliver $100,000 to anyone who could find "any studies which indicate that researchers used methods capable of detecting cases of chronic fluoride poisoning in any U.S. city in the past, but failed to find them."

We know. You have to read it twice. But double negatives and all, it does seem to offer a cash reward for something. So why didn't anybody ever try to claim it? Could it really be that U.S. cities are rife with fluoride-poisoned people? "Bosh," says Stephen Barrett on his Quackwatch website, where he mocks the offer as a crude publicity stunt. He notes that the sponsors have never stated how any response would be judged or who would make the judgment. He suspects that the anti-fluoridationists themselves would have the right to appoint the judges. The offer also requires that the claimant post a bond to cover any costs that the offerers of the reward might incur if the proof is deemed invalid. Barrett makes the observation that if a lawsuit were filed to collect the reward, such a suit would probably require at least $25,000 for the bond and legal fees. Even if the suit were won, there would be no assurance that the money would be recovered from those who sponsored the reward. Barrett notes with tongue in cheek that the Stop Fluoridation website often carried a plea for help in defraying the $19.95 per month that it costs to maintain the site, not exactly a harbinger of solvency. In late 2001, a note appeared on the Stop Fluoridation website stating that the $100,000 offer had been withdrawn. There was no indication as to whether the cold feet arose from technical, economic, or legal pressures.

As it turns out, Barrett didn't need to claim the reward to get involved in a legal battle with the anti-fluoridationists. He and Sherrell have already tangled in a lawsuit. Two of them, in fact. Or rather, the same one twice. On April 12, 1999, a decision was rendered in the U.S. District Court for the Eastern District of Pennsylvania on a suit brought by Stephen Barrett against Darlene Sherrell for defamation of character.[12] The Eastern District is the federal court that has jurisdiction in Allentown, Pennsylvania, where Barrett lives. Also named in the suit were the author of a book quoted by Sherrell on her website, the publisher of that book, and the server that delivered Sherrell's message around the world. As examples of the defamatory statements on Sherrell's website, Barrett asserted that Sherrell referred to him as a "bogus consumer watchdog" and a "big liar." Moreover, she stated that Barrett's true purpose on the Quackwatch website is to eliminate competition in the health care field and pander to anticonsumer special interests.

Barrett claims that he first became aware of the existence of Darlene Sherrell after she joined a health-fraud discussion group cosponsored by the Quackwatch site. Later, she attempted to engage Barrett in private e-mail discussions about fluoridation. Later still, the alleged defamatory statements began to appear on Sherrell's website. Barrett states that he has good reason to believe that Sherrell posted at least 90 messages to at least 12 other network newsgroups, and that many of these messages encouraged people to visit one or more of the websites that contained defamatory statements about him.

As it turns out, Barrett's suit was dismissed without prejudice by the Pennsylvania court on procedural grounds. In his lengthy order dismissing plaintiff's complaint, the judge cited many precedents to support his finding of a lack of jurisdiction in the case. The primary reason was Sherrell's lack of connection with the state of Pennsylvania. She was living in Grenada in the West Indies at the time of the suit, and other than some peripheral involvement in a fluoridation case in Pennsylvania in the early 1980s, she has no ties to the state. Sherrell's lawyers argued successfully that "the presumed defamatory statements made by the Defendant attacked the Plaintiff in his national capacity as an advocate against health-care fraud, and in favor of the fluoridation of water sources. ... Plaintiff cannot point to any defamatory statements that attack him in his capacity as a Pennsylvania psychiatrist, or to any postings by the Defendant that intended to target Internet users in Pennsylvania."

In one of his e-mail interactions with Sherrell, Barrett says: "If you want to attack what I say, you have a right to do so. ... I am not thin skinned and have no objection to people disagreeing with my ideas. But attacking me as dishonest is quite another matter. ... I regard libel as a serious matter." Proof of the latter statement can be found in the fact that Barrett has brought several other libel suits against others over the years. However, a judgment handed down recently in a northern California court on one of his cases may give him pause. In that case, Barrett sued an anti-breast-implant activist named Ilena Rosenthal for libel after she called the Quackwatch team "a power-hungry, misguided bunch of pseudoscientific socialist bigots." The judge dismissed the claim on the grounds that Barrett was a public figure and the online discussion was protected by the Constitution's right to free speech.[13]

Undaunted, Barrett refiled his defamation case against Darlene Sherrell in the U.S. District Court in Medford, Oregon. This venue was selected because Sherrell was apparently in Oregon visiting her daughter at the time the alleged defamatory statements were posted on her website. In 2004, an Oregon judge dismissed Barrett's defamation claim. In her first submission to the Oregon court,[14] Sherrell alleged that Barrett's lawsuit "has no purpose other than creating fear in the minds of consumers who have legitimate concerns about matters of public interest." She also noted that Barrett finds epithets that are tossed his way libelous, yet he refers to his own opponents as "poisonmongers." Ignoring the intended slur, she instead played the fussy schoolmarm and took Barrett to task on his English usage. "Mongers" are sellers, she explained (as in *fishmonger*), and as the anti-fluoridationists are certainly not trying to "sell" fluoride, poison or no, they can hardly be classed as "poisonmongers." In her eyes, the label fits the pro-fluoridationists far better.

AS ONE VOICE

Table 2.2 presents a selection of U.S. national organizations that support and oppose fluoridation. The pro-fluoridation list is taken from a much longer list that appears on the American Dental Association website, entitled "National and International Organizations that Recognize the Public Health Benefits of Community Water Fluoridation for Preventing Dental Decay." By now it won't come as any surprise to learn that a similar list appears on an anti-fluoridation website[15] under the title "Organizations Colluding in the Use of Mind-Numbing Fluorides."

The pro-fluoridation list in Table 2.2 is led by the American Dental Association. The ADA represents some 75% of the nation's 200,000 dentists (a higher percentage membership than the 44% of doctors who belong to the American Medical Association or the 50% of lawyers who belong to the American Bar Association).[16] The ADA provides a fourfold service to its members (and indirectly to the public). First, it establishes standards for materials, drugs, and devices used by dentists and consumers; some 1300 products carry the ADA Seal of Acceptance. Second, it sets the rules for accreditation of dentists, dental hygienists, dental assistants, and dental laboratory technicians. Third, it hosts scientific meetings at the local, state, and national levels, and publishes a variety of technical and professional journals. Fourth, and most pertinent to our undertaking, it searches out consensus positions on public policy issues among its membership and promotes these positions within public health agencies and to the public at large.

The leaders of the American Dental Association have endorsed fluoridation of community water supplies for more than 50 years.[17] They support the position that all communal water supplies that are below the optimum fluoride level recommended by the U.S. Public Health Service (0.7 to 1.2 ppm) "should be adjusted to the optimum level in order to provide a safe, beneficial, and cost-effective public health measure for preventing dental caries." The ADA emphasizes that its policies are based on "generally accepted scientific knowledge." They define this body of knowledge as that which "is validated by the efforts of nationally recognized scientists, who have conducted research using the scientific method, have drawn appropriate balanced conclusions based on their research findings, and have published their results in

TABLE 2.2   Selected U.S. National Organizations That Support and Oppose Fluoridation

Pro-fluoridation

Alzheimer's Association	American Public Health Association
American Academy of Allergy, Asthma and Immunology	American School Health Association
American Academy of Family Physicians	American Society of Clinical Nutrition
American Academy of Pediatrics	
American Academy of Pediatric Dentistry	American Society for Nutritional Sciences
American Association for Dental Research	American Veterinary Medical Association
American Association of Community Dental Programs	American Water Works Association
American Association for the Advancement of Science	Chocolate Manufacturers Association
American Association of Orthodontists	Consumer Federation of America
American Association of Public Health Dentistry	National Association of Community Health Centers
American Cancer Society	National Association of Local Boards of Health
American College of Dentists	National Dental Hygienists Association
American College of Physicians	National Association of County and City Health Officials
American Council on Science and Health	National Confectioners Association
American Dental Association	National Down Syndrome Congress
American Dietetic Association	National Down Syndrome Society
American Hospital Association	National Head Start Association
American Medical Association	Oral Health America
American Nurses Association	U.S. Public Health Service: Centers for Disease Control and Prevention
American Osteopathic Association	U.S. National Institutes of Health: National Institute of Dental and Craniofacial Research
American Pharmaceutical Association	

Anti-fluoridation

Center for Science in the Public Interest	
Citizens for Health	National Health Federation
Citizens for Safe Drinking Water	National Nutritional Foods Association
Earth Island Institute	Natural Resources Defense Council
International Academy of Oral Medicine and Toxicology	Preventive Dental Health Association
Leading Edge International Research Group	International Society for Fluoride Research

peer-reviewed professional journals that are widely circulated." The implication is clear that they do not think that the anti-fluoridationist position has similar backing.

It is difficult to ignore the unanimity of the American medical establishment. When it comes to fluoridation, they speak as one voice. The pro-fluoridation list in Table 2.2 (and the longer list on the ADA website) includes just about every national association of dentists, doctors, nurses, pharmacists, nutritionists, and public health officials in the land. The list could be made even longer and more impressive if it were to include similar organizations from other countries, such as Canada, Australia, New Zealand, and Britain, and such international medical organizations as the World Health Organization. Indeed, it is difficult to understand why this issue continues to produce controversy at all given the strength of the endorsement by the medical establishment. After all, doctors and dentists are held in almost universally high regard in American society. On almost every health issue except this one, the public places its unwavering trust in medicine. There is an anomaly here that is deserving of our attention.

Fears of adverse health impacts from the ingestion of fluoridated drinking water do not find resonance in any mainstream branch of the medical establishment. While anti-fluoridationists worry about the impact of fluoride on cancer, heart disease, allergies, Down's syndrome, and many other illnesses, the national health organizations that represent the sufferers of these diseases almost all support the fluoridation of community water supplies. Much is made in anti-fluoride literature that the National Kidney Foundation (NKF) no longer supports fluoridation as they once did. However, careful reading of the NKF position makes it clear that they do not support *or oppose* fluoridation. Their position is one of no position.

Several anti-fluoridation websites post lists of many other organizations that they claim were once on the list of fluoride supporters but no longer appear there. The implication is that support is soft and that former adherants to the cause are scurrying away like rats from the *Titanic*. On careful examination, however, it appears that these claims do not deserve much weight. Most of the purported backsliders (organizations such as the National Institute of Municipal Law Officers) no longer take a public position on this issue because their interest in fluoridation is so peripheral that a position need not be taken, or because they wish to avoid the political conflict that a public position engenders.

If you look carefully at Table 2.2, you will find a couple of unexpected, nonmedical organizations in the list of pro-fluoridation parties. We have included the Chocolate Manufacturers Association and the National Confectioners Association on the list just to remind us that there are self-interested parties on all sides of all issues. Sugar manufacturers and those who would like to ply our children with sugar-filled delights have always supported fluoridation. It can't be bad for business to get the public thinking that the guilt of a cavity-enhancing sugar fix can be wiped out with a little dose of fluoride.

If we return to Table 2.2 and look at the list of organizations that *oppose* fluoridation, it is clear that the anti-fluoridation camp simply cannot match the pro-fluoridation camp with respect to the number of supporting organizations, their size and influence, or their credibility. Most of the anti-fluoridation organizations represent limited constituencies, and in some cases, their position could be seen as self-interested. Several of the organizations exist solely as agents of an anti-fluoridation message (Citizens for Safe Drinking Water, Preventive Dental Health Association). Many of the others represent devotees of alternative medicine and nutritional health. The National Nutritional Foods Association, for example, is an organization that represents the health food industry. It supports herbal remedies and organically grown foods, and opposes food additives and chemical agriculture.

One of the most persistent opponents to fluoridation has been an organization known as the National Health Federation (NHF). It is a consumer organization that works to guarantee "your right to use the doctor, nutrition, or therapy of your choice." The NHF lobbies for passage of effective health-freedom legislation and advocates the cessation of a mixed bag of "dangerous practices," including fluoridation, smallpox and polio vaccination, pasteurization of milk, and toxic spraying of agricultural crops.[18] The NHF was founded by a man named Fred J. Hart, who had a long history of run-ins with the Food and Drug Administration (FDA).[19] In the early 1950s, he was the president of a company that sold electronic devices for diagnosis and treatment of a variety of diseases. Practitioners of alternative medical therapies would send him dried blood specimens from their patients, and he would use his electronic equipment to analyze the blood, following which he would mail back his diagnosis by postcard. The FDA investigated his equipment and found that they contained circuits that resembled those of an electric doorbell or small radio transmitter. In 1954 a U.S. district court ordered Hart to discontinue offering his treatment devices for sale. He ignored the order and was prosecuted for criminal contempt in 1962. The early years of the NHF were also fraught with legal problems. Between 1957 and 1963, several officers of the NHF were convicted of labeling products with false medical claims. In 1963, the FDA released a report that stated that "the Federation has been a front for promoters of unproved remedies, eccentric theories, and quackery." Throughout all of this, Hart, the NHF, and their supporters in the world of alternative medicine, cried foul, claiming that the

FDA provocations and pronouncements were nothing more than harassment from the establishment against well-tested and effective alternative medical therapies.

It would be unfair to the anti-fluoridation camp to imply that the NHF is representative of the entire movement. For example, two of the anti-fluoridation organizations listed in Table 2.2 come from the environmental community (the Earth Island Institute and the Natural Resources Defense Council). The Earth Island Institute was founded by David Brower, one of the world's leading environmentalists, and it has a strong positive image in the environmental world. It is clearly in the anti-fluoridation camp, having published some very provocative articles in its journal and serving as a charter member of the Fluoride Action Network. The Natural Resources Defense Council has been involved in much anti-fluoridation litigation over the years.

Other environmental organizations are more circumspect. Greenpeace doesn't mention fluoridation on its website. The Sierra Club recently posted a statement that could be viewed as neutral, but leans toward opposition. It reads in part: "The Sierra Club understands the historic reason that fluoridation of public water supplies has been promoted and that it may have been historically justifiable. There are now, however, valid concerns regarding the potential adverse impact of fluoridation on the environment, wildlife, and human health. The Sierra Club therefore supports giving communities the option of rejecting mandatory fluoridation of their water supplies." The statement goes on to recommend a national review of fluoridation by the National Academy of Sciences and the U.S. Geological Survey to provide more "reliable information for forming future public policy." There are some groups within the Sierra Club with an even stronger agenda. The Pennsylvania chapter has a fluoride committee that has put together a document that is strongly anti-fluoride.[20]

We have placed the Center for Science in the Public Interest on the anti-fluoridation list in Table 2.2. Although their literature does not emphasize their position, the opposition of the center's founder, Ralph Nader, is well known, and they have also published books with a strong anti-fluoride stance.[21] We have also placed the International Society for Fluoride Research (ISFR) on the anti-fluoridation list, despite a disclaimer in their journal, *Fluoride*, that they take no official position. The reasons for this decision will be clear to the reader after perusing the material in Chapter 11, which traces the history of the ISFR and documents the clear one-sidedness of its membership. It belongs in the anti camp in the same sense that the ADA and the AMA belong in the pro camp.

Despite the views of such credible opponents as the Natural Resources Defense Council, the Center for Science in the Public Interest, and the International Society for Fluoride Research, any fair-minded assessment of the information in Table 2.2 leads to the conclusion that anti-fluoridationists are clear losers in the war of organizational endorsements. To offset this situation, anti-fluoridationists have tried to gain credibility through personal endorsements of well-known scientists and public figures, but here too it is difficult to judge their campaign a great success. The opposition of a presidential candidate such as Nader is somewhat underwhelming when balanced against the fact that every sitting president since Kennedy has publicly supported fluoridation.[22]

The fall 1983 issue of the *National Fluoridation News*, an anti-fluoridation newsletter, is widely quoted for a list published there of 14 Nobel prizewinners who object to fluoridation. On closer examination, however, it turns out that most of these Nobel laureates won their awards long before the evidence for and against fluoridation could be fairly judged. The list is probably based on a survey of Nobel prizewinners carried out by the *Christian Science Monitor* in 1954. The editors contacted the 81 living laureates in the fields of chemistry, medicine, and physiology, and received replies from 52 of them. They found 11 to be in favor of fluoridation, 12 opposed, and 29 uncommitted. In other words, Nobel laureates at that time were just as evenly divided on the issue as was the general public. Presuming that the lists quoted on current anti-fluoridation websites have been updated, it appears that only one Nobel prizewinner since 1963 has publicly stated his objection to fluoridation. He is Arvid Carlsson, who won a Nobel Prize in Medicine for the year 2000 for his work on the brain, and who also played a role in the rejection of fluoridation in Sweden. His views deserve weight, but they must be balanced against those of the hundreds of other Nobel prizewinners since 1963 who support or remain neutral with respect to this issue.

There are many individual dentists, doctors, and scientists who have publicly stated their opposition to fluoridation. The Fluoride Action Network (Table 2.1) is currently sponsoring a "Professional's Statement Calling for an End to Water Fluoridation," which has been signed by over 1800 scientific and medical professionals (although it is clear that a fairly large number of signees, perhaps a majority, come from the alternative health realm, which has historically opposed fluoridation). Undoubtedly, many of these men and women are highly respected medical scientists, but they are not household names that are likely to impress the average citizen. And for every opponent of fluoridation in the medical–dental community, there are hundreds, perhaps thousands, of supporters. The American Dental Association alone has 144,000 members, and only a handful of them publicly oppose fluoridation. The American Medical Association has twice as many members as the ADA, and only a very few dissenters have declared themselves. In this light, a list of 1800 dissidents is hardly Earth-shattering. What is perhaps more surprising, given the controversy that has swirled around the issue for so long and the eccentricities of human nature, is that so few medical practitioners have come forward to take an anti-fluoridation position.

There is one anti-fluoride statement that comes from high up in the medical establishment, and it is widely quoted in the anti-fluoridation literature. Charles Gordon Heyd, a past president of the American Medical Association (AMA), is quoted as saying: "I am appalled at the prospect of using water as a vehicle for drugs. Fluoride is a corrosive poison that will produce serious effects on a long-range basis. Any attempt to use water this way is deplorable."[23] What is not made clear, however, is that Heyd was president of the AMA from 1935 to 1936, long before widespread fluoridation had been undertaken and well before the evidence of its effectiveness was available for examination. No AMA president since Heyd has ever taken a stand against fluoridation. And even if one were inclined to give much weight to Heyd's hoary pronouncement, pro-fluoridation forces can point to the more compelling fact that every Surgeon General since 1945 has publicly supported fluoridation.

When it comes to endorsements, both organizational and individual, the pro-fluoridationists can claim a clear victory. Anti-fluoridationists, of course, see this as evidence of an establishment conspiracy: sheep following sheep without proper analysis of the available evidence. They claim that many of the organizational endorsements were pushed through without due process, in order to get on the bandwagon. They point to a lack of independent evaluations, the interlocking memberships of a small number of influential scientists in the various societies, and the close ties between many of the endorsing organizations and the main proponents, the American Dental Association and the Public Health Service.[24] In later chapters we examine the dynamics of public opinion and how it is influenced by these contrary interpretations. For now, however, we would expect the neutral observer to be fairly impressed with the unanimity in the medical and scientific communities in favor of fluoridation.

WHO DRINKS FLUORIDATED WATER AND WHO DOESN'T

Table 2.3 traces the growth in the number of U.S. residents who have gained access to fluoridated drinking water since 1945. The total numbers have grown steadily, and by 2005 there were 170 million Americans using fluoridated water supplies, approximately 67% of the total population.[25] Most

TABLE 2.3 Growth of Fluoridated Population in the United States, 1945–2000

Date	Fluoridated Population (millions)
1945	0
1951	5
1954	22
1960	41
1967	62
1969	90
1977	105
1988	122
2000	151
2005	170

of these users receive artificially fluoridated water from community water systems. Some receive naturally fluoridated groundwater from wellfields that tap aquifers that are already rich in fluoride. A few communities actually have to remove fluoride from their water because the natural concentrations exceed the drinking water standards set by the Environmental Protection Agency or the concentrations specified as optimal by the Public Health Service. The great majority of fluoridated water systems are in the cities and larger towns of the nation. People in smaller communities and rural areas are much less likely to have access to fluoridated water than those in larger cities and towns.

The growth indicated in Table 2.3 has not been as smooth as a first glance at the numbers might suggest. The apparent steady rise in the fluoridated population, as indicated in the right-hand column, hides a plethora of setbacks and reversals suffered by the pro-fluoridation forces in hundreds of individual fluoridation battles fought out over the years in the polling booths of the nation. Many communities stumbled back and forth between fluoridation and no fluoridation with each passing election. Some years saw more defections from the fluoridation column than additions. Nevertheless, over time the trend is clear. When it comes to numbers, the pro-fluoridation camp may not have won all the battles, but they are winning the war.

As indicated in Table 2.4, almost all major U.S. cities are now fluoridated. Only six of our larger cities remain unfluoridated (Fresno, California; Honolulu, Hawaii; Portland, Oregon; San Diego, California; San Jose, California; and Wichita, Kansas), and San Diego is scheduled to come off this list by May 2010. In fact, the two largest cities in North America that are still not fluoridated are actually in Canada (Montreal, Quebec; and Vancouver, British Columbia). Mind you, several of the cities listed in Table 2.4 are relatively

TABLE 2.4   Fluoridation Status of Major U.S. Cities

Fluoridated

Albuquerque, NM	Houston, TX	Omaha, NB
Atlanta, GA	Indianapolis, IN	Philadelphia, PA
Austin, TX	Kansas City, MO	Phoenix, AZ
Baltimore, MD	Las Vegas, NV	Pittsburgh, PA
Boston, MA	Long Beach, CA	Sacramento, CA
Buffalo, NY	Los Angeles, CA	St. Louis, MO
Charlotte, NC	Memphis, TN	Salt Lake City, UT
Chicago, IL	Miami, FL	San Antonio, TX
Cincinnati, OH	Milwaukee, WI	San Francisco, CA
Cleveland, OH	Minneapolis, MN	Seattle, WA
Columbus, OH	Nashville, TN	Toledo, OH
Dallas, TX	New Orleans, LA	Tulsa, OK
Denver, CO	New York, NY	Virginia Beach, VA
Detroit, MI	Oakland, CA	Washington, DC
Fort Worth, TX	Oklahoma City, OK	

Naturally Fluoridated

Colorado Springs, CO	Jacksonville, FL	Tucson, AZ
El Paso, TX		

Not Fluoridated

Fresno, CA	Portland, OR	San Jose, CA
Honolulu, HI	San Diego, CA[a]	Wichita, KS

[a]Not fluoridated as of 2008, but funding is now available and the city is required by the California mandate to begin fluoridating its public water supply by May 2010.

recent additions to the fluoridated column. Las Vegas, Nevada; Los Angeles, California; Salt Lake City, Utah; and San Antonio, Texas all approved fluoridation for the first time in the years since 1999.

When it comes to *worldwide* fluoridation statistics, the situation is somewhat surprising. We suspect that it is quite different from what most Americans might expect. Until we saw the statistics, we had always assumed that fluoridation was moving forward in the other countries in the world, or at least in the other developed countries in the world, at more or less the same rate as in the United States. As indicated in Table 2.5, this is not the case.[26] There are only a few countries in the world where more than 50% of the population use fluoridated water. These include the United States; the British Commonwealth countries of Australia, Canada, and New Zealand; and the small but prosperous Asian countries of Hong Kong and Singapore. In fact, apart from these few, it seems that there are no other countries in the world

TABLE 2.5   Fluoridation Status of Developed Countries of the World

Countries with Greater Than 50% of the Population Using Fluoridated Water

Australia	Ireland	Singapore
Canada	Malaysia	United States
Hong Kong	New Zealand	

Countries with 5–20% of the Population Using Fluoridated Water

Brazil	Czech Republic[a]	Russia[a]
Chile[b]	Israel[b]	United Kingdom
Colombia[b]	South Africa	Venezuela

Countries with Less Than 5% of the Population Using Fluoridated Water (Most Essentially 0%)

Argentina	Greece	Netherlands
Austria	Guatamala	Norway
Belgium	Hungary	Paraguay
Bulgaria	India	Peru
China	Indonesia	Philippines
Cuba	Iran	Poland
Denmark	Italy	Portugal
Egypt	Japan	Romania
Equador	Korea	Spain
Finland	Libya	Sweden
France	Luxembourg	Switzerland
Germany	Mexico	Taiwan

[a]Before the fall of the iron curtain in 1989. Current situation unknown.
[b]ADA *Fluoridation Facts* claims "extensive fluoridation" in these countries. Actual population percentages unknown.

where more than 20% of the population is serviced with fluoridated water. Most of the countries in the world do not fluoridate their drinking water supplies at all. In particular, it is noteworthy that none of the democracies of Western Europe give more than token attention to public water fluoridation. This has led anti-fluoridationists to charge that fluoridation is "an American obsession."

It turns out that there have been many attempts to fluoridate drinking water supplies in Europe and that these attempts led to the same types of political battles as those that were fought in the United States. Sometimes, they may even have been fought with more *panache*. In Scarborough, England, during a fluoridation battle there, opponents built a giant allegorical sand castle on the beach which featured the "truth fairy" being chased by an evil fluoride-flaunting ogre.[27] The fact is that in European countries, community water fluoridation simply never attracted the support that it received in North America. The primary reason given by American fluoridationists for the European failure is the impracticality of fluoridating the multitude of small, complex, multisource water systems that are common in Europe. They also point to lower levels of decay and higher levels of natural fluoride in European waters. The American Dental Association, trying to put the best possible light on the situation, notes that "no European country has specifically imposed a ban on fluoridation." They conclude, somewhat vaguely, that "it has simply not been implemented for a variety of technical or political reasons."

Anti-fluoridationists have a different take on the European situation. They argue that scientific advisors to European governments are better educated regarding the dangers of fluoridation and that they are not subject to the ostracizing pressures of the U.S. Public Health Service lobby. In Sweden, for example, the Nobel Medical Institute recommended against fluoridation of Sweden's water supplies. In reality, however, it is hard for anti-fluoridationists to make too much hay out of this issue. Although it is true that Europeans have rejected the fluoridation of their water supplies, they have not rejected fluoride as an aid to dental health. The European dental community uses topical fluoride treatments, and the public consumption of fluoride supplements in one form or another is especially high in Western Europe.

The question of whether any European country has actually "banned" fluoridation is hotly contested among the pros and antis. Anti-fluoridation literature lists many countries as having instituted a "ban." The ADA categorically states the opposite. The most complete information on this issue (at least up to 1991) can be found in Brian Martin's book *Scientific Knowledge in Controversy: The Social Dynamics of the Fluoridation Debate.*[28] As one might expect, the answer depends on one's interpretation of the word *ban.* Sweden, for example, passed a law in 1962 that made it possible for municipalities to seek permission for local fluoridation, but this law was repealed in 1971. Sweden still has no law permitting fluoridation, and this might be viewed as a ban, but in fact there is no Swedish law that specifically bans fluoridation. In the Netherlands, early fluoridation efforts were halted by a court decision which ruled that there was no acceptable legal basis in place to permit the practice. Political opposition has prevented the passage of legislation to promote fluoridation, but there has been no move to declare it illegal. In Germany, sources replying to Martin's inquiries from within different government departments differed as to whether or not fluoridation is legally permissible. The closest thing to an outright ban uncovered by Martin is a 1977 statement by the Danish Minister of the Environment that fluoridation "should not be allowed" in Denmark.

For now, it is fair to summarize the situation by noting that many countries that often follow the lead of the United States have not done so in the case of community water fluoridation. This is not necessarily a strong argument against fluoridation, but it is nevertheless a fact that deserves our further attention as we move through the historical record.

FEAR AND LOATHING

The case *in favor of* fluoridation is relatively straightforward. It goes as follows. Fluoride has proven itself an effective agent in reducing dental decay in children's teeth. There are no known side effects of any importance. The optimal concentration has been determined through experience over the years. It is relatively simple and inexpensive to introduce fluoride into drinking water supplies at the optimal concentration. It is a safe and efficient public health measure that has effectively brought an end to the pain and distress of childhood dental caries. Case closed.

For better or for worse, it is the case *against* fluoridation that sets the agenda. From the very beginning, those who espouse fluoridation have had to fight a rearguard action against the claims of those who oppose this public health measure. Over the years there have been many objections to fluoridation. One study of the anti-fluoridation movement identified 255 separate objections that have been raised at one time or another against fluoridation.[29] Although it may be possible to produce a list of this length, it is also possible to group the objections under a much smaller set of headings. In Table 2.6 we identify the seven main elements of the anti-fluoridationist case. These are the issues that arise over and over again, in city after city, in book after book. These are the issues that claim the most prominent billing and the most accessible links on the network of anti-fluoridation websites. These issues represent the *creed* of those opposed to the fluoridation of drinking water supplies.

The anti-fluoridationist claims are arranged in Table 2.6 with the most rational objections at the top and the most paranoid at the bottom. At the top are questions that relate to whether fluoridation is effective and cost-efficient, and whether it is prone to engineering failures. At the bottom are the conspiracy theories that accuse government and industry of purposely duping the public into accepting the disposal of toxic wastes into our water supplies. In the middle are the issues that have proven to be the real battleground: whether fluoridation is a health hazard and whether its implementation constitutes a form of involuntary mass medication that represents an unacceptable intrusion of government into private life.

TABLE 2.6   Summary of Objections to Fluoridation

Anti-fluoridationist Claims	Questions That Need to Be Answered
Fluoridation is not effective. It is not responsible for the historical reduction in the occurrence of dental caries.	How strong is the evidence for a cause–effect relationship between water fluoridation and reduced dental caries? What other drivers could be responsible for the historical reductions observed?
Fluoridation is not cost-efficient. Cheaper and more effective fluoride delivery systems are available.	What are these alternative delivery systems, and what are their pros and cons relative to drinking water fluoridation? Is it possible to carry out comparative cost–benefit analyses?
Fluoridation systems are prone to engineering failures that could release toxic concentrations of fluoride into public water supply systems.	Is there any evidence in the historical record of toxic releases due to engineering failures? If so, how do the risks associated with such failures compare with other widely accepted technological risks?
Fluoridation is a health hazard. It causes increased incidence of dental fluorosis, skeletal fluorosis, hip fractures, bone diseases, heart problems, allergic reactions, and certain types of cancer. It is implicated in Down's syndrome, Alzheimer's disease, diminishment of IQ, and premature aging.	What is the status of current medical research into the impact of fluoride on human health? What conclusions can be drawn on the basis of toxicological and epidemiological evidence currently available with respect to each potential impact or disease?
Fluoridation constitutes a form of socialized medicine, involuntary mass medication, and/or human medical experimentation.	How does fluoridation compare with other widely accepted health-based delivery programs, such as chlorination of water, pasteurization of milk, iodinization of salt, and school vaccination?
Fluoridation is an infringement on personal freedoms and liberties. It is an unacceptable governmental intrusion into private life.	How does fluoridation compare with other intrusive but apparently widely accepted governmental programs, such as tax collection or the setting of speed limits?
Fluoridation is a planned conspiracy against the populace: (a) by certain industries as a cheap method of disposing of their toxic fluoride wastes, or (b) by government, as a method of pacifying the public chemically.	Is there any basis for these apparently fluorophobic conspiracy theories?

One can also identify a historical time line associated with these objections, wherein each issue mirrors the tenor of its times. In the 1950s, wary citizens worried about communist plots. The 1960s saw a growth in concern over military–industrial conspiracies. The 1970s placed fluoridation in an environmental context. The issues of the 1980s and 1990s reflected societal obsessions with personal health, beauty, and aging. Even the diseases targeted by anti-fluoridation forces reflect the fears of the day, as early concerns over Down's syndrome gave way to anxiety over heart disease, then cancer, and now AIDS.

In the right-hand column of Table 2.6 we have identified the questions that have to be addressed if one is to meet the anti-fluoridation arguments. These questions have set the public agenda, and to some degree they set the agenda for this book. In later chapters, each of these questions is addressed in as objective a manner as can be mustered. The goal is to uncover the facts as best we can, identify the most defensible current thinking, and emphasize the viewpoints that seem to be supported by the strongest weight of evidence.

FLUORIDATION FACTS, DR. Y, AND THE *LIFESAVER'S GUIDE*

On October 8, 2000, the anti-fluoridation forces lost one of their most effective and charismatic spokesmen, John Yiamouyiannis, known among both his supporters and his opponents as Dr. Y. He died at the relatively young age of 58 after a long fight with cancer. It was the disease he most feared and the one he linked throughout his life to fluoridated drinking water. After his death, a eulogy posted by the anti-fluoride website of the Fluoride Action Network described him as "a man of true honor and integrity" and "one of those rare kind of scientists who has the courage and commitment to take scientific truth to political power."

John Yiamouyiannis was a biochemist who served as an editor of the respected journal *Chemical Abstracts*. He abandoned the safe and easy career path that was available to him, and chose instead to dedicate his life to the anti-fluoridation movement. He wrote pamphlets and brochures by the dozens and made sure that they were widely distributed in every community facing a fluoridation referendum. He visited many of these cities and towns personally and campaigned tirelessly on behalf of the anti-fluoridation forces. Calling himself "the world's leading authority on the biological effects of fluoride," he attracted attention wherever he went by persistently claiming that fluoridation is linked to an increased incidence of cancer. He testified to this effect on several occasions before subcommittees of the U.S. Congress. When the National Institute of Dental Research (NIDR) carried out a survey of U.S. schoolchildren in 1986–1987, Dr. Y used the Freedom of Information Act to obtain copies of the original data, which he then used to try to refute the claims made in the NIDR report about the benefits of fluoridation. His book *Fluoride: The Aging Factor: How to Recognize the Devastating Effects of Fluoride* is perhaps the most widely quoted anti-fluoridation treatise ever published.[30]

Dr. Y's anti-fluoridation activities cost him his job at at the American Chemical Society, publishers of *Chemical Abstracts.* He brought a wrongful-dismissal lawsuit against his employers, claiming in the suit that the federal Department of Health, Education, and Welfare had threatened to cut off annual grants of $1.1 million to the ACS unless his anti-fluoridation views were silenced.[31] In 1974, he landed in the bosom of Fred Hart's National Health Federation (NHF). It was in that year that the NHF decided to mount a national campaign to "break the back" of the pro-fluoridation movement. They hired John Yiamouyiannis as science director and asked him to lead the charge. They couldn't have picked a better man. Yiamouyiannis produced a report claiming that fluoridation of drinking water supplies was responsible for 25,000 excess cancer deaths per year in the United States. Mainstream medical agencies, including the NCI, slammed the report, both for its methodology and its conclusions. But Yiamouyiannis continued to press his viewpoint forcefully in fluoridation campaigns across the nation. Dr. Y's cancer scare is credited for the defeat of a fluoridation initiative in Los Angeles in 1975 and for countless others over the years. The Yiamouyiannis studies even had an impact on European campaigns, especially those in England and the Netherlands.[32] In 1979, Dr. Y had a falling-out with the NHF and left to form his own Center for Health Action, from which base he continued his anti-fluoridation efforts until his death.[33]

John Yiamouyiannis was an enigma to the pro-fluoridation camp. Unlike many others who trekked the anti trail, Dr. Y was not strident in the pulpit. He was forceful but sincere in debate, and was generally liked, even by his opponents. His written material, on the other hand, was shrill and alarmist. The quiet Dr. Jekyll became the ferocious Mr. Hyde when he took pen in hand. Opponents pilloried him over his cancer claims, accusing him of shamelessly playing on people's fears to advance his anti-fluoridation agenda. In 1978, *Consumer Reports* published a two-part article on fluoridation that was critical of Yiamouyiannis's claims.[34] He filed suit for libel, but the suit was dismissed both in a lower court and on appeal. In 1995, the *British Dental Journal* was so exercised at his involvement in British fluoridation battles that they felt the need to publish a denigrating article entitled "Putting Yiamouyiannis into Perspective." Michael Easley, commenting on his passing and apparently looking for something positive to say, noted somewhat patronizingly that if Yiamouyiannis had only chosen a more productive topic for his life's work, he could surely have had an enormous positive impact on human affairs. On the Quackwatch homepage, the best that Stephen Barrett could bring himself to say was that John Yiamouyiannis was "personable and appeared sincere" and "to the uninformed he seemed credible." In a final irony, his home town of Delaware, Ohio, approved fluoridation just a few months before he died there.

Perhaps Dr. Y's most influential piece of writing is a short pamphlet that he wrote in 1993 entitled the *Lifesaver's Guide to Fluoridation*. It was written as a counterpoint to the information package put out by the American Dental Association under the title *Fluoridation Facts*. Both monographs are in question-and-answer format. *Fluoridation Facts* answers 58 questions in 69 pages using 358 references to the scientific literature. The *Lifesaver's Guide* answers 17 questions in 8 pages using 220 references. Many of the questions are the same, but the answers are certainly not. It is difficult to imagine two documents that could provide more polarized information to the public. Here are some selected excerpts from *Fluoridation Facts* (FF) and the *Lifesaver's Guide* (LG):[35]

What Is Fluoride?

> FF: Fluoride is a naturally occurring element that prevents tooth decay systemically when ingested during tooth development and topically when applied to erupted teeth.

> LG: Fluoride is more poisonous than lead and just slightly less poisonous than arsenic. It has been used as a pesticide for the control of mice, rats, and other small pests.

Does Fluoridation Reduce Tooth Decay?

> FF: Yes. In the United States, an epidemiological survey of nearly 40,000 schoolchildren was completed in 1987. Nearly 50% of the children in the study aged 5 to 17 years were decay-free in their permanent teeth, which was a major change from a similar survey in 1980 in which approximately 37% were decay-free. This dramatic decline in decay rates was attributed primarily to the widespread use of fluoride. ...

> LG: No. The largest U.S. study examining the effect of fluoridation on tooth decay found that fluoridation does not reduce decay in permanent teeth. Examination of the dental records of 39,207 schoolchildren, ages 5 to 17, from 84 geographical areas around the United States showed the number of decayed, missing, and filled permanent teeth per child was 2.0 in fluoridated areas, 2.0 in nonfluoridated areas, and 2.2 in partially fluoridated areas.

Does Fluoride Cause Genetic Damage?

FF: No. Following a review of generally accepted scientific knowledge the National Research Council of the National Academy of Sciences supports the conclusion that drinking optimally fluoridated water is not a genetic hazard.

LG: Yes. A study by Procter & Gamble showed that as little as half the amount of fluoride used to fluoridate public water supplies resulted in a sizable and significant increase in genetic damage.

Are there any links between Fluoridation and Cancer?

FF: No. According to generally accepted scientific knowledge, there is no connection between cancer rates in humans and adding fluoride to drinking water.

LG: Yes. In animal studies, water fluoridated at 1 part per million has been shown to increase tumor growth rate by 25%, to produce melanotic tumors, and to transform normal cells into cancer cells.

And so on. The ADA assures us that everything is okay, while Dr. Y warns us that everything is amiss. Both claim that they are relying on references from the scientific literature, but the two documents have very few references in common. The ADA relies heavily on the "weight of evidence." If there are 10 experimental studies whose results are favorable to the fluoridation case and two that raise doubts, the ADA extols the 10 and questions the methodology of the two. Dr. Y doesn't even mention the 10; he quotes only the two, as if they represented the total sum of knowledge on that issue. *Fluoridation Facts* refers regularly to supporting statements from august bodies in the medical establishment. The *Lifesaver's Guide* gives them no mention. *Fluoridation Facts* belittles the motives and reputations of those researchers whose results call into question the establishment position. The *Lifesaver's Guide* treats them as messiahs.

In 1985, a group of four scientific editors from well-known state and federal dental-research agencies, with the help of 14 contributing research scientists, published a stinging attack on the *Lifesaver's Guide* in a publication entitled *The Abuse of the Scientific Literature in an Antifluoridation Pamphlet.*[36] The report carries a preface by Michael Easley and a foreword by Stephen Barrett. The authors accuse Yiamouyannis of misleading and inappropriate use of the scientific literature in the *Lifesaver's Guide*. First, they note that many of the references cited are impossible to locate or come from obscure foreign journals that are far from the scientific mainstream. Some even come from journals that the authors claim were set up specifically to provide an outlet for anti-fluoridation papers that would never have been accepted by established medical journals. They found further that the only articles quoted on a given subject were those few that provided some ammunition to anti-fluoridation claims. The much larger number of more reputable articles that refuted these positions were not referenced. More damaging yet, the authors accuse Yiamouyiannis of "selectively interpreting a number of scientific articles" to make them look more supportive of his position than they actually are. In many cases, they claim, the authors of articles quoted in the *Lifesaver's Guide* qualified their conclusions carefully "to avoid impugning water fluoridation," but these disclaimers were ignored. Overall, they castigate Yiamouyiannis for using "a pseudo-scientific approach that could, at first glance, fool the casual reader." They accuse Dr. Y. of darkening the fluoridation debate with "half-truths," "innuendo," and "deception."

Trying to look at the two documents objectively, it is difficult not to side with those who attack Yiamouyiannis's methods. The *Lifesaver's Guide* is indeed propaganda masquerading as science. The information that it provides to the reader is selective, incomplete, and in that sense, dishonest. *Fluoridation Facts* suffers some of the same flaws, but at least the (anonymous) authors inform the reader that there is another side to some of the arguments. They usually proceed to trash the opposing arguments as if they were an evil smell, but in the street fight that passes for dialogue in the fluoridation wars, one must give credit where it is due, even if that credit is for the most token nod to fairness and civility.

Perhaps recognizing the lack of sophistication in the original *Lifesaver's Guide*, an anti-fluoride group has recently posted a new and somewhat fairer response to *Fluoridation Facts*. The language is more conciliatory, but the arguments remain unresolved. It can be found at the website www.fluoridedebate.com.

WHAT WE HAVE HERE IS A FAILURE TO COMMUNICATE

The battle of the pamphlets is just one aspect of a massive failure to communicate. There seems to be no common ground at all between the two sides. Neither side even tries to engage the other side in dialogue. There is no move toward compromise. Each side continues to appeal to its own narrow constituency by refusing to move off its fixed positions. Even minor differences over language seem to be insoluble. Both sides agree that fluoridation involves the addition of a chemical to the water, but anti-fluoridationists refer to this augmentation as "forced medication," whereas pro-fluoridationists speak of the "enhancement" of the natural water chemistry.

The two sides seldom interact, even at the level of scientific research. One would think that a scientific journal called *Fluoride* would be an outlet where scientists could set out their experimental results and let the chips fall where they may. Not so. It turns out that *Fluoride* was founded in 1966 by George Waldbott, a Detroit physician who specialized in allergies, and in particular in "chronic fluoride toxicity syndrome." He was quite highly regarded in his field, having served as vice-president of the American College of Allergists, but like John Yiamouyiannis, he chose to devote much of his energy to active opposition of community water fluoridation, and in doing so he squandered some of his credibility with his medical peers. He was the senior author of one of the first anti-fluoridation books to hit the public consciousness,[37] and he and his wife Edith started the first widely circulated anti-fluoridation newsletter, the *National Fluoridation News*. He also founded a scientific society, the International Society for Fluoride Research, that he hoped would provide a home for fluoride researchers of all stripes. Alas, the ISFR and its journal, *Fluoride*, were considered from the beginning as a vehicle for anti-fluoridation propaganda and were never taken seriously by the mainstream medical–dental fraternity. The ISFR still exists, still holds regular meetings, and still publishes *Fluoride*, but most of the scientists who attend meetings of the ISFR and publish their results in *Fluoride* are also active in the political struggle against fluoridation.

Unfortunately, the shoe fits the other foot almost as well. The medical establishment has not exactly welcomed dissident researchers to its bosom. Research papers that brought the value or safety of fluoridation into question were systematically denied publication by mainstream medical–dental journals, and the authors of such papers were often shunned by their peers. Pro-fluoridation scientists also have their own closed-shop meetings. The National Fluoridation Summit held in Sacramento in September 2000 featured only speakers that supported fluoridation. The sponsors of the meeting included the American Medical Association, the California Dental Association, and the National Center for Fluoridation Policy and Research. Participation in the meeting was by "invitation only."

The National Fluoridation Summit was a magnet for anti-fluoridation activists. They secured a permit to demonstrate on the sidewalk outside the hotel, then violated their permit by entering the hotel property and verbally assaulting several of the meeting attendees. They attempted to invade closed meetings and had to be evicted by conference organizers. At the close of the conference, protesters attempted to blockade the hotel driveway to prevent conference attendees from getting to their scheduled airline connections. These attempts failed when police were called by hotel security, and protesters fled the scene to avoid arrest.[38]

During the 1970s, 1980s, and early 1990s, in the pre-Internet era, the fluoridation battles were fought in print. Anti-fluoridation authors put out books by the bushelful, usually self-published, highly inflammatory, and having limited sales, mostly to the already converted. The press took scant interest in these tracts. Waldbott's book, which appeared in 1978, and Yiamouyiannis's in 1983, had somewhat broader circulation and received more press interest, probably because of the stronger medical credentials of the authors. The pro-fluoridation forces took the high road, releasing heavy scientific tomes under the imprimatur of the Public Health Service, the National Academy of Sciences, and the World Health Organization.[39] Few Americans actually read these studies, but their results usually made the news, and they formed the basis for many articles in women's magazines and *Reader's Digest* that touted the benefits of fluoride on children's teeth.

It was only in the 1990s that investigative journalists discovered the fluoridation question. In its February 5, 1990 issue, *Newsweek*, For example, carried an article with the provocative title "The Fluoride Risk: Evidence of a Link to Cancer."[40] Despite the title, the article covered the topic in a balanced manner with quotes from all the players, both pro and anti. The response of the two camps to these "balanced" articles is interesting. The pro-fluoridation camp is extremely displeased with any article that does not toe the establishment line fully and completely. They dislike ifs and buts. It is their position that there is no scientific controversy. In their view, all opposition to fluoridation is heresy and paranoia. They go ballistic when the mainstream press strives for "balance" on the fluoridation issue. In their eyes there is no need for balance. One side is right and the other side is wrong. "They're flat-Earthers," says Michael Easley, "I don't bother trying to convince them. They're uneducable." When the author of a lengthy article for the Sunday supplement of the *Cleveland Plain Dealer* interviewed him for her piece, his advice was blunt. "Don't do the article," he said. "It will only scare people. Just bringing it up makes people think there's something wrong."[41]

The anti-fluoridation camp, on the other hand, tends to be tickled pink with "balanced" articles, because to them, half a loaf is better than no loaf at all. Their message may be diluted, but at least it gets out to the lay public. They see these articles as an antidote to the one-sided viewpoint that is delivered to the public by the American Dental Association and the Public Health Service. They are so used to being held up to ridicule by the medical establishment that they are pleased to be taken even semiseriously by the popular press.

One of the most influential popular articles to appear on fluoridation was published in the August 1, 1988 issue of *Chemical and Engineering News*.[42] It was written by one of the editors of this journal as a special report entitled

"Fluoridation of Water: Questions About Health Risks and Benefits Remain After More Than 40 Years." *Chemical and Engineering News* is a journal of the American Chemical Society. The article in question may have been the first to present a "balanced" treatment of the issue in the mainstream scientific press. As such, it created quite a furore. The article generated news stories in the popular press around the country. Anti-fluoridation organizations quoted selectively from it and played up its establishment credentials. Pro-fluoridation groups were livid and accused the American Chemical Society of giving credibility to half-baked scientific criticisms. They demanded that the American Chemical Society clarify the fact that it did not have an official stand on fluoridation, nor was it in any position to take such a stand, given its admitted lack of expertise in dental science. In the issues following the one that contained the contentious article, the journal printed 38 letters to the editor, most of them quite long, and many of them authored by some of the principal public figures in the fluoridation battle. Twenty-one of the letters took a clear anti-fluoridation stance, and almost all of them were complementary to the article and commended the authors for its "balance." Seven of the letters took a clear pro-fluoridation stance, and every one of them claimed that the article was severely biased.

All of these books and articles still rest on the shelves of your local library (or perhaps your nearest university library). But they probably haven't been checked out in years. The Internet is with us now, and the battleground has gone electronic. All the naughty bits are now posted on somebody's website. And the really naughty bits are posted on *everybody's* website. The Internet is usually touted as a great liberating force in society: infinite information on call, and instant communication at our fingertips. But there is a downside. A recent book by Cass Sunstein,[43] a law professor at the University of Chicago, raises troubling questions. He argues that Internet technology, with its instantaneous links to other websites, encourages people to limit their exposure to like-minded viewpoints. In this sense, the medium tends to polarize rather than broaden thinking. It offers a powerful pulpit for fringe groups and extremists, a chance for them to reach much larger audiences than they ever reached before, and an opportunity for them to draw in new recruits with greater ease. Such groups use the Internet as a tool for propaganda, not as an aid to education.

We worry that the fluoridation controversy supports Sunstein's thesis. We enter the new millennium with the two sides pulling ever farther apart. The relative success of the fluoridation movement seems to have driven its opponents to take even more extreme positions than they have in the past. Not only that, but anti- and pro-fluoridationists alike are circling the wagons, building networks of like-minded anti- and pro-establishment thinkers, and closing the door to meaningful dialogue across the great divide. ADA spokesman John Stamm recognizes the standoff. "We've all tried hard to persuade each other," he says, "but the evidence appears to be that we haven't persuaded each other very much. On both sides a certain level of futility sets in that we're never going to persuade the other side. There's a feeling that not much is going to change."[44] In a 1991 study, a social scientist interviewed 18 of the leading scientific proponents and opponents of fluoridation in Australia.[45] He found the representatives of each camp to have a strikingly "monolithic perspective" that features total rejection of all the arguments of the other side. Most interviewees claimed that their position was based totally on the scientific evidence while denying that there is any rational basis for a contrary view. In explanation, he found that contact between partisans on opposite sides was uncommon, whereas interaction between those on the same side was frequent and intense. He speculated that peer pressure within the group may discourage "breaking ranks" and promotes a clonish viewpoint. He suggested that "those with intermediate, complex, or ambivalent positions" received little encouragement to take leading roles. Followers seldom openly criticized the "inaccuracies, exaggerations, and simplifications" made by their leaders, even though they may have privately deplored these shortcomings.

There is a telling anecdote in a recent article describing a fluoridation campaign in a small community in western Canada.[46] At the end of a public meeting with 100 or so people in attendance, the moderator asked if anyone present had changed his or her mind after hearing the night's speeches and discussion. Not one hand was raised.

REFERENCES

1. M. W. Easley, Fluoridation: a triumph of science over propaganda, *Priorities*, 8(4), 1996.

2. U.S. Public Health Service, Centers for Disease Control and Prevention, Ten great public health achievements, United States, 1900–1999, *MMWR* 48(12), 241–243, 1999; U.S. Public Health Service, Centers for Disease Control and Prevention, Achievements in public health, 1900–1999: fluoridation of drinking water to prevent dental caries, *MMWR* 48(41), 933–940, 1999.

3. A. L. Gotzsche, *The Fluoride Question: Panacea or Poison*, Davis-Poynter, London, 1975; P. R. N. Sutton, *The Greatest Fraud: Fluoridation*, Factual Books, West Yorkshire, UK, 1994; G. Caldwell and P. E. Zanfagna, *Fluoridation and Truth Decay*, Top Ecology Press, Reseda, CA, 1974.

4. E. M. Whelan, *Toxic Terror: The Truth Behind the Cancer Scares*, Prometheus Books, Amherst, NY, 1993.

5. A. J. Lieberman and S. C. Kwon, *Facts Versus Fears: A Review of the Greatest Unfounded Health Scares of Recent Times*, 3rd ed., American Council on Science and Health, New York, 1998.

6. American Dental Association, Fluoridation Facts, http://www.ada.org.

7. National Center for Fluoridation, http://www.fluoridationcenter.org.

8. The quotes and biographical material on Stephen Barrett are taken from the curriculum vitae that appears on the Quackwatch homepage, http://www.quackwatch.com, and from the transcript of an interview with Barrett by Marjorie Rosen of Biography magazine, which is also reproduced on that website.

9. S. Barrett and S. Rovin, eds., *The Tooth Robbers: A Pro-Fluoridation Handbook*, George F. Stickley, Philadelphia, 1980.

10. The quotes attributed to Darlene Sherrell in this section are taken from her opinion piece on the Stop Fluoridation website, http://www.rvi.net/~fluoride/, entitled "What is quackery? What is fraud? And who decides?"

11. S. Barrett and W. T. Jarvis, *The Health Robbers: A Close Look at Quackery in America*, Prometheus Books, Amherst, NY, 1993.

12. All of the facts and quotes about the Barrett–Sherrell lawsuit come from the opinion and order filed by U.S. District Judge F. S. Van Antwerpen on April 12, 1999 in the U.S. District Court for the Eastern District of Pennsylvania in the matter of *Stephen Barrett, M. D. v. The Catacombs Press, James R. Privatera, M. D., Alan Stang, M. A., Darlene Sherrell, and CDS Networks*.

13. Quackbuster busted, *Chiropract. J.*, as posted by the World Chiropractic Alliance, http://www.worldchiropracticalliance.org, September 12, 2001.

14. Letter dated March 3, 2001, from Darlene Sherrell to the Office of the Clerk, U.S. District Court for the District of Oregon; as posted by Stop Fluoridation, http://www.rvi.net/~fluoride/.

15. As posted at http://www.trufax.org.

16. B. A. Burt and S. A. Eklund, *Dentistry, Dental Practice, and the Community*, W. B. Saunders, Philadelphia, 1999.

17. American Dental Association, *Statement on Water Fluoridation Efficacy and Safety*, http://www.ada.org.

18. National Health Federation, http://www.thenhf.com.

19. Fluoridation: the cancer scare, *Consumer Reports*, July 1978, pp. 392–396, and August 1978, pp. 480–483.

20. The Sierra Club statement can be found at http://www.fluoridealert.org. The Pennsylvania position paper is authored by L. Landes and M. Bechis, and is titled "America: over-dosed on fluoride." It is posted by the Leading Edge International Research Group, http://www.trufax.org.

21. M. J. Prival and F. Fisher, *Fluorides and Human Health*, Center for Science in the Public Interest, Washington, DC, 1972.

22. R. R. Harris, *Dental Science in a New Age: A History of the National Institute of Dental Research*, Montrose Press, Rockville, MD, 1989.

23. California Citizens for Safe Drinking Water, http://www.nofluoride.com.

24. B. Martin, *Scientific Knowledge In Controversy: The Social Dynamics of the Fluoridation Debate*, State University of New York Press, Albany, NY, 1991.

25. The historical fluoridation statistics in Table 2.3 represent a kind of smoothed average of the (not always in agreement) values garnered from a variety of articles and books on the history of fluoridation. The 2005 value is from the American Dental Association, *Fluoridation Facts*, op. cit.

26. Information in Table 2.5 has been integrated from several sources, including American Dental Association, *Fluoridation Facts*, op. cit.; Burt and Eklund, 1999, op. cit.; Martin, 1991, op. cit.; J. J. Murray, A. J. Rugg-Gunn, and G. N. Jenkins, *Fluorides in Caries Prevention*, 3rd ed., Butterworth-Heinemann Publishers, Boston, MA, 1991; J. R. Mellberg and L. W. Ripa, *Fluoride in Preventive Dentistry*, Quintessence Publishing, Hanover Park, IL, 1983.

27. J. Wynbrandt, *The Excruciating History of Dentistry: Toothsome Tales and Oral Oddities from Babylon to Braces*, St. Martin's Press, New York, 1998.

28. Martin, 1991, op. cit.; M. E. Bernhardt, Fluoridation international, *J. Am. Dent. Assoc.*, 80, 731–734, 1970; R. Scobie, Water fluoridation: a survey of the international picture, *Alabama J. Med. Sci.*, 12(3), 225–229, 1975; World Health Organization, *Experience on Water Fluoridation in Europe*, WHO, Geneva, Switzerland, 1987.

29. K. R. Elwell and K. A. Easlick, *Classification and Appraisal of Objections to Fluoridation*, University of Michigan School of Public Health, Ann Arbor, MI, 1960.

30. J. Yiamouyiannis, *Fluoride: The Aging Factor—How to Recognize the Devastating Effects of Fluoride*, Health Action Press, Delaware, OH, 1983.

31. Caldwell and Zanfagna, 1974, op. cit.

32. *Consumer Reports*, 1978, op. cit.

33. The quotes and information on John Yiamouyiannis are taken from his obituary in the *Columbus Dispatch*, October 10, 2000; the Fluoride Action Network, http://www.fluoridealert.org; Quackwatch, http://www.quackwatch.com; and the paper by J. Hunt, S. Boulton, M. A. Lennon, R. J. Lowry, and S. Jones, Putting Yiamouyiannis into perspective, *Br. Dent. J.*, 179(4), 121–123, 1995.

34. *Consumer Reports*, 1978, op. cit.

35. American Dental Association, Fluoridation Facts, op. cit.; J. Yiamouyiannis, *Lifesaver's Guide to Fluoridation*, Safe Water Foundation, Delaware, OH, 1982. The wording of the questions in the two documents is not identical. We have edited the wording in a way that we believe is fair to the sense of both documents.

36. C. A. Wulf, K. F. Hughes, K. G. Smith, and M. W. Easley, *The Abuse of the Scientific Literature in an Antifluoridation Pamphlet*, American Oral Health Institute Press, Columbus, OH, 1985.

37. G. L. Waldbott, A. W. Burgstahler, and H. L. McKinney, *Fluoridation: The Great Dilemma*, Coronado Press, Lawrence, KS, 1978.

38. M. W. Easley, Antifluoridation zealots resort to criminal acts in Sacremento, News Bulletin posted by NCFPR, http://fluoride.oralhealth.org.

39. U.S. Public Health Service, *Review of Fluoride, Benefits and Risks*, U.S. PHS, Washington, DC, 1991; National Academy of Sciences, National Research Council, Board on Environmental Studies and Toxicology, *Health Effects of Ingested Fluoride*, National Academics Press, Washington, DC, 1993; World Health Organization, *Fluorides and Oral Health*, Report of the WHO Expert Committee on Oral Health Status and Fluoride Use, WHO Technical Series 846, WHO, Geneva, Switzerland, 1994.

40. *Newsweek*, February 5, 1990.

41. F. Henry, The invisible fear, *Cleveland Plain Dealer*, Sunday supplement, March 26, 2000.

42. B. Hileman, Fluoridation of water: questions about health risks and benefits remain after more than 40 years, *Chem. Eng. News*, 66, 26–42, August 1, 1988.

43. C. Sunstein, *Republic.com*, Princeton University Press, Princeton, NJ, 2001.

44. Quoted in Henry, 2000, op. cit.

45. Martin, 1991, op. cit.

46. C. Clark and H. J. Hann, A win for fluoridation in Squamish, B. C., *J. Pub. Health Dent.*, 49(3), 170–171, 1989.

CHAPTER 3

A TALE OF TWO CITIES

On November 7, 2000, the first presidential election night of the new millennium unfolded like a surrealistic dream. Americans of all stripes remained tethered to their TV sets as the networks lurched from one pronouncement to the next, first declaring George W. Bush to be the new president, then Al Gore, then Bush again, and finally admitting after we had all gone to bed that it was too close to call. The next morning, and indeed for the next 36 days, we learned more than we needed to know about the frailties of exit polls, the arcane niceties of Florida election law, and the partisan passions that could be aroused by a hanging chad.

Of course, passions are not reserved solely for presidential politics. State and local measures often fan the flames of community discord even more than national contests. On the night of November 7, 2000, voters also hung on the results of 204 statewide referendums and initiatives that were on the ballot in 42 states.[1] Voters in Maine were deciding if they wanted to sanction doctor-assisted suicide. In Alaska, the legality of marijuana was on the ballot. An Oregon initiative asked voters to ban the promotion of homosexuality in public schools. In Virginia and North Dakota, voters were set to declare hunting a constitutional right. In Alabama, voters considered the repeal of that state's constitutional ban on interracial marriage, the last such ban in the nation.

At the local level, voters in Ventura, Minnesota, which was named for Governor Jesse Ventura, considered renaming their town St. Augusta. In Greensboro, West Virginia, voters were deciding whether an elegant resort should be allowed to turn a fallout shelter built for Congress into a fancy underground casino. And in 26 U.S. cities and towns, there were fluoridation

The Fluoride Wars: How a Modest Public Health Measure Became America's Longest-Running Political Melodrama By R. Allan Freeze and Jay H. Lehr
Copyright © 2009 John Wiley & Sons, Inc.

measures on the ballot. Would Las Vegas take the gamble? Would the ghost of Davey Crockett sip fluoridated water from the taps of the Alamo in San Antonio? What about those free-spirited westerners in Abilene, Texas; the Silicon Valley bedroom commuters of Sunnyvale, California; and the academic literati of Ithaca, New York?

In the months leading up to election day, activists on both sides of the fluoridation issue worked hard to coin names for their civic action teams that they hoped would put them on the high ground in voters' eyes. In Las Vegas, the Citizens for Healthy Smiles faced off against the Citizens for Safe Drinking Water. In Spokane, Washington, it was People for Healthy Teeth versus the Fluoride Awareness Coalition. In nearby Yakima, the Yakima County Children's Oral Health Coalition squared off against the Yakima Safe Water Coalition.

The level of engagement in Connersville, Indiana, was representative.[2] Connersville is the largest city in Indiana without fluoridated water, and John Roberts, the local dentist who led the fluoridation fight there, could point to studies that showed that the Connersville population has a 20% higher rate of cavities than the state average. He brandished the unimpeachable evidence of reduced tooth decay with fluoridation and called on the endorsements of the national and local medical establishment to defend the safety of fluoridation against charges of adverse health impact. Mary Hendershott of the Citizens for Safe Water accused government and industry of colluding on a toxic waste scam and charged that organizations that support fluoridation get government kickbacks. As proponents and opponents both pressured reluctant local candidates to take a stand, outgoing councilman Virgle Carey sat in a smoke-filled barbershop amid a group of men loudly voicing their opinions. "It's the number one issue around here," he says. "I'm sure glad I won't have to deal with it."

In Salt Lake City, an election-day bomb threat delayed vote tabulation of absentee ballots for all the election races and propositions, including a fluoridation initiative.[3] The threat came in to the Salt Lake County office about 11 A.M., and workers were not allowed to return until 4:30. Although no group claimed responsibility, and the perpetrators were never apprehended, the stewards of the website for the pro-fluoridation National Center for Fluoridation Policy and Research couldn't resist a little speculation. "Were anti-fluoride zealots responsible for this?" they ask. The level of acrimony runs deep, at least among the cadres of committed activists. Among the voters themselves, things are a bit less intense. "Are you going to vote for fluorine?" runs the apocryphal one-liner. "I don't know," comes the answer. "What's she running for?"

SPOKANE, WASHINGTON

One of the cities that hosted a fluoridation plebiscite on the night of the Bush–Gore dead heat was the city of Spokane, Washington. Hailed in tourist pamphlets as the "Heart of the Inland Empire," Spokane lies in the piney rangeland of eastern Washington, almost in Idaho and just 100 miles south of the Canadian border. With a population of 184,000 and a county total that runs upward of 400,000, Spokane is the second-biggest metropolitan area in the state of Washington, and it is advertised by local boosters as the biggest city between Minneapolis and Seattle. There are 76 lakes within a 50-mile radius of the city, more than 1600 miles of hiking trails in the area, and 13 ski resorts within 250 miles. People arrive here on assignment from their firms in San Francisco or Los Angeles or Seattle, and many never leave. They come to escape the crowds, or the high cost of living, or the earthquakes, and they fall in love with a land of contrasts. Rolling wheatfields give way to snowcapped mountains, lush forests to near-desert, and pristine lakes to raging rivers.[4]

The Spokane River runs right through the center of town, and it was on the banks of the river, not far from a spectacular set of rapids known as "The Bowl and Pitcher," that John Jacob Astor's Pacific Fur Company established a trading post in 1810 known as Spokane House. In 1881, the Northern Pacific Railroad arrived, and by 1910 the population of Spokane had grown to 140,000, despite the great fire of 1889, which wiped out the entire business district. In 1974, Spokane hosted Expo '74, a world's fair that was only modestly successful in attracting exhibits from the international community but which placed the city's name in the nation's consciousness. The red-tile-topped campanile (just like the one in St. Mark's Square in Venice) that was built for the fair remains the centerpiece of the city. The old Expo grounds have become Riverfront Park, one of the loveliest city-center parks in the nation and a gorgeous backdrop for the nearby Spokane Opera House, the Performing Arts Center, the Memorial Arena, and the historic Flour Mill shopping district.

In case this all sounds a bit too tasteful for the usual image of a gun-totin', beer-slingin' western town, let it be known that Spokane also hosts an annual event known as "Hoopfest," the largest three-on-three basketball tournament in the world, during which time the beer joints in town do a booming business. And if we are to believe the dark vision set out in a recent *noir* novel, the city even has a serious underbelly.[5] In his book *Over Tumbled Graves*, Jess Walter, a veteran Spokane journalist, invents a disquieting serial killer who preys on drugged-out prostitutes plying their trade in Riverfront Park. He describes Spokane as "the trailer park of the Pacific Northwest" and his book is populated with trashy losers. It is a pessimistic image of the city, and to be fair, it is an image that doesn't square with any other source of information on the city. It certainly doesn't fit with the Chamber of Commerce statistic which claims that 85% of Spokane residents over 25 have completed high school, or with the presumed cultural impact of three university campuses in a tight-knit midsize city. Spokane hosts the campuses of Washington State University at Spokane, Eastern Washington University, and Gonzaga University. (Yes, this is *the* Gonzaga University, home to the perennial cinderella basketball squad that always seems to upset some powerhouse team in the first round of the NCAA basketball tournament during "March Madness" every year.)

Spokane has been through the fluoridation wringer three times. In 1969, voters approved fluoridation in an advisory vote to the city council, but then rejected it in a binding vote. In 1984, the city council approved fluoridation without going to the people, but opponents subsequently forced a public vote and the voters spurned the initiative yet again.

In the spring of 2000, a bill that would have mandated the use of fluoride in all community drinking water systems in Washington was introduced in the state senate, but it stalled in the senate budget committee. The state representative for Spokane, Republican Linda Schindler, opposed the bill. Washington is one of the few states that have formally rejected a statewide fluoridation mandate.

With the failure of the statewide mandate, the dental community in Spokane decided to revive the issue at the local level. A public action committee was formed under the title "People for Healthy Teeth." Mary Smith, a Spokane dentist and the first woman ever elected as president of the Washington State Dental Association, was named chairperson. The PFHT approached the city council and requested them to place a question on the November ballot that would permit the addition of fluoride to the Spokane water supply. The council scheduled a hearing on the ballot measure for June 26.[6]

Technically, there were only two issues on the agenda at the June 26 council meeting. The first entailed consideration of the specific wording of the ballot measure, and the second revolved around whether the council would place the measure on the ballot immediately or would require the proponents to go through a petition process to prove that there was a sufficient level of support in the community to warrant the ballot question. Not surprisingly, the speakers at the meeting did not feel constrained by the technicalities. Comments ranged over the full suite of fluoridation arguments, pro and con. Kim Thorburn, director of the Spokane Regional Health District, informed council of fluoridation's ranking as one of the top 10 public health accomplishments of the twentieth century. Betty Fowler of the Washington

State Safe Water Coalition called studies supporting fluoride "junk science." Opponent Robert Stockton said that fluoridation violated his right to choose what he drinks. "All I want in my water, is water," he said.

On the question of the ballot title, People for Healthy Teeth argued for wording that strongly emphasized dental health benefits. Betty Fowler argued that a correct ballot title would say that the city is planning to introduce "an industrial waste poison" into the city's water system. In the end, the city council approved placing the measure on the ballot by a vote of 6 to 0. They made minor adjustments to the wording of the title, editing some of the language proposed by People for Healthy Teeth, which they felt was biased toward the fluoridation proponents. The final wording was: "Shall the city of Spokane periodically adjust the fluoride content of its water supply within the range prescribed by the Washington State Administrative Code, as provided by ordinance C32655?" The council refused to waive the petition process, a decision that ultimately forced the proponents to hire a professional signature-gathering organization to scour Spokane's shopping malls on their behalf in order to find 8500 fluoride supporters in the two-week period between the June 26 meeting and a specified deadline of July 10.

The signature-gathering team did their job. The final petition presented to the Spokane city council contained 12,742 signatures, considerably more than the 8500 required. However, this did not stop opponents from demanding a judicial audit of the signatures. On the weekend of August 26, groups of supporters and opponents hung silently in the background in a room in the Spokane County courthouse staring tensely at one another as professional auditors carefully checked the signatures. Very few signatures were deemed unsuitable, and the petition was approved. The cost of the professional signature gatherers (borne by PFHT) was about $25,000, and the cost of the auditors (borne by the taxpayers) was about $6000.

On September 18, Spokane city council added the fluoridation initiative to the November ballot as Proposition 1. In doing so they had to reject a legal argument presented by the opponents that the wording of the initiative was "slanted, biased, misleading and manipulative." The city attorney advised opponents to go to court over this issue if they desired. On September 29, they accepted his challenge. Betty Fowler and two other women filed a lawsuit in superior court against the city of Spokane, stating that the title of the fluoridation initiative "does not give a true and impartial statement of the purpose of the measure." The suit alleged that the ballot title is deceiving because it states that the fluoride level of the water will be "adjusted" and does not make it clear to voters that fluoride will be "added" to the water supply. John Robideaux, a spokesman for People for Healthy Teeth, countered that the word "adjust" was chosen carefully because there is already a certain level of naturally occurring fluoride in the water.

One of the two other women who joined Betty Fowler in bringing suit against the city was Rose Waldram, the founder of a small group, Citizens Allergic to Fluoride. She herself suffered from chronic rashes, flulike symptoms, painful joints, and bladder irritation, which she ascribed to the presence of fluoride in the environment. Some doctors in the past had apparently labeled her claims of fluoride allergy as hypochondria, but her then-current physician was willing to state publicly that her complaints were legitimate. Ms. Waldram claimed that she would have to move from her home if the fluoridation measure passed.

On October 10 Judge Linda Tompkins of the Spokane Superior Court handed down her ruling on the suit. She rebuffed the plaintiffs' demand for a change in wording on the ballot measure, ruling that Proposition 1 should go onto the ballot in its current form. She found nothing wrong with the language. "It doesn't create prejudice for or against the measure," she said.

Meanwhile, the campaign got into gear. Diane Eve and her husband, Michael Southworth, stood on street corners holding signs that said: "Fluoridation Will Cost Millions. Vote No." The League of Women Voters sponsored a public debate that attracted 50 people, most of whom seemed to have their mind made up before they got there, given the prevalence of lapel pins that read "Stop Fluoridation Before It Stops You," or "Fluoride: The Natural Solution. Vote Yes." Mary Smith, chairperson of People for Healthy Teeth, spoke for the proponents. Don Caron, a local healthy-living advocate and leader of the newly formed Fluoride Awareness Coalition, spoke for the opponents. In one interesting exchange, the moderator asked whether claims that fluoride could cause mottled teeth were true. Mary Smith replied that such a claim was "absolutely false," whereas Don Caron stated that two out of three children who lived in cities with fluoridated water developed such fluorosis. (The exchange is interesting because both these answers are incorrect.)

The fluoridation question posed a difficult problem for many of the politically appointed lay members of the Spokane Regional Health District. They were buffeted on the one hand by requests for support from their medical staff, including Kim Thorburn, the district director, and on the other hand by active lobbying from the anti-fluoridation community. Heated discussion of the issue erupted at the September 29 meeting of the regional health board. One board member argued that it is a moral responsibility of the health district to provide the best scientific information to the public. Another argued that it would be illegal for the health district to advocate a particular political position. In the end it was decided that the Spokane Regional Health District would take no official position in the fluoride controversy, while allowing Dr.

Thorburn to publicly express her personal endorsement of the fluoridation initiative. The pro-fluoridation camp left the meeting angry over their failure to gain the support of the primary health care agency in the region. The anti-fluoridation camp left the meeting angry that Dr. Thorburn had been given so much rope.

Throughout the campaign, the local newspaper, *The Spokesman Review*, maintained full and balanced coverage of the fluoridation initiative. On October 21 the paper published an editorial strongly recommending the passage of Proposition 1. The editorial closed with the clear instruction to "Vote to fluoridate Spokane's water." However, the very next day *The Spokesman Review* published a much longer article on the fluoridation fight that may have served to buttress the anti-fluoridation case. The article quoted Brad Blegan, director of the city water department, as one who would prefer to leave things as they are. "We've been blessed with clean water," he is quoted as saying, "so it's foreign to our thinking to start putting new chemicals in it." He is also quoted as estimating a $1 million capital cost for the installation of fluoridation equipment and annual maintenance costs of about $300,000 per year. There is information later in the article on the cost of filling a cavity, and it is mentioned that dental savings might therefore arise from fluoridation, but the cost–benefit relationship between these two sets of dollar figures is not clarified for the reader. The article also refers to the potential malfunctioning of fluoridation equipment, and it highlights the fluoride-allergy claims of Rose Waldron, who is quoted to the effect that she can't even shower or bathe in cities with fluoridated water.

On Saturday, October 28, Paul Connett came to town. Paul Connett is a professor of chemistry at St. Lawrence University in Canton, New York. He is one of a small cadre of nationally known anti-fluoridation spokesman. During the election campaign leading up to the November 2000 elections, Connett traveled to several cities that had fluoridation initiatives on the ballot, including San Antonio, Salt Lake City, and Spokane. He and his wife, Ellen, are politically active on *two* fronts. On the first front, they are coeditors of the newsletter *Waste Not* ("The Reporter for Rational Resource Management"), which is concerned primarily with the reduction of dioxin releases from incinerators and the promotion of sustainable alternatives to mega-landfills. Ralph Nader has described Paul Connett as "the only person I know who can make waste interesting." The second front is fluoridation. Paul and Ellen Connett were instrumental in creating the Fluoride Action Network, which is described as a "collective, international volunteer effort ... to counteract the misinformation spread by fluoridation spokespeople from the American Dental Association and the Centers for Disease Control." Paul Connett claims to have made over 1200 public presentations and radio and TV appearances, most of which have involved the fluoride controversy. He is very much at home in his radio appearances, because back in Canton, in another facet of his life, he hosts a weekly program of classical music on North Country Public Radio.

Paul Connett was brought to Spokane by Don Caron and the Fluoride Awareness Coalition as part of a ploy designed to embarrass the pro-fluoridation forces. Caron publicized Connett's visit as a debate. He booked Hughes Auditorium at Gonzaga University, and then, knowing full well that they would not agree to attend such a setup, he invited the leaders of People for Healthy Teeth to participate as well as several well-known national pro-fluoridationists, including Michael Easley of the National Center for Fluoridation Policy Research in Buffalo, New York. On the night of the "debate," Connett spoke alone in front of a big screen with a row of eight empty chairs behind him. Each chair was labeled in large print with the name of one of the people who had been invited to the debate but who had declined to show, including Kim Thorburn, Mary Smith, and Michael Easley.

In his presentation, Connett admitted that he is in the minority among scientists, dentists, and doctors when it comes to opinions on fluoride, but he accused the majority of failing to study the issue carefully and simply accepting endorsements made by the Surgeon General and other establishment medical organizations. "We're getting a wedge driven between good science and public policy," he said. When tracked down by the press, those leading the fight for Proposition 1 were not impressed with their opponents' gambit. Mary Smith questioned Connett's qualifications to speak on public health policy. "He's a chemist, not a dentist," she said.

On November 7, 2000, the voters of Spokane got their say. The final tally was 30,256 in favor, 31,865 against. Spokane voters had rejected fluoridation for the third time, this time by a margin of 51% to 49%. The only good news for the proponents was that the percentage of citizens supporting fluoridation has increased in each of the three elections: 35% in 1969, 45% in 1984, and 49% in 2000. People for Healthy Teeth spent $100,000 on the campaign ($25,000 for the petition and $75,000 on mailings and TV). The Fluoride Awareness Coalition spent only $5000, mostly on billboards and flyers. They claim that Paul Connett paid his own way to visit Spokane. Among the excuses offered by People for Healthy Teeth for their failure to convince the electorate to their point of view was their inability to gain a clear endorsement from the Spokane Regional Health District, the deflection of their energies into the litigation over the wording of the initiative, and the dollars spent on signature gathering for the petition that should have gone into "public education."

The leaders of People for Healthy Teeth vow they will try again in a future election. "We're not going to stop because of this election," said Mary

Smith. "We're not going to wait another 16 years." Rose Waldron of Citizens Allergic to Fluoride had a simpler response. "Praise the Lord," she said, when informed of the result.

CUMBERLAND, MARYLAND

The voters of Cumberland, Maryland, didn't have to wait until November to get their say on fluoridation. The issue was on the ballot in their local civic election on May 16, 2001. Well, sort of.

In actual fact, the ballot measure didn't even mention the word *fluoridation*, but everyone in town knew what the fuss was all about. What the ballot measure actually said was: "Do you support the repeal of section 226 of the Cumberland city code?" It was this section of the city charter that prevented fluoridation of the Cumberland water supply. Section 226 states: "No substance shall be added to the water supply of the city of Cumberland for preventive health care purposes. ..." It had been made clear to the voters that only if section 226 were repealed would the Cumberland city council be able to take the necessary steps to fluoridate the town water supply.

Cumberland is the county seat of Allegany County in western Maryland on the border with Pennsylvania. It is a small city with a population approaching 25,000, nestled in a lovely Appalachian valley a few miles from the fabled Cumberland Gap. The orderliness of tree-lined streets is interrupted here and there by tall church spires and blocky red-brick buildings, some of which date back to the late eighteenth century. The Chesapeake & Ohio Canal, which runs through downtown Cumberland, used to carry barge traffic to Washington, DC, a little over 100 miles away, during the late nineteenth and early twentieth centuries. Canal Place in downtown Cumberland is now a heritage site. Antique shops display sepia pictures of old barges plying the narrow canal, with genteel couples strolling along the towpath in their suits and Easter bonnets.

Modern-day Cumberland is the takeoff point for Allegany Expeditions, whose owners satisfy their clients' craving for the wilderness by taking them into the hills for a day of rock climbing, kayaking, caving, fly-fishing, or backpacking. Until recently, Cumberland hosted the national headquarters of Kelly-Springfield tires, but the plant is now closed and young people are forced to head off to Baltimore, or Pittsburgh, or Washington to find work. Like many other Appalachian communities, the economy in Cumberland is less than vibrant.

Section 226 of the Cumberland city code has a long and tortured history. It first appeared in the city charter in 1963, and the citizens followed up in the same year with a vote that would prevent their water being treated with "fluoride, fluorides, or any derivative or derivatives of fluoride or fluorides." Twenty-five years later, in 1988, the city council rescinded section 226, and the voters approved its repeal in the November elections of that year. Anti-fluoridationists challenged the repeal in court unsuccessfully, and the Cumberland water supply was fluoridated in early 1989. However, less than a year later, opponents again launched a campaign to return section 226 to the city code. In the civic elections that year, voters approved this step while at the same time defeating a popular mayor who had campaigned in favor of fluoridation and against section 226. The fluoridation equipment was mothballed.

In the spring of 2001, the Allegany/Garrett Dental Society, under the leadership of William Tompkins, 42, a prominent local dentist, decided to revive the issue once again. They sent out 13,000 letters to registered voters in Cumberland, together with a stamped self-addressed postcard which was to be signed and returned to the society if the recipient supported the repeal of section 226. They also placed an advertisement in the Cumberland *Times-News* to remind people to sign and return their postcards. On March 14, Tompkins presented 3300 signed postcards to the city clerk. He argued that the postcards, taken in total, constituted a petition, and that the 3300 signatures exceeded the 2619 (20% of all registered voters) needed for council to pass a resolution placing the repeal issue on the May 16 ballot.

That same evening, the city council meeting was packed with fluoridation supporters expecting to speak in support of the proposed referendum. However, they were rebuffed by mayor Ed Athey. "Being that the petition was only submitted this afternoon, we will have no discussion on fluoridation this evening," he said. Tomkins protested, saying that he believed he had the right to speak. Athey replied, "Thank you anyway, we will not be discussing that issue tonight."

However, one week later at its next meeting, the city council accepted the postcards as a valid petition, and the following week, they voted to place repeal of section 226 of the city code on the May 16 ballot. In announcing the ballot measure, city solicitor Jack Price emphasized that repeal of section 226 would not mean that fluoride would be added to the water supply automatically. That issue would have to be decided by the incoming council.

As the campaign commenced, the pro-fluoridation forces got an immediate lift from public statements of support from the Cumberland Rotary Club, the Allegany County Chamber of Commerce, the Allegany County Health Department, the Mountainside Community Coalition Health Task Force, the Upper Potomac Dental Hygiene Society, the Maryland State Medical Society, and the medical staff of the Western Maryland Health

System (representing doctors and nurses at both Cumberland hospitals, Memorial and Sacred Heart). Throughout the campaign, William Tomkins maintained a scholarly and noncombative tone. He insisted that people should treat the issue as a "public health matter" and not a political one, and that the fluoridation of Cumberland's water supply should "not be an emotional argument but a thoughtful discussion." He made repeated reference to a study carried out by the University of Maryland Department of Pediatric Dentistry which indicated that western Maryland had the worst dental decay rates in the state and that the children in Allegany County had 50% more decay than did those living in fluoridated counties. Throughout the campaign, the *Cumberland Times-News* provided balanced coverage of the events, treating both sides with respect. However, a careful reading of the articles suggests a pro-fluoridation stance, and this position was confirmed in an editorial a few days before the election "strongly urging city residents to vote in favor of fluoride, by voting YES on the referendum question."[7]

Opposition was provided by the Pure Water Committee of Western Maryland. The president of this organization was a colorful iconoclast, Virginia Rosenbaum, 79 years old and proud to be in her sixth decade of battling the addition of fluoride to drinking water. During the campaign, she told audiences that she had been called every name imaginable in her 60 years of anti-fluoride efforts, but that it doesn't bother her—she sees fluoride as a toxic industrial waste. "It eats through glass jugs," she says. "It leaches the lead out of plumbing. It's against the will of the people. Our government is laughing at us for buying into the scam. Somebody is getting rich on the sale of fluoride." Other members of the Pure Water Committee had their own objections. "It's another freedom being taken away, another government intrusion into people's lives," said Ed Taylor. Mary Miltenberger warned that a national class action lawsuit was brewing over childhood fluorosis. "It will be bigger than the tobacco suit," she said.

Outgoing mayor Ed Athey was also a strong opponent of fluoridation, but his opposition did not influence the electorate significantly because he was not running for reelection. Athey's opposition to fluoridation had a sad genesis. Forty years earlier, he and his wife lost their two-and-a-half-year-old son as a result of a fatal reaction to a smallpox vaccination. It is understandable that in later years he found it difficult to support state-run medical prevention programs.

There were four men running to replace Ed Athey in the mayor's chair. Two of them were ardently anti-fluoridation. The eventual winner, Lee Fiedler, former president of the defunct Kelly-Springfield Tire Company, was one of the two who stayed on the fence. He stated that he would await the result of the ballot measure and then follow the wishes of the people. During the campaign he consistently downplayed the fluoridation issue, stating that jobs and downtown redevelopment were far more pressing issues than fluoridating the water supply.

Within days of the city council's decision to place the code amendment on the civic ballot, the Pure Water Committee filed an injunction in Allegany County Circuit Court claiming that the postcards presented to the council did not constitute a valid petition. Joyce Kenney, secretary-treasurer of the Pure Water Committee, argued that a petition is a piece of paper on which a person prints and signs his name, and gives his address. "They sent out postcards; they are not a petition," she said. City solicitor Price immediately filed a motion to dismiss plaintiff's complaint, calling the suit "frivolous, filed in bad faith, and solely for the purpose of causing a delay in the implementation of the legislative decision." The *Times-News* editorialized that "for years the Pure Water Committee has loudly proclaimed that the will of the people should prevail on the issue of fluoride. In challenging the petition, the group betrayed its true motivation: that the will of the people should be subverted to the group's blind opposition to fluoride."

On May 9, Allegany County Circuit Court Judge J. Frederick Sharer dismissed the injunction filed by the Pure Water Committee against the city of Cumberland, thus allowing the proposed repeal of section 226 to go to the voters. On the question of the postcards, Sharer's decision was clear: "Because collectively the postal cards fulfill the affirmative requirements of the law, they clearly suffice as a petition."

On May 16, the citizens of Cumberland voted to repeal section 226 of the city code, thus opening the door to fluoridation of their water supply. The vote was 2525 to 1633. In a letter to the *Times-News*, William Tompkins of the Allegany/Garrett Dental Society expressed his thanks to the electorate. He also made indirect reference to the scare tactics of the anti-fluoridation camp. "The voters of Cumberland showed some courage today," he said. Virginia Rosenbaum of the Pure Water Committee vowed to continue the fight. "We're going to regroup," she said. "This isn't over by any means."

At its May 23 meeting, the outgoing city council unanimously approved a proclamation repealing section 226 of the city charter. After doing so, mayor Ed Athey immediately went to the next agenda item without comment.

At the first meeting of the incoming city council, new mayor Lee Fiedler stated that the fluoridation process would move forward. He instructed staff to file the necessary permit applications and investigate equipment costs. There was an obvious mood in the new council that it was time to move on. During the campaign, Fiedler had argued that Cumberland's long-running political fight over fluoridation was hurting the city's business image. "The major disadvantage is not that we don't have it," he said at one point. "It's that we can't quit fighting about it."

FLUORIDATION, 2000

In all, 26 U.S. cities went to a referendum over fluoridation in the year 2000, and another 11 made decisions through administrative action (i.e., through direct action of city council or regional health board, without going to the people). Table 3.1 summarizes the results.[8] In 12 of the 26 referendums, fluoridation was approved; in the other 14, it was defeated. In Las Vegas, the Citizens for Healthy Smiles were triumphant; in Spokane, the People for Healthy Teeth suffered defeat. The lunch pail city of Abilene, Texas approved fluoridation; the ivy-walled university town of Ithaca, New York did not. In the 11 cities that reached a decision by administrative action, 10 approved a fluoridation program and only one rejected such a program. In terms of population, over 7.5 million people affected by these decisions will have a fluoridated water supply, whereas fewer than 500,000 will not. Using these population statistics as the ultimate measure, it is clear that the year 2000 was a very good year for the pro-fluoridation camp.

It is rare to have so many large cities contesting the fluoridation issue in the same year, and even rarer to have such unanimity in the results. Spokane was the largest city in the nation to reject fluoridation. Eight cities larger than Spokane approved it. Of the five largest cities that approved fluoridation, three of them (Las Vegas, Salt Lake City, and San Antonio) got there through referendum, and two of them (Sacramento and San Diego) got there by administrative action.

In the decisions for the year 2000 that are summarized in Table 3.1, the success rate by way of administrative action is much higher than by way of referendum. This is in keeping with a trend that has held throughout the history of civic decision making on fluoridation. A study carried out in 1969 based on data from 515 cities with a population greater than 10,000 found that 391 of the cities made their decision through administrative action while 124 cities went to referendum. The success rate for the adoption of fluoridation was 50% in those cities that made decisions through administrative action and less than 30% in those cities that used a referendum.[9] It was estimated in 1970 that less than one-third of the 900 referendums that took place in the first 25 years of fluoridation were successful.[10] Between 1977 and 1982, only one ballot measure out of four led to the approval of fluoridation. In 1980 alone, 33 fluoridation referendums were defeated and only eight approved.[11] Between 1989 and 1994, there were only 19 approvals through referendums. During the same period, 318 fluoridation programs were approved by

TABLE 3.1   Fluoridation Decisions, 2000

By Public Referendum				
City	Population	Pro	Anti	Result
Abilene, TX	108,995	54%	46%	Approved
Cumberland, MD	23,901	61%	39%	Approved
Davis County, UT	239,364	52%	48%	Approved
Dover, ME	2,400	73%	27%	Approved
Gilbert, AZ	97,590	54%	46%	Approved
Las Vegas, NV	1,321,319	57%	43%	Approved
Leavenworth, KA	39,123	60%	40%	Approved
Mesa, AZ	288,091	62%	38%	Approved
North Attleboro, MA	25,908	59%	41%	Approved
Salt Lake City, UT	850,243	58%	42%	Approved
San Antonio, TX	1,147,213	52%	48%	Approved
Sunnyvale, CA	127,324	65%	35%	Approved
Brattleboro, VT	12,136	44%	56%	Defeated
Hyrum, UT	5,631	38%	62%	Defeated
Ithaca, NY	29,401	45%	55%	Defeated
Logan, UT	40,778	46%	54%	Defeated
Nibley, UT	1,849	37%	63%	Defeated
Ozark, MO	9,787	41%	59%	Defeated
Pequannock, NJ	12,218	48%	52%	Defeated
Providence, UT	4,513	46%	54%	Defeated
River Heights, UT	1,492	41%	59%	Defeated
Shawano, WI	8,199	49%	51%	Defeated
Smithfield, UT	6,979	44%	56%	Defeated
Spokane, WA	184,323	49%	51%	Defeated
Wenatchee, WA	24,733	47%	53%	Defeated
Wooster, OH	24,308	44%	56%	Defeated

By Administrative Action			
City	Population	Council Vote	Result
Boynton Beach, FL	46,194	4–0	Approved
Colorado Springs, CO	281,140	no formal vote	Approved
Connersville, IN	15,550	5–2	Approved
Loch Lynn, MD	500	unanimous	Approved
Modesto, CA	164,730	4–3	Approved
Mountain Lake Park, MD	1,938	5–0	Approved
Sacramento, CA	1,741,000	5–0	Approved
San Diego, CA	1,110,549	8–1	Approved
Superior, CO	1,000	unanimous	Approved
Wellington, FL	20,670	4–1	Approved
Frostburg, MD	8,075	2–3	Defeated

administrative action.[12] As of 1986, there were approximately 7000 central water supplies in the United States that had been fluoridated, and it is estimated that only 8 percent of these were approved by referendum.[13]

The difference in likely outcome between referendum and administrative action has not escaped the attention of strategists for either the pro- or anti-fluoride movements. The pro-fluoridation camp prefers administrative action. They argue that referendums are inappropriate because the public is not qualified to judge scientific and medical evidence. One widely used dental textbook puts it baldly: "Public referenda should be avoided because they can distort the democratic decision-making process by encouraging the circulation of misleading and/or false information, which can profoundly confuse the public."[14] This elitist statement seems to assume that only the "other" side is likely to circulate misleading information and that all those who don't share your position on a given issue must be "confused."

The anti-fluoridation camp tends to favor referendums. They have always claimed that they do so out of respect for the American tradition of strong community participation in political decision making. Historically, this has been an easy stand for the anti-fluoride community to take, because referendums have turned out to be such an effective way to stop fluoridation. However in recent years, as referendums have become more of a turkey shoot (witness the 2000 results on Table 3.1), anti-fluoride claims of democratic purity are open to question. We have seen in the Cumberland campaign how anti-fluoride forces opposed a referendum in a case where the outcome was unlikely to be favorable to their cause.

Proponents of fluoridation like to see city councils make their administrative decisions on the basis of recommendations from advisory committees of experts. The experts they have in mind, of course, are those that would be supplied by the medical–dental establishment. The opponents of fluoridation tend to oppose expert panels because they feel that the choice of experts is usually biased. As one anti-fluoridationist proclaimed: "Inquiries are not set up for science, they're set up to keep people quiet."[15] It is probably true that many of the expert panels set up to advise city councils on fluoridation in past years have been biased toward adoption. In recent years, however, anti-fluoridation councils have not been above setting up expert panels that are loaded in *their* direction. The reports of such panels in Natick, Massachusetts and Escondido, California are widely available on anti-fluoridation websites. There is one company based in Tennessee that seems to specialize in providing anti-fluoridation advice to receptive councils.

In short, neither side has a monopoly on virtue. Both sides fight for the decision-making milieu that is most likely to meet their ends. While most of the arguments between the antagonists revolve around scientific and medical issues, neither side is naive enough to see the public decision-making process as a search for scientific truth. It is politics: pure and simple; down and dirty.

THE PUSH FOR STATEWIDE MANDATES

In the past few years, the pro-fluoridation movement has taken a different tack in trying to bring fluoridated water to the people. Rather than continuing to ride the roller coaster of local politics in individual communities, they have tried to promote legislation at the state level. Such state legislation usually mandates the use of fluoridated water across the state or at least in cities and towns above a certain size. In some cases, these state mandates have been approved by state legislators without going to the people. Pro-fluoridation forces have fared better in winning the hearts and minds of legislators than they have with the voting public in local referendums. Table 3.2 indicates that 11 states and the District of Columbia have approved fluoridation mandates.[16] At least three states have rejected mandates in a public vote: Kansas, Pennsylvania, and Washington. As of 2008, two additional states are in the process of developing mandates: Louisiana and Oregon.

State mandates have succeeded in bringing fluoridated water to several large cities that had consistently rejected fluoridation under local referendums. Most of the California cities noted in Table 2.4 (including Los Angeles and Sacramento, and soon to include San Diego) have arrived in the fluoridation column in response to passage of the 1995 California mandate. One of the unfluoridated cities in Table 2.4 (San Jose, California) has so far avoided the institution of fluoridation by invoking a loophole in the California mandate that allows cities to postpone the step until outside funding is made available, but sooner or later San Jose will have to fluoridate or suffer the penalties imposed by the law for noncompliance.

Of course, the anti-fluoridation forces are not pleased by the trend toward statewide mandates. They feel that the use of state mandates circumvents the

TABLE 3.2   Fluoridation Mandates

States That Have Approved		
California	Georgia	Nebraska
Connecticut	Illinois	Nevada
Delaware	Kentucky	Ohio
District of Columbia	Minnesota	South Dakota

true grassroots democracy that takes place at the local level. They argue that those cities that have already approved fluoridation now get a say in what happens in other cities in their state, and that this represents an undemocratic type of coercion and double-counting. They feel broadsided and perhaps somewhat outmaneuvered by this new statewide strategy. They see themselves placed at a disadvantage in that most anti-fluoridation organizations are based in local communities and are not experienced in campaigning at the state level, whereas most pro-fluoridation organizations are national in scope and better able to mount statewide campaigns.

However, you can be sure that they are not simply going to quit. Anti-fluoridation forces have quietly been reorganizing, integrating local chapters into state and national networks, and preparing to fight on this new battleground. In California and in other mandated states, they have already attempted to put anti-fluoridation propositions on the state ballot. In Pennsylvania, mandated statewide fluoridation has been rejected three times, but there *is* a law on the books in Pennsylvania that prevents communities from changing their minds once fluoridation is approved. Anti-fluoridation forces are currently pushing a "pro-choice" bill in the state legislature that would repeal this law. It seems clear that the never-ending battle will continue, regardless of which battlefield is selected by the opposing forces.

ON THE PHONE AND IN THE BOOTH

When we examine the voting percentages in Table 3.1 we find that in only one case (the small town of Dover, Maine) did the vote favoring fluoridation exceed 70%. There are four results in the 60–70th percentile, seven in the 50–60th percentile, 12 in the 40–50th percentile, and two that are less than 40%. If anything, the 2000 statistics are more favorable to fluoridation than in most earlier years. Few successful referendums in past years posted percentages above the mid-50s.

At first glance, it is hard to reconcile this low level of support with the results of opinion polls that have been carried out over the years. In 1968, a Gallup poll posed the question to 1000 adults: "Do you believe community water should be fluoridated?" The results were: yes: 70%; no: 18%; don't know: 12%. In 1991, a Gallup poll asked 1200 parents: "Do you approved or disapprove of fluoridating drinking water?" The results were: approve: 78%; disapprove: 10%; don't know or refuse to answer: 12%.[17] In five polls carried out during the period 1959–1972 by the National Opinion Research Center, fluoridation was deemed "desirable" or "very desirable" by 65 to 77% of the population. It was deemed "undesirable" or "very undesirable" by only 12 to 14%.[18] In a study carried out in Massachusetts in 1985, 60% of voters contacted in a telephone survey claimed to favor fluoridation, but 61% of them voted against it in the actual referendum.[19]

On second thought, however, these figures lead to a simple conclusion. At the beginning of most fluoridation campaigns, the great majority of voters (perhaps upward of 75% of them) expect to vote in favor of fluoridation, but by the time they get into the voting booth a few months later, many of them have changed their mind. The question is: Why? Are the campaigns run by anti-fluoridation groups that much more effective than those run by pro-fluoridation groups? If so, is this due to misleading fear-mongering, as pro-fluoridationists charge; or do anti-fluoridation arguments have some resonance with the electorate? If we assume that voters in Spokane and Cumberland both started at 75% support, why did Spokane drop all the way to 49%, while Cumberland arrested the decline at 61%?

Social scientists have leapt into the breach on these questions. There is a huge bibliography of academic studies relating to the sociopolitical aspects of the fluoridation question. For our purposes, it is probably best if we divide them into an early period (the 1960s, 1970s, and early 1980s) and a later period (since the mid-1980s).

THE EARLY STUDIES: SOCIAL DYNAMICS AND POP PSYCHOLOGY

Most of the early studies were carried out with an unstated, and probably unconscious, establishment bias. The most comprehensive and widely quoted of these studies[20] was actually funded by the U.S. Public Health Service. These authors, and others of the day, accepted the word of their medical and dental colleagues that fluoridation was a well-established and proven preventive health measure. People who opposed fluoridation were seen as self-interested, irrational, or misled. Psychologists and sociologists were interested in the anti-fluoridation leadership and how they had come to their iconoclastic position. Political scientists were interested in how this undistinguished leadership was able to persuade respectable voters to their side.

These early analyses of the social dynamics of the fluoridation issue led to two notions of what constituted the "anti-fluoride personality."[21] The first became known as the *alienation hypothesis*[22] and the second as the *confusion hypothesis*.[23] Initially, these labels were applied to both leaders and followers, but later synthesis of these ideas[24] found that it is the leaders who are alienated and followers who are confused. The alienation hypothesis holds that many of the anti-fluoridation leaders are men and women who come from outside the professional mainstream and who feel a sense of deprivation with respect to economic status, political power, and social prestige. They disdain the medical establishment and exploit society's current fears and phobias about health and disease. They fear further government intervention in their lives and are easily frustrated at what they see as arbitrary decisions made by remote and untrustworthy decision makers. They tend to be poorly integrated into the social life of the community. They see the fluoridation proponents as elitist and arrogant.

It is certainly possible to find evidence of alienation in many of the anti-fluoridation leaders if one looks for it, especially in the early years of the movement. It is easy to point to bona fide cranks such as C. Leon de Aryan of San Diego (whose real name was Constantine Leganopol), the publisher of an anti-Semitic weekly, who felt that fluoridation was a Jewish plot to "weaken the Aryan race mentally and spiritually."[25] Even the more reputable early leaders were indeed "a melange of strange bedfellows."[26] They included naturopaths, who found fluoridation incompatible with their nutritional philosophy; chiropractors, who did not wish to follow the dictates of organized medicine; members of the Christian Science religion, who opposed forced medication; members of the John Birch Society, who suspected a communist plot; and those involved in the natural food industry, who worried that fluoridation would "poison" their food and water.[27]

However, not all of the early anti-fluoridation leaders were alienated, unless of course one takes opposition to the medical dictates of the day as prima facie evidence of alienation. Even in the early days, there were many reputable dentists and physicians who felt that fluoridation proponents were moving too fast. Such leaders as George Waldbott and John Yiamouyiannis were active in their professional societies and were considered reputable researchers. They were not considered alienated until after their views on fluoridation became known. In a later chapter we look at the experiences of several dental researchers and practitioners who were shunned by the medical establishment after they changed their mind about fluoridation. Many of these men and women ended up alienated from their professional colleagues, but it could be argued that their alienation was to some degree forced upon them.

The second half of this sociopolitical argument holds that a significant segment of voters begin the campaign with a pro-fluoridation stance but become "confused" by the emotionally charged anti-fluoridation rhetoric and end up casting a "safe" vote opposing fluoridation. To be sure, there is some evidence of confusion on the part of the electorate. In the National Opinion Research Center polls taken between 1959 and 1977, 18 to 30% of those polled knew nothing about fluoridation. Of those that claimed they did know something about it, 49 to 76% correctly identified the purpose of fluoridation as preventing tooth decay, but 23 to 29% thought its purpose was to purify the water supply.[28] One of the central themes of the confusion hypothesis is that voters are easily confused by scientific evidence and technical arguments. It is felt that the public is unable to distinguish between legitimate, reputable health professionals and those with equally impressive titles who have only marginal status in their profession. The confused voter is viewed as being very vulnerable to scare propaganda served up by the anti-fluoride side. Many voters may feel that they are being called upon to decide whether or not fluoridation is safe, and they don't feel qualified to judge.

The final strand of the argument developed in the early social studies comes from the political analysis of voting blocs in fluoridation referendums. All the early studies found a clear correlation between a voter's social status and his or her stance on the fluoridation question. Election districts that tended to vote against fluoridation had a higher proportion of voters with lower education, lower income, and lower-class occupations.[29] It was felt that such voters may be more distrustful of authority and more receptive to the freedom-of-choice argument.[30] Such groups may harbor more true fluoro-phobics and more voters who accept the conspiracy theories put forward by some anti-fluoridation leaders.[31] In short, the implication is that such voters are more likely to be "confused."

Reading these early articles leaves one with the impression that this establishment theory of alienated leaders and confused voters is a bit too glib. Surely it is a touch arrogant to assume that there cannot exist any legitimate political opposition to fluoridation. Pro-fluoride authors are always drawing attention to the near-religious fervor of the anti-fluoride leaders, but the tenor of all these early studies displays a level of obsession that is not all that different in kind. Having said that, there are many valid observations of merit hidden in the elitist interpretations. If we replace the loaded word *confused* with the more appropriate appellation *risk-averse*, we can, without impugning the intelligence of the voters, understand why support for fluoridation is so often lost during a campaign. It is not surprising that anti-fluoridation campaigners are successful in planting seeds of doubt in the electorate through their constant warnings of potential harm. No matter how far-fetched some of these warnings may sound, it is difficult for voters to disregard them completely. As noted ruefully in an early study,[32] it is "not irrational to draw back from taking an action where there is some evidence that great harm will result." Most voters probably don't believe the scare stories, perhaps giving them a 1% probability of being true. But in many voters' minds a 1% chance of cancer may outweigh a 99% chance of reduced cavities. The doubt, coupled with the feeling that the matter is not one of great importance, may be enough to make many voters play it safe. One study found that 80% of those voting against fluoridation would vote for it if they were sure that it was safe.[33] Anti-fluoridation forces only have to create doubt; pro-fluoridation forces have to create a guarantee of safety. Given their inability to judge the scientific arguments, the doubts created by the scare tactics of the anti-fluoridationists, and the relatively small upside, many voters who would like to vote yes may in fact vote no, feeling that the safest course is to postpone their approval until the situation becomes clearer.

As for the polling results, it is clear that there is a difference between an opinion poll and a referendum. Stating your opinion in a poll has no consequences; voting in a referendum carries responsibility for the action that will result.

THE LATER STUDIES: JUST PLAIN POLITICS

As the years have gone by, it has become clear that the early social studies linking anti-fluoridation attitudes with poverty and ignorance were more wishful thinking than fact. The demographics are more complicated than that.[34] Modern electoral analysis and polling techniques have identified many new constituencies that apparently vote against fluoridation for a variety of reasons not related to poverty and ignorance. Chief among them is the environmental constituency, whose members have exhibited a growing reluctance to have chemical agents of any type added to the environment. They are joined by the growing numbers of people who subscribe to healthy-living doctrines that value good nutrition and oppose the use of synthetic chemicals in food production. The disdain that these groups feel for pesticides, food additives, and genetically altered meats (to name just a few of their concerns) may in some cases translate into a vote against the addition of fluoride to drinking water. There is also evidence that the elderly, whose "gray power" is now recognized to form an effective voting bloc, are unlikely to be supportive. Fluoridation does them no good; their children are long gone; and it sounds expensive. There has also been a growth in the number of people who question increased government regulation and increased government intervention in our lives. It is not just alienated cranks who sometimes doubt the wisdom of government-recommended programs.

More important than their votes, perhaps, is the fact that all these diverse groups have provided the anti-fluoridation movement with more creditable and credentialed leaders than in earlier years. Their backgrounds are more mainstream, and their arguments are more sophisticated. It may not be politically astute, as perhaps it was in earlier years, for the pro-fluoride camp to treat these leaders with ridicule.

On the other side of the fence, the pro-fluoride movement has finally realized that they are involved in a political battle, not a program of scientific education. Fluoridation referendums are not won or lost on the quality of scientific discourse. They are won in the trenches: by ensuring favorable wording on the ballot question; by developing reliable sources of funding; by getting media endorsements and the support of community organizations; and by assessing past voting records, targeting key areas, identifying supporters, and getting out the vote. Complicated scientific explanations are out; simple, catchy slogans are in.

A 1973 analysis of 16 fluoridation referenda in Massachusetts[35] used a Political Activity Advantage Index (PAAI) to rank the extent to which proponents outcampaigned opponents (or vice versa). The percentage of voters in favor and opposed to fluoridation was highly correlated with the PAAI. Fluoridation ballot measures were much more likely to pass in communities where the pro-fluoride camp outcampaigned the anti-fluoride camp (and vice versa).

One of the primary reasons for the failure of fluoridation referendums has been the failure of dental and medical professionals to get their hands dirty in the political scuffle. It has been shown over and over again that any weakness in support from local health authorities is the kiss of death in a fluoridation campaign. Endorsements from national bodies such as the American Medical Association and the Public Health Service are less important. Voters are generally not impressed with high-falootin' experts who are parachuted into their local contests. It is the local health authorities they want to hear from, people whose opinions they know and trust.

Even more important is the support of local politicians. The voters seldom support fluoridation if popular local politicians are opposed or even neutral. One study suggests that the stance of the mayor or mayoral candidate is the major determinant of the outcome. This study showed that in cases where the mayor favored fluoridation, it was adopted in 155 cities and rejected in 103. In cases where the mayor was neutral or opposed to fluoridation, there were only 19 adoptions and 219 rejections.[36] Unfortunately for the pro-fluoridation forces, getting the support of politicians is not easy. Local politicians and community leaders view fluoridation as a no-win situation. They often refuse to take a stand: not because they don't have an opinion, but because a stand on fluoridation brings controversy, a possible loss of votes from one-issue voters, and the threat of litigation from trigger-happy truebelievers. A politician who is willing to stand up and be counted on the fluoridation issue is money in the bank.

There is one thing that all pro-fluoridation strategists agree on. They want to avoid public debate. As Michael Easley puts it:[37] "Almost nothing can be gained by debating. An opponent can present more misinformation in five minutes than can be refuted in five hours." In Easley's eyes there are no valid grounds for opposing fluoridation; therefore, any debate only gives credibility to the opponents. Regardless of who fares best in the debate, "the fact that the debate even took place conveys to the public that a legitimate scientific controversy exists." In his opinion, there is little to gain and much to lose from debating such an emotional issue. In any case, meetings are packed with supporters of both sides. There is nobody there to "educate."

In most elections, money talks. We are all familiar with the obscene sums of money that are generated by politicians for their election war chests. The press is rife with post-election analyses that indicate that the candidate who spends the most money often wins the election. Surprisingly, perhaps, fluoridation referenda do not seem to follow this rule. In most campaigns, the pro-fluoridation camp outspends the anti-fluoridation camp several times over, but as we have seen, their record of success does not reflect their investment. It is likely that the explanation lies in our previous discussion of the "seeds of doubt." It doesn't cost much to plant the seeds, but it costs a lot to try to whisk them away.

It is common for both sides to use radio and TV sound bites during a campaign. Given their larger budgets, one would think that the pro-fluoridation camp would be able to saturate the airwaves and overwhelm the anti-fluoridation message. To their chagrin, however, the pro-fluoride forces have found that they can't get a leg up in this way. The reason is a little-known policy of the Federal Communications Commission (FCC) known as the Cullman doctrine.[38] This policy is an FCC interpretation of the broadcast fairness regulations that require TV and radio stations to afford reasonable opportunities for the presentation of contrasting views by spokespersons of responsible opposition groups on political questions. The doctrine does not specify the amount or value of free time that must be provided to opponents, other than it be "reasonable" to inform the public of both sides of the issue. In Portland, Oregon in 1980, pro-fluoride groups spent $25,000 on TV spots promoting the defeat of a ballot measure aimed at repealing fluoridation. The anti-fluoride camp demanded and got a significant amount of free airtime under the Cullman doctrine (about 20% of the time paid for by the pro-fluoridationists, or $4500 worth).

The dental literature is filled with anecdotal articles describing fluoridation campaigns in U.S. cites both successful and unsuccessful. Most of the more recent campaigns that describe successful outcomes emphasize the campaign strategy. There is no crying over the spilled milk of "alienated" or "confused" voters. The emphasis is on the creation of an efficient and inclusive coordinating committee, a strong volunteer effort in direct voter contact, a savvy political assessment of past voting records, and concerted last-minute action to get out the vote in targeted key areas. In Seattle in 1975, victory was achieved by deemphasizing scientific issues, avoiding all confrontation with opponents, and saturation doorbell ringing.[39] In Phoenix in 1989, pro-fluoridation forces targeted the media, gained their trust, and rode the strong editorial support to success.[40] In Oakland in 1980, proponents had to enter the seamy side of political give-and-take to reach their goal. To get union support, they had to use some of their funds to make contributions to other political causes, a practice euphemistically known as a "piggyback effort."[41]

SPOKANE AND CUMBERLAND: REPRISE

So why did fluoridation pass muster in Cumberland and not in Spokane? Do all these academic studies tell us anything? We think they do. Not everything fits like a glove, of course, but many of the generalizations reached by the social scientists, especially in their more recent studies, apply to our two test cases.

In Spokane, one might say that everything went wrong. The referendum was carried out in the glare of negative publicity from the recently defeated state mandate, and local state politicians were known to be opposed. The wording of the ballot question was too complicated for voters to grasp at a glance, referring as it did to administrative codes and ordinances with long meaningless numbers. The unwillingness of the pro-fluoridation camp to debate was turned back on them cleverly by the opposition in a way that guaranteed coverage on prime-time local TV. And although the local newspaper supported the fluoride initiative editorially, it also published many articles that highlighted the views of opponents with respect to allergic reactions to fluoride, the possibility of equipment malfunction, and the potential for cost overruns. The pro-fluoride campaign was also hampered by the two months that were lost between June 26 and August 26 in the petition effort that was demanded by the city council. A savvier political group would have seen the need to have the petition in hand before going to council. Overall, one must judge the political aspects of the pro-fluoride campaign a failure; they outspent the opposition 20 times over and they got less than half the votes. Yet even with all these missteps, the pro-fluoride forces might have carried the day had they been able to gain the strong unequivocal support of the local health agencies. The unwillingness of the Spokane Regional Health District to endorse the fluoridation initiative was the shot to the heart that scuttled fluoridationist hopes in Spokane. If they couldn't even convince the agencies that are charged with looking after our well-being, they could hardly expect to convince the voters.

In Cumberland, the pro-fluoride forces were better organized, more politically savvy, and luckier. They had a strong leader in William Tomkins, who was reasonable and noncombative and who made his case in a straight-forward constructive manner. The leader of the opposition, on the other hand, was an old school anti-fluoridationist who sang the same old songs. The pro-fluoride camp received strong and immediate support from all local medical–dental agencies. They used local doctors and dentists to endorse their program, and local statistics to back up their claims of poor dental health in the community. They had their petition ready before approaching council. The outgoing mayor was opposed to fluoridation, but because he was not running for reelection, his opposition was not a factor. The leading candidate to replace him did not go on record as a supporter, but he made it clear that he was willing to abide by the decision of the people in the matter. The local newspaper was supportive editorially and in the tenor of the news articles that it published about fluoridation during the campaign. By gaining the support of all the important factions of the community power structure, the pro-fluoride camp also gained the trust and support of the voters.

REFERENCES

1. This anecdotal summary of statewide and local measures on the election 2000 ballot is taken from an Associated Press release that appeared in the Spokane, Washington *Spokesman-Review* on November 2, 2000.

2. Connersville story taken from a posting at http://www.CNN.com, November 1, 1999.

3. Salt Lake City *Deseret News*, November 8, 2000.

4. Information on Spokane comes from the Spokane Chamber of Commerce, http://www.spokanechamber.org, and from the article: Spokane: Northwest's best-kept business secret, *Skywest Magazine*, Spring 2001.

5. J. Walter, *Over Tumbled Graves*, ReganBooks/HarperCollins, New York, 2001.

6. The description of the Spokane fluoridation battle of 2000 is taken from news articles in the Spokane *Spokesman-Review* during the period March 12–November 9, 2000.

7. The description of the Cumberland fluoridation battle of 2000 is taken from news articles from the Cumberland *Times-News* during the period March 3–September 26, 2000.

8. The information in Table 3.1 was compiled from a fairly diligent search of a large number of pro- and anti-fluoride websites on the Internet.

9. R. L. Crain, E. Katz, and D. B. Rosenthal, *The Politics of Community Conflict: The Fluoridation Decision*, Bobbs-Merrill, Indianapolis, IN, 1969.

10. J. W. Knutsen, Water fluoridation after 25 years, *J. Am. Dent. Assoc.*, 80, 765–769, 1970.

11. P. J. Frazier and E. Newbrun, Legal, social and economic aspects of fluoridation, Chapter 5 in *Fluorides and Dental Caries: Contemporary Concepts for Practitioners and Students*, edited by E. Newbrun, Charles C Thomas, Springfield, IL, 1986, pp. 115–154.

12. American Dental Association, *Fluoridation Facts*, http://www.ada.org.

13. Frazier and Newbrun, 1986, op cit.

14. Newbrun, 1986, op. cit.

15. Quoted in B. Martln, *Scientific Knowledge In Controversy: The Social Dynamics of the Fluoridation Debate*, State University of New York Press, Albany, NY, 1991.

16. M. H. K. Greer, Community water fluoridation mandates: state statutes, presented at the National Fluoridation Summit, Sacramento, CA, September 2000; National Center for Fluoridation, http://www.fluoridationcenter.org.

17. American Dental Association, *Fluoridation Facts*, op. cit.

18. P. J. Frazier, Fluoridation: a review of social research, *J. Publ. Health Dent.*, 40, 214–233, 1980; R. J. Hastreiter, Fluoridation conflict: a history and conceptual synthesis, *J. Am. Dent. Assoc.*, 106, 486–490, 1983.

19. J. A. Wientraub, G. N. Connolly, C. A. Lambert, and C. W. Douglass, What Massachusetts residents know about fluoridation, *J. Publ. Health Dent.*, 45, 240–246, 1985.

20. Crain et al., 1969, op. cit.

21. The term *anti-fluoride personality* comes from M. W. Easley, The new anti-fluoridationists: Who are they and how do they operate? *J. Publ. Health Dent.*, 45, 133–141, 1985.

22. A. L. Green, The ideology of anti-fluoridation leaders, *J. Social Issues*, 17, 13–25, 1961; W. A. Gamson, The fluoridation dialogue: Is it an ideological conflict? *Publ. Opin. Q.*, 25, 526–537, 1961; W. A. Gamson and P. H. Irons, Community characteristics and fluoridation outcome, *J. Social Issues*, 17, 66–74, 1961; A. Simmel, A signpost for research on fluoridation conflicts: the concept of relative deprivation, *J. Social Issues*, 17, 26–36, 1961; M. Pinard, Structural attachments and political support in urban politics: the case of fluoridation referendums, *Am. J. Sociol.*, 68, 513–526, 1963; H. D. Hahn, Fluoridation and patterns in community politics, *J. Publ. Health Dent.*, 25, 152–157, 1965; L. K. Cohen, A sociologist looks at fluoridation, *Oregon Dentl. J.*, 35, 26–30, 1966; C. T. Shaw, Characteristics of supporters and rejectors of a fluoridation referendum and a guide for other community programs, *J. Am. Dent. Assoc.*, 78, 339–341, 1969.

23. H. M. Sapolsky, The fluoridation controversy: an alternative explanation, *Publ. Opin. Q.*, 33, 244–248, 1969; H. M. Sapolsky, Science, voters, and the fluoridation controversy, *Science*, 162, 427–433, 1968.

24. Hastreiter, 1983, op. cit.

25. D. R. McNeil, *The Fight for Fluoridation*, Oxford University Press, New York, 1957.

26. Ibid.

27. Easley, 1985, op. cit.; McNeil, 1957, op. cit.; Fluoridation: the cancer scare, *Consumer Reports*, July 1978, pp. 392–396, and August 1978, pp. 480–483.

28. Frazier, 1980, op. cit.; Hastreiter, 1983, op. cit.

29. B. Mausner and J. Mausner, The anti-scientific attitude, *Sci. Am.*, 192, 35–39, 1955; Green, 1961, op. cit.

30. R. C. Faine, J. J. Collins, J. Daniel, R. Isman, J. Boriskin, K. L. Young, and C. M. Fitzgerald, The 1980 fluoridation campaigns: a discussion of results, *J. Publ. Health Dent.*, 41, 138–142, 1981; R. Isman, Public views on fluoridation and other preventive dental practices, *Community Dent. Oral Epidemiol.*, 11, 217–223, 1983.

31. E. Newbrun, The fluoridation war: a scientific dispute or religious argument, *J. Publ. Health Dent.*, 56, 246–252, 1996.

32. Crain et al., 1969, op. cit.

33. Gamson, 1961, op. cit.

34. Gamson, 1961, op. cit.; Martin, 1991, op. cit.; S. Rovin, Reaction paper, *J. Publ. Health Dent.*, 45, 146–148, 1985.

35. J. M. Frankel and M. Allukian, Sixteen referenda on fluoridation in Massachusetts: an analysis, *J. Publ. Health Dent.*, 33, 96–103, 1973; as reported in Frazier, 1980, op. cit.

36. Crain, et al., 1969, op. cit.

37. Easley, 1985, op. cit.

38. R. Isman, The FCC, F, and fairness, *J. Publ. Health Dent.*, 40, 247, 1980.

39. P. K. Domoto, R. C. Faine, and S. Rovin, Seattle fluoridation campaign 1973: prescription for a victory, *J. Am. Dent. Assoc.*, 91, 583–588,1975.

40. K. G. Smith and K. A. Christen, A fluoridation campaign: the Phoenix experience, *J. Publ. Health Dent.*, 50, 319–322, 1990.

41. J. M. Boriskin and J. I. Fine, Fluoridation election victory: a case study for dentistry in effective political action, *J. Am. Dent. Assoc.*, 102, 486–491, 1981.

CHAPTER 4

TWO WOMEN

On October 9, 1995, most newspapers in California carried a front-page story announcing that the California Fluoridation Act had been signed into law by Governor Pete Wilson. The act mandates the fluoridation of all community water supplies in the state of California for cities with more than 10,000 users. In many of the newspapers, the article was accompanied by a photograph of Jackie Speier, a Democratic assemblywoman from San Mateo, a Bay Area suburb. She was identified as the prime sponsor of the new law, the architect and catalyst of California's long-delayed march into the fluoridation age. In fact, Speier's picture is often in the paper. She is an active politician with a remarkable record of getting substantive legislation signed into law. She is so popular that in 1994, when she ran for her fifth term in the state assembly, she ran unopposed, endorsed by Democrats and Republicans alike.[1]

On the same day in 1995, Darlene Sherrell sat in a lawn chair on the patio of her recently completed cottage on a hillside on the remote south coast of Grenada. In the foreground, she surveyed her well-tended garden, the okra plants thriving without benefit of modern chemical sustenance. The Caribbean shone in the distance. The cottage is self-built, certainly not ostentatious, a cinder-block construction that Sherrell calls her "concrete tent." She had just returned from a cyber-café in St. Georges, where she sent and received a slew of e-mails from her far-flung correspondents in the anti-fluoridation subculture. She also checked her Stop Fluoridation website. There were hundreds of new hits in the past week alone; people from all over the world were reading her dispatches. She settled down with a Guinness, "snug as a bug, and happy as a lark."[2]

Two women as different as two women could be: Speier, stylish and coifed, a lawyer and politician, used to moving in the highest circles of San

The Fluoride Wars: How a Modest Public Health Measure Became America's Longest-Running Political Melodrama   By R. Allan Freeze and Jay H. Lehr
Copyright © 2009 John Wiley & Sons, Inc.

Francisco society; Sherrell, with her long gray hair tied unceremoniously at her back, a streetsmart gadfly, living in cyber-connected seclusion on a Caribbean island. Yet, much as they might shudder at the thought, they have much in common. Each has been a major influence in the fluoridation controversy. Each of them has attained success in middle age: on her own terms and likely as not, beyond her wildest youthful dreams. Each was influenced by life-changing experiences in her youth. Somehow, through the mix of similarities and differences, they came to hold diametrically opposed positions on the fluoridation question. How did that come to pass? Here are their stories.

DARLENE SHERRELL: THE CANARY IN THE MINE

Darlene Sherrell was born in January 1941 near Detroit, Michigan. As a teenager in the Detroit suburbs she suffered from stiff joints and painful limbs. In 1959, at the age of 18, while working as a clerk in a Detroit steel plant, she collapsed in front of the company drinking fountain. She experienced stomach cramps, chest pains, and puffed-up eyes. She felt she was going blind. She passed out and was rushed to a hospital, where she was diagnosed as having suffered anaphylactic shock, a potentially fatal allergic reaction to the drugs she had been taking for her arthritic problems. She altered her medicinal recipe, but in subsequent years she suffered two similar attacks, experienced bouts of narcolepsy, and endured recurrent allergic reactions. In time, she found herself working with an allergy doctor who suggested an alternative diagnosis. He suggested that Sherrell's troubles could be due to an aversion to certain chemicals in food and drinking water. In response to this diagnosis, Sherrell made radical changes to her diet. Under her new regimen, her allergic reactions abated and her painful symptoms disappeared. She has adhered to these changes ever since, and her health problems have remained largely under control for over 40 years. She drinks only distilled water and avoids all fruits, vegetables, and grains that are not organically grown. "With a very few exceptions," she says, "nothing on my plate comes from boxes, cans, or bottles. There are no artificial colors, flavors, or preservatives. Everything is made from scratch."

The 1960s were as turbulent for Darlene Sherrell as they were for the rest of the country. She went through three marriages, finally settling in Lansing, Michigan with her fourth husband and two daughters from earlier marriages. The success of her new diet led her to take an activist role in the fight to ban the artificial sweetener saccharin, and against many other food additives which she felt might have contributed to her allergic attacks. She established a nonprofit foundation called Orenda, and published a weekly newsletter, the *Golden Thread*, that highlighted the virtues of natural foods, organic gardening, and herbal remedies. She wrote many letters about these issues to the editor of her local newspaper. In 1976, a local anti-fluoride activist named Martha Johnson saw one of Sherrell's letters about Red Dye No. 2. They made contact. Sherrell remembers Johnson as "a heavyset woman with a shopping bag full of papers." She told Sherrell about a government plot to dull our minds through the fluoridation of public water supplies. Sherrell thought she was crazy, but it got her thinking. She began to frequent the Michigan State University library, studying up on fluoride and learning about the toxic effects of very high doses. She read about mottled teeth in the United States and crippling skeletal fluorosis in India. She began to view fluoride as a drug, and at higher doses as a poison. She reviewed her own health history and came to the conclusion that her own allergic reactions may well have come from a supersensitivity to fluoride. She began to worry that there could be many people in the country suffering ill effects from the same reaction to fluoride that she had experienced.

Throughout the late 1970s, Sherrell continued her library research, focusing on fluoride dosage issues. She began to hector the medical establishment. She wrote many letters to the National Institute for Dental Research, the Centers for Disease Control, and her local Congress members and state legislators. At that time, the state of Michigan had a mandatory fluoridation law, and she began badgering the Michigan State Health Department over the lack of choice engendered in such a law. In 1978, due largely to Sherrell's public campaign against the inflexibility of the mandatory law, the state legislature passed a bill granting municipalities the right to shut down their fluoridation systems if they desired. It was Sherrell's greatest success, but also her greatest disillusionment, as hardly any Michigan municipalities took advantage of the new provisions.

In the course of her library research, Sherrell uncovered many examples of what she saw as collusion between government health agencies and industrial corporations. She began to suspect a systematic cover-up of the true facts about the toxicity of fluoride in human health. The first case involved a book of scientific abstracts given to her by a state agency.[3] When she went to the library and located the original full-length articles, she found that the abstracts were systematically more favorable toward fluoride than the original articles. More damning yet, there were discrepancies that appeared to have arisen through the shifting of decimal points in the results of numerical calculations. The collection of abstracts had been prepared by the Kettering Lab of the University of Cincinnati, and Sherrell uncovered the fact that this laboratory received heavy funding from many large corporations, such as Alcoa, du Pont, and Kaiser. She was aware from the burgeoning underground anti-fluoridation literature that these same companies were thought to be looking for a profitable secondary market for the fluoride wastes that come from their primary industrial operations. She felt that the lack of correspondence between the abstracts and the papers was proof of malfeasance. She was convinced that the abstracts had been doctored by the publisher in cahoots with the fluoride-producing industries and their government supporters.

It wasn't long before Sherrell found her second smoking gun. She uncovered a letter written some years earlier addressed to a government health agency. It was written by Donald Kennedy, then a professor at Stanford University, offering his support for the views expressed in the Ph.D. dissertation of Edward Groth III, which indicated the need for "a serious reappraisal of the wisdom of mass fluoridation."[4] Sherrell found out that Kennedy was now a commissioner with the Food and Drug Administration, an agency on record as a strong supporter of community fluoridation. She wrote Kennedy asking him whether he now supported fluoridation, and if so, why he had changed his mind. She never received a reply, but she later learned that the Centers for Disease Control had sent a memo to many state and local health departments warning them not to listen to Sherrell's claim that Kennedy had ever questioned the value of fluoridation.

Sherrell's greatest coup came with the discovery of a serious error in *Fluoridation Facts*, the information booklet distributed by the American Dental Association. The booklet recommended that the intake of fluoride should not exceed 20 to 80 milligrams per day per person (depending on body weight). In presenting this range of values, the ADA implied that if you kept below this maximum dosage you would be ensured against any and all potential chronic toxicity effects of fluoride. The booklet quoted the deliberations of a 1953 National Academy of Sciences panel meeting on fluoride dosage as the source of their figures. Sherrell thought this number looked high and wrote to the National Academy of Sciences asking for more information. After considerable delay, she was informed that the calculations leading to these intake values were performed by Harold C. Hodge, the former chairman of the National Academy of Sciences Committee on Toxicology. He prepared the chart in 1953 and offered it in testimony at congressional hearings on fluoride in 1954. His calculations were based on values that were first published by a Danish researcher named Kaj Roholm in 1937 in his classic textbook *Fluorine Intoxication*.[5] Roholm's dosage recommendations were given in milligrams of fluoride per kilogram of body weight per day. Hodge wanted to take the body weight out of the equation and present the values in milligrams (mg) per day, which he thought would be more easily grasped by the public. He therefore converted Roholm's figures to milligrams per day using body weights in the range 100 to 229 pounds. However, Sherrell was able to show that in making his calculations, Hodge neglected to convert the body weights from pounds to kilograms, and thus overstated the maximum acceptable dosage by a factor of 2. The error remained in print for almost 40 years, not only in *Fluoridation Facts*, but in many other articles and pamphlets prepared by the ADA and other agencies. Sherrell still bristles over the fact that these values misled the public to such a degree for so long.

She is even more upset by what she views as a willful and deliberate cover-up. It turns out that Hodge himself recognized his error in 1979 and corrected it publicly. However, the incorrect figures continued to appear in *Fluoridation Facts* until 1993, and it was only under pressure from Sherrell [with the help of Robert Carton, a former Environmental Protection Agency (EPA) scientist who had fought his own fluoride battles within the EPA] that the corrected figures were published. When these values appeared for the first time in a U.S. government report in 1993,[6] it brought an end to the 40-year mistake that many anti-fluoridationists think was ignored with malicious intent. Throughout this period, the World Health Organization published maximum daily acceptable fluoride dosages that were in the range 2.5 to 5 mg/day, almost 10 times lower than those that appeared in *Fluoridation Facts*. They were correctly calculated from Roholm's data, and they were based on a longer period of exposure than that used by ADA (40 to 80 years rather than 10 to 20 years).[7]

During this period, Sherrell was also involved in two court cases that were fought over the fluoridation issue, one in Pennsylvania and one in Illinois. As we will see in a later chapter, the courts have not been kind to the anti-fluoridation movement, rejecting their arguments at almost every turn. However, in 1978, in Pittsburgh, Pennsylvania, in one of the cases in which Sherrell was involved, Judge John P. Flaherty gave the antis one small morsel to chew on when he stated in his decision that the evidence presented in the case (which challenged the right of the borough of West View to fluoridate its public water supply) convinced him that the addition of fluoride was "deleterious to the human body." His judicial opinion is now highlighted in bold type on every anti-fluoride website (without mention, of course, of the almost universal judicial preference for the pro-fluoride arguments, nor of the fact that Judge Flaherty's decision was overturned on appeal, albeit on jurisdictional, not evidentiary grounds). Sherrell became involved in the Pennsylvania lawsuit at the invitation of the prominent anti-fluoridationist John Yiamouyiannis, who had learned of her Michigan activism. She assisted him in his role as the leading expert witness for the anti-fluoridation case. There is no doubt that Sherrell's involvement with the famous Dr. Y deepened her commitment to the anti-fluoride crusade.

In 1982, Sherrell became disillusioned with the life of a housewife in Lansing. She left her fourth husband and hit the road to begin a life of adventure. At the age of 41 she took trucking lessons, got her license, and began driving an 18-wheeler back and forth across the country. She found that her income from a few coast-to-coast trucking hauls each year was more than enough to pay for a life of ease in Jamaica and the Grand Cayman Islands, where she could live for a few dollars a day. "For six years," she says, "I traveled, living outdoors most of the time, sleeping in a rain- and mosquito-proof hammock, making whole-grain breads and cooking fresh vegetables on an open fire or kerosene stove. I became accustomed to using a machete; walking and swimming distances measured in miles, not yards; and could carry everything I owned in a backpack. I was an international bag lady and I loved it!"

In 1988 she met a man, and the two of them moved to Florida. They spent a few years island hopping through the Caribbean on their 36-foot sailboat *Seafever*. By 1993, they found themselves based in Grenada, the beautiful "Spice Island" at the southern end of the West Indies, between Trinidad and Barbados. In October of the following year, they sailed to Chaguaramas, Trinidad, where they planned to spend a few months while the boat was repainted, repaired, and outfitted with a new anchor windlass and wind generator. "We arrived," she writes, "in time to ride the shifting currents through the Boca de Monos, check in with Customs and Immigration, and dinghy over to the Lifeline Bar for a cold drink." Idyllic it may sound, but it was here, after 25 years of excellent health, that she experienced a recurrence of her problems from the distant past. She suffered pounding headaches, hands that were stiff and sore, and aching legs. After just a few weeks in Trinidad, she couldn't hold a pen, and could barely dress herself. She experienced numbness in her left arm. "My left shoulder and arm felt like fine wires with hooks were being dragged through the flesh."

It was not long before Sherrell discovered a cause for her relapse. It turns out that she and her partner were anchored downwind from a bauxite transfer station that was part of Alcoa's aluminum mining operations on the island. Sherrell began talking to the local citizens. Many of them suffered from the same symptoms as she did. They blamed the aluminum dust from the transfer station, which settled in every nook and cranny of their homes. It turned out that Sherell had just missed a noisy public meeting the month before on the "Alcoa dust case." She agreed with the locals that Alcoa was to blame, but she told them that in trying to pin the blame on the aluminum dust itself, they were barking up the wrong tree. In her opinion, the "fine particles of bauxite dust could easily contain enough fluoride to cause the problem." After six weeks in Trinidad, the boat was ready and they returned to Grenada. Sherrell's health slowly improved and her complaints faded away.

In 1996, Sherrell spent a few months in the United States visiting her daughters in Oregon and Michigan. Here again she experienced what she felt was fluoride-induced pain, despite "remaining true to my carefully-controlled diet, and drinking only distilled water." In one case, she blamed airborne fluorides, and in the other, her carelessness in drinking a Bloody Mary mix and beer that was brewed with fluoridated water.

It is natural to wonder whether Darlene Sherrell might simply be a hypochondriac. However, the long period between her early and later attacks, during which she was in good health and had no complaints, would seem to argue against hypochondria. Furthermore, there seems little doubt that the physical pain that she suffered was real. Her allergy diagnosis seems reasonable. The symptoms she describes are quite common in society, and they are often ascribed to allergic reactions of one kind or another. However, the question as to whether the source of the allergic reactions is *fluoride*, as Sherrell devoutly believes, remains open. Sherrell's evidence for her diagnosis is anecdotal. She does not provide any medical support to prove her case. As we shall learn in a later chapter, there are some allergists who support the possibility of allergies to fluoride, but they are in the minority. The symptoms of those who claim an allergy to fluoride, including those described by Darlene Sherrell, are very similar to those associated with allergies to many other potential sources.

Throughout her years of travel and adventure, Sherrell kept in touch with the anti-fluoridation subculture through e-mail correspondence with people of like-minded views. In 1995 her partner left, and she built her hut on the Grenadian hillside. At first she didn't have power in the cottage, so she worked from a cyber-café in St. George's. Then, in 1997, she got a laptop, wired the cottage, and discovered the Internet. She first found a home among the fluoride pages at www.trufax.org, the website of the Leading Edge International Research Group. However, she found her virtual neighbors to be too far into left field, and she soon moved to a site at www.rvi.net/~fluoride, where she became the webmaster of the Stop Fluoridation pages. Sherrell is a clear and colorful writer. She peppers her dispatches with stories from her own experience. Some of her tales have become part of the anti-fluoridation mythology across the web. One finds references to the Kettering Lab, the Kennedy letter, the Hodge error, and Judge Flaherty's ruling on site after site. As her anti-fluoride contributions multiplied, the hit rate on her website swelled. Over the years, e-mails arrived by the dozens seeking her help and solace. She has been asked to provide information to anti-fluoride groups in towns facing fluoride referendums. She has heard from worried parents, from concerned government bureaucrats, and from allergy victims like she once was.

As the years went by, Darlene Sherrell did not soften. The fluoridation of public water supplies, she has said, "is the most bizarre conspiracy of modern times." It is a scheme that "demonstrates, like no other issue before us, the infiltration of politics into science, a cancerous corruption of our health-care system which must be removed." She sees conspiracy and cover-up everywhere. "During the last 20 years, Uncle Sam's experts have had a great deal to say about the nature of fluoride, things everyone should know. The problem is that policy requires that these things never see the light of day. They lie buried under executive summaries and official interpretations handed out in press releases. Most of what you know about fluoride just isn't so."

Recently, ill-health has taken Darlene Sherrell to the sidelines. She has returned to the United States and has put her Stop Fluoridation website on hiatus. But there is no question of her impact. She has been an ongoing burr in the side of pro-fluoridationists for over 25 years. As Michael Easley declaimed in frustration during Sherrell's most active years, "I'm not going to believe a word that Darlene Sherrell says. I give her no credit for knowing anything."[8]

Roger Masters, a Dartmouth professor who is the author of academic papers that often find resonance in the anti-fluoridation community, has a different take. "If some people take extreme positions," he says, "you can say they aren't educated and their science is no good. Or you can say their passion is understandable. I call them canaries in the mine. They tell you there's something we ought to spend more time studying. Darlene Sherrell is one of those people. Darlene is a canary in the mine."[9]

JACKIE SPEIER AND THE LEGACY OF JONESTOWN

The event that shaped Jackie Speier's life took place on November 18, 1978, on a muddy jungle airstrip in South America, near the village of Port Kaituma, Guyana. She saw at first hand the apocalyptic ending of the People's Temple commune in Jonestown. She watched in horror as her mentor, Congressman Leo J. Ryan, was cut down on the tarmac. And she nearly lost her own life.

Jackie Speier is a native of San Francisco. After completing high school in the Bay Area, she took a B.A. at the University of California at Davis, and then in 1976 completed a law degree at the University of California's Hastings College of Law.[10] She was interested in politics, so after graduation, rather than apprenticing with a law firm, she decided to join the office of Congressman Ryan as his personal assistant and legal counsel. Leo Ryan was a former teacher who was first elected to Congress in 1964 after serving a term as the mayor of South San Francisco. He was a handsome and well-spoken man of firm resolve, used to the limelight, and known for his attraction to political issues that would draw media attention. He once spent a well-publicized day as a teacher in Watts, and on another occasion spent a day as an inmate in Folsom Prison. In the fall of 1977 he became aware of the People's Temple through an article that appeared in the *San Francisco Examiner*. It was the story of Bob Houston, a People's Temple member who died under questionable circumstances a day after announcing his decision to leave the Temple. Shortly after that, Houston's two daughters were spirited off to Jonestown without the knowledge of the rest of the family. By chance, Bob Houston was a former pupil of Leo Ryan, and when Ryan saw the article, he offered his help to the Houston family.[11]

The People's Temple was the creation of a charismatic religious leader named Jim Jones and his wife, Marceline. They began their ministry in Indianapolis, Indiana and met with some success there, but in 1965, the Joneses and a flock of 70 adherents decided to move west. They selected Redwood Valley, California, near Ukiah, as their new home, apparently in part because Jones had seen an article in *Esquire* magazine listing Redwood Valley as one of the safest places on earth in the event of a nuclear holocaust. Jim Jones was a white man, handsome, with jet-black dyed hair. He was neat and well groomed and a powerful speaker in the evangelical mode. His ministry spread, and in the early 1970s he opened churches in San Francisco and Los Angeles that soon attracted large congregations of downtrodden urban blacks. His message combined the ethical teachings of Christianity with the socialistic leanings of Marxism. He preached a social gospel of human freedom, love, and equality, with emphasis on the care for the marginalized members of society, especially blacks and the elderly. However, this message of love was mixed with a call for humiliating physical punishment for those who transgressed against his teachings, and ever-increasing warnings of approaching apocalyptic disaster due to nuclear war, racial hatred, or fascist takeover.

In the mid-1970s, Jones began to believe that his dream of an egalitarian, apostolic community could only be achieved through communal living in a promised land of security and peace far away from the corrupting influences of American society. He approached the government of Guyana, a former British colony but by then a socialist republic, and arranged to lease almost 4000 acres of land from the government in the western part of the country, 25 miles from the Venezuelan border, 150 miles northwest of the capital of Georgetown, and 10 miles south of the small village of Port Kaituma. In 1974, the first small group of "pioneers" began clearing land for what would become the People's Temple Agricultural Project, now known to the world as Jonestown. In the summer of 1977, construction began in earnest, and in the following year, Jones and over 1000 of his followers relocated to Jonestown.

Meanwhile, back in San Francisco, the People's Temple was under attack. The Bob Houston case simmered. An article in the July 1977 issue of *New West Magazine* exposed the use of disciplinary beatings within the cult. San Francisco District Attorney Joseph Freitas investigated charges that the Temple leadership was administering drugs to its congregation for the purpose of mind control. The California Department of Health investigated the misuse of public funds in Temple-operated care facilities. Former members told of armed guards at Temple services, and grotesque, faked, faith-healing demonstrations.

The families of Temple members who had relocated to Jonestown were becoming very nervous. They formed an organization called Concerned Relatives and issued a 50-page document entitled *Accusation of Human Rights Violations by Reverend James Warren Jones Against Our Children and Relatives at the People's Temple Jungle Encampment in Guyana, South America.* They accused Jones of brainwashing, sleep and food deprivation, mail censorship, prohibiting outside contact with family, and stationing guards around the compound to prevent escape.

The final blow to the People's Temple came in June 1978 with the revelations of Deborah Layton, a Jonestown defector who had previously been part of the leadership team there. She painted a picture of Jim Jones as "a good man gone bad," increasingly paranoid, psychotic, and dangerous. More prophetically, she described his chilling dry runs for a mass suicide that would allow the cult members to escape their persecutors and come together again on the "other side."

Layton's avowal of impending disaster at Jonestown galvanized Leo Ryan and Jackie Speier into action. They received approval from the State Department to carry out a fact-finding visit to Guyana. After flying to Georgetown and fighting the delaying tactics of Jim Jones and his American lawyers, the party finally set out on Friday, November 17, 1978, on a Guyanese Airways plane from Georgetown to Port Kaituma. On board were Ryan and Speier, the two People's Temple lawyers (one of whom was Mark Lane of Kennedy assassination fame), nine media personnel, four members of Concerned Relatives, one representative of the U.S. Embassy in Georgetown, and one Guyanese government official.

When Jackie Speier entered the Jonestown compound with the other members of the investigative team, what she saw was a village of prefab cottages and dormitories surrounding a large central plaza. The plaza featured a huge open-air pavilion that resembled a livestock barn at a county fairground.[12] There were also drying sheds for food, a large communal kitchen, an infirmary, an office building, a radio shack, two school buildings, and a nursery. The buildings were connected by muddy roads and wood-slatted walkways. One observer likened the compound to a Boy Scout summer camp,[13] another to a southern plantation before the Civil War.[14] In back of the buildings were the gardens, where eddoes (a tropical tuber), sweet potatoes, yams, casava, bananas, and papaya were cultivated, along with other vegetables, fruits, and nuts. Behind the gardens, and indeed all-around the compound, was dense and treacherous jungle.

Over three-quarters of the people in the camp were black, two-thirds were female, and almost a third were children. Jones claimed that Jonestown society was classless, although it soon became clear to Ryan and Speier that the original mostly white members from Indiana and the young educated whites who joined the People's Temple in Redwood Valley were very much in charge. Within hours of their arrival, the party began receiving surreptitious notes from Temple members asking for help in escaping Jonestown. Surprisingly, most of the requests came from the white community. It seems that many of the poor black members of the Temple really had nowhere to go. Ryan assured all who asked that they would be allowed to leave Jonestown with the investigating party if they desired. Jones's behavior swayed in a disturbingly volatile fashion from gracious host to persecuted demagogue.

The following day there was almost unbearable tension in the compound, with much crying and hysteria, as families were torn apart, some wishing to defect and others to stay. When all was said and done, there were only 15 defectors who decided to make the break.

In the late afternoon of Saturday, November 18, 1978, several trucks took the expanded party of investigators and defectors back to the airstrip at Port Kaituma, where two planes awaited their arrival, a large twin-engine Otter and a small six-passenger Cessna. As everyone spilled out onto the airstrip, Jackie Speier acted as the traffic director, moving between the groups, clipboard in hand, assigning seats on the two planes.[15] The small plane was quickly loaded with a mix of concerned relatives and defectors. One of the defectors on the Cessna was Larry Layton, the brother of Deborah Layton, whose revelations in San Francisco had acted as the catalyst for the investigative operation. As the Cessna prepared to taxi down the runway, Larry Layton pulled out a gun and began firing at his fellow passengers.

As the rest of the party was making their way onto the Otter, more gunshots suddenly rang out. A group of young men from the People's Temple leaped off a haywagon, from where they had been observing events, and began firing into the boarding party. Bodies fell on the mud-packed runway. Congressman Ryan went down. People were screaming and diving for cover. Jackie Speier found herself "near the cargo hatch of the Otter. She hung onto the edge of the hatch with one arm; her other arm and one leg were soaked with blood, nearly shattered."[16]

In the Cessna, Larry Layton was overpowered and pushed out of the plane. Some of those who were hit by his bullets were critically injured, but no one died in the Cessna. The young men that had attacked the Otter disappeared back into the jungle. They left five dead on the runway: Congressman Ryan, one of the defectors, and three of the media personnel. Jackie Speier took five bullets, but she lived through the ordeal.

Back at the compound, Jim Jones told his followers that their cause had been betrayed, that the People's Temple was under siege by CIA mercenaries and would not survive. The vats of deadly purple liquid were prepared: Fla-Vour-Aid laced with potassium cyanide and tranquilizers. The next day, horrified journalists and rescue forces found 911 bloated, mosquito-infested bodies rotting in the tropical sun, 260 of them children. Jim Jones and his wife took their lives by gunshot.

Eighty-five members of the People's Temple survived the holocaust by escaping into the jungle. When they returned to the United States, they faced prejudice, harassment, and shunning. They made no attempt to reestablish the Temple. In the years since 1978, "Jonestown" has become a watchword for "the madness of charismatic leadership, the vulnerability of religious devotees," ... and the dangerous "alchemy of love, loyalty, and rebellion" that is intrinsic to communal cult societies.[17] On October 17, 1989, the Loma Prieta earthquake demolished the former headquarters of the People's Temple on Geary Street in San Francisco.

Jackie Speier and the other survivors of the Port Kaituma massacre were flown to Georgetown, then airlifted back to the United States by a U.S. Air Force evacuation team. Back in San Francisco, Speier picked up the pieces of her life. She did not lick her wounds for long, returning quickly to the political arena, where Leo Ryan could no longer tread. In 1980, she won her first election for public office, beating a 20-year incumbent in a race for the San Mateo County Board of Supervisors. In 1986, after six years as a supervisor, she was elected to the California State Assembly, running as a Democrat. She was reelected five straight times. In her final assembly election in 1994, she was nominated by both the Republican and Democratic parties. In 1998, she moved to the state senate, were she became senator for the Eighth District (northern San Mateo County and the western half of San Francisco), running up a plurality of 79% in her first senate election. In her 20 years in the legislature, Speier put together a remarkable legislative record. Between 1986 and 1996, two Republican governors signed 181 of her bills into law. The *Los Angeles Times* calls this legislative record "Ruthian." The *San Jose Mercury News* said: "No one comes close to Speier's remarkable record of getting substantial legislation signed into law."[18]

Her bills run the gamut from women's health issues, through consumer protection, to the environment. On the health front, she has put
together the necessary nonpartisan support in the assembly and senate to
ensure passage of laws that create a statewide office of women's health,
introduce a tax checkoff for breast cancer research, require health plans
to cover prescription contraceptives, require osteoporosis screening for all
women, and mandate that clinical drug trials must include women and
minorities. Her consumer protection bills protect Californians from misleading Internet transactions, travel frauds, telemarketing scams, unfair
funeral practices, illegal stock transactions, inaccurate credit reports, and
gender discrimination in the pricing of services. She has supported environmental initiatives to create sea-life reserves, control offshore drilling,
protect wild and scenic rivers, and reauthorize bottle-recycling programs.
She was also the prime author of bills to curb domestic violence and to
increase the collection of delinquent child support payments. And she
was the guiding light behind bill AB733, the California Fluoridation Act,
signed into law in 1995.

During her period in the state assembly, Speier married and had two
children. She was the first member of the California legislature to give birth
while in office. But in 1994, tragedy struck again. She lost her husband in a
tragic car accident while pregnant with her second child.

Speier weathered Jonestown and she weathered widowhood. In 2001 she
remarried, and in 2008 she entered and won a special election that placed her
on the national stage in the U.S. House of Representatives. The early trag-
edies in her life, she says, have "absolutely molded my philosophy and my
zest for work and for life," and Jonestown will remain forever in her memories as a daily reminder that "no one is guaranteed tomorrow."

THE CALIFORNIA MANDATE

In the early 1990s, as Jackie Speier's reputation grew as a legislator who was
interested in public health and who knew how to get things done, many
groups brought a variety of health issues to her attention. One of those that
caught her interest was the fluoridation issue. Her own district in the Bay
Area was already fluoridated, and as the mother of a young family, she
had always felt comforted by this form of dental protection. However, she
quickly learned that this protection was shared by only 17% of Californians.
In fact, California ranked forty-seventh among all the states in terms of
progress toward full water fluoridation. She learned that 73% of California
children experienced tooth decay, over twice the national average. She was
made aware of a three-year study in the state that showed that 71% of adults

favored fluoridation. She also learned that despite these figures, California voters had rejected fluoridation over 70 times in local initiatives, apparently under the influence of what she saw as emotionally charged anti-fluoridation propaganda. She knew that a mandatory fluoridation bill would be a tough sell. She was aware of the conservative nature of southern California voters and their seeming disdain for social regulation, and of the popularity of alternative medicine and environmental causes in the more liberal North, which sometimes fostered anti-fluoridation attitudes. Speier's reaction to these facts is described by one of her admirers: "She was dismayed that fluoridation was not available to all Californians and viewed its persistent denial to most Californians as an issue of equity; she insisted that statewide legislation was appropriate because of California's slow adoption of this public health measure; she argued that it was achievable; she was convinced that the timing was perfect; and she was determined to make it happen on her watch."[19]

The push for fluoridation in California in the early 1990s grew at least in part out of a report that was published by the U.S. Surgeon General's office in 1991 entitled *Healthy People, 2000*. It assessed the state of the nation's health and set a number of public health goals for the decade 1990–2000. The report identified 22 priority areas and outlined 319 specific objectives. These objectives were designed to increase longevity, reduce health disparities, and increase preventive health services across the nation.[20] One of the most prominent objectives was the one relating to fluoridation, wherein it was resolved that 75% of Americans should be hooked up to fluoridated community water systems by the year 2000.

In 1991, the California Department of Health Sciences signed a contract with an organization known as the Dental Health Foundation to determine where California stood on this national public health objective. The results, which were determined largely on the basis of examinations and questionnaires received from 6643 children from 156 California schools, were published in 1994 in a report entitled *California Oral Health Needs Assessment*. Its major conclusion focused on the need for increased fluoridation of water supplies.[21]

With the tabling of bill AB733 in the California legislature, the fight was on for the hearts and minds of California legislators. The pro-fluoridation forces formed a coalition of advocacy groups known as the California Fluoridation Task Force. Among its members were the California Dental Association, the California Medical Association, the California Public Health Association, and the dental faculties from the University of California at Los Angeles, the University of California at San Francisco, and the University of Southern California. The California

Dental Association devoted considerable staff and financial resources to the campaign. They set out to counter anti-fluoridation "misinformation" aimed at the public, media, and legislators, and they tried to reassure the legislators and the governor that the overwhelming majority of Californians supported fluoridation. The American Dental Association aided in the media and public relations efforts and provided expert testimony for public and legislative hearings.

The task force took the view that most legislators were probably familiar with the dental benefits of fluoridation. They decided to zero in on the economic arguments, thinking that this was an angle that might catch the representatives' attention. They offered a figure of $4 billion per year as the amount spent by Californians on dental care and noted that $600 to 700 million of this total was paid out by the Denti-Cal program, a government-funded dental care system for the poor. They provided documented cost data from other parts of the country showing that fluoridation costs only "pennies per person per year," whereas the cost of filling one cavity can run as high as $140. They projected that the overall economic benefit of fluoridation to Californians, both public and private, would be on the order of hundreds of millions of dollars.

The anti-fluoridation forces were led by the Citizens for Safe Drinking Water under the leadership of the well-known anti-fluoridation activist David Kennedy and the organization's executive director, Jeff Green. Their first volley was against the *California Oral Health Needs Assessment.* They charged that the Dental Health Foundation (DHF), the organization that produced this report, was demonstrably biased and had been awarded the contract from the California Department of Health Sciences (CDHS) without competitive bidding. They noted that the CDHS and the DHF were now both members of the California Fluoridation Task Force and that it was inappropriate in the extreme to award a contract of this nature to an organization whose founding purpose is to promote the very issue being investigated. Green and Kennedy also peppered legislators with documentation of the usual anti-fluoridation arguments: loss of freedom, forced medication, and the threat of allergies, bone disease, kidney disease, cancer, and AIDS. They called fluoridation "the politically protected poison," and charged that "the same material that goes into fluoridating water would otherwise go into an industrial hazardous waste site."[22]

Apparently, the economic arguments had greater impact on the legislators than the scare tactics. They passed bill AB733, and on October 8, 1995, Governor Pete Wilson signed the California Fluoridation Act into law. It requires all California cities with more than 10,000 water connections to fluoridate their water supplies if funds are available for implementation from a source other than local ratepayers. The act specifies fines up to $25,000 per day to any community that does not take steps to fluoridate within two years after outside funds become available. It requires that the fluoridation systems be under local control, and that such control include constant and automatic monitoring of fluoride concentrations every minute of every day, to ensure against overdose. The act also recognizes that water demand (and hence the total amount of fluoride delivered to water users) changes with the weather. The act requires seasonal adjustment of fluoride concentrations so that they are reduced in summer months when temperatures are higher and drinking water usage increases.

Even with the passage of the California Fluoridation Act, Jackie Speier's contributions to the dental health of Californians were not complete. She recognized that without the requisite outside funding, her victory would be hollow. She took up the further challenge of developing the necessary financial support and was instrumental in finding donors for the newly established California Endowment, a private charitable foundation whose mission is "to expand access to affordable quality health care for California's underserved individuals and communities, and to promote fundamental improvements in the health status of all Californians." In May 1996 the California Endowment announced a $10 million grant to provide support to 13 cities for the fluoridation of their water systems. The grant was announced from the steps of the state capitol by Speier, together with representatives of the Dental Health Foundation and the California Endowment.

As one might expect, the anti-fluoridation forces were far from happy with these developments. They immediately tried to place an initiative on the 1996 state ballot that would reverse the mandatory law. This led to a quarrelsome dispute with the State Attorney General's office. By law, the Attorney General must provide an unbiased title and summary to accompany any proposed ballot measure while it is circulated to get the necessary supporting signatures. Anti-fluoridationists were livid when the summary came back stating that the cessation of fluoridation would cost the state at least $15 million annually and that there was no scientific evidence to suggest that drinking fluoridated water increases the incidence of cancer in humans. They claimed that such statements were severely biased, and they threatened to take the state to court to settle the issue.[23] The delays caused by these events saw the 1996 election pass without an anti-fluoridation initiative on the ballot. The Citizens for Safe Drinking Water tried to mount another campaign before the 1998 election, but they failed to get the requisite number of signatures (almost 1 million) before the deadline of October 1997. Undoubtedly, these efforts to rescind the law will continue.

SAN DIEGO, ESCONDIDO, AND THE GOLDEN FLEECE

One of the cities that took advantage of the California Fluoridation Act was San Diego. However, even with the statewide mandate in place, it was not an easy process.[24] As with so many other cities, San Diego has a long and checkered history on the fluoridation front. In November 1952 the San Diego city council voted unanimously in favor of fluoridation, and in January 1953 began adding fluoride to the city water supply. The anti-fluoridation camp immediately took up the cudgels and was successful in placing an anti-fluoride proposition on the June 1954 civic ballot. Proposition A, which referred to fluoridation as a "dangerous experiment" on a "captive population," was approved by the electorate by 53% to 47%. It required the establishment of a city ordinance forbidding the addition of fluoride to the city water supply, thus effectively ending this early fluoridation experiment. In 1969, voters continued their anti-fluoride stance, rejecting an initiative to repeal this ordinance.

And so things sat for 27 years, until passage of the 1995 statewide mandate. By that time, San Diego and Los Angeles were the two largest cities in the United States without fluoridation. In 1996, the San Diego city council tried to bring the fluoridation issue to the fore once again, but they found that they were still stymied by the 1954 civic ordinance. It was not clear to the city's attorneys which of the conflicting laws took precedence: the 1954 municipal law, which was put in place by a vote of the electorate, or the 1995 state law, which came from a higher jurisdiction but which did not have the imprimatur of the ballot box. It took four years to get a ruling. In February 2000, after much legal skirmishing, California Attorney General Bill Lockyer issued his opinion that the 1995 state law takes precedence over municipal law even if such municipal law resulted from a ballot measure passed by the electorate.

A few months prior to Lockyer's proclamation, the San Diego County science advisory board, consisting of three medical doctors and eight Ph.D.'s, issued the findings of their five months of "exhaustive study" of the fluoridation issue, which included listening to hundreds of presentations by both pro-fluoridation and anti-fluoridation partisans. They recommended fluoridation of the county's water supply. The report was welcomed by Ellie Nadler, executive director of the newly active San Diego Fluoridation Coalition, and decried by Jeff Green, the long-time director of Citizens for Safe Drinking Water.

On April 11, 2000, mayor Susan Golding, the mother of two young children and a longtime supporter of local fluoridation initiatives, asked the San Diego city council to approve a plan to add fluoride to the city's drinking water under the auspices of the 1995 statewide mandate. She had previously announced the availability of a $4 million grant from the California Endowment to cover the costs of the program. The same day, the *San Diego Union Tribune* published a guest editorial by Golding entitled *Why San Diego Should OK Fluoridation.*[25] Then, after hearing more than four hours of emotional rhetoric from supporters and opponents, the city council voted 8 to 1 in favor of fluoridation and instructed the city management team to prepare a fluoridation plan.

Two months later, another supporting voice was heard. The San Diego County grand jury recommended that local cities and water districts seek the necessary grants to fluoridate their drinking water. Many Californians were probably surprised to hear from this quarter. It is widely known that grand juries have the authority in criminal matters to issue indictments charging one or more persons with the commission of a crime, but a less publicized duty involves the investigation of the operations of governmental programs of the county, cities, and special districts under their jurisdiction. It was in the latter capacity that the jury worked for many months, interviewing knowledgeable sources on both sides of the issue and then publishing their recommendation. In the San Diego fluoridation battle, proponents and opponents had at least three opportunities to make their views known: to the science advisory board, to the city council, and to the grand jury. All three of these bodies ultimately came down in favor of a fluoridation program.

In the summer of 2000, the Citizens for Safe Drinking Water went to court to challenge San Diego's fluoridation plans. They argued that the city council action violated the 1954 law. On September 6, 2000, Superior Court Judge William R. Nevitt concurred with Attorney General Lockyer's earlier ruling: that the 1995 state law requiring fluoridation takes precedence over the 1954 municipal law banning fluoridation.[26] However, San Diego's march toward fluoridation has continued to be beset by legal, political, technical, and economic problems. As this book goes to press in 2009, the implementation plans for fluoridation of San Diego's water supply are still in the works. Under the requirements of the California Fluoridation Act, the city must implement their program by May 2010 or face the stiff penalties outlined in the act.

As the city of San Diego stutter-stepped toward fluoridation, a fluoridation sideshow erupted in the neighboring suburb of Escondido. The city council in that community was irrevocably split on the fluoridation issue, with three of the five councilors strongly opposed. In March 1999, this group took advantage of their majority status, voting 3 to 2 to defy the 1995 mandatory fluoridation law. To back up their decision, they commissioned a $5000 review of the original 1994 *California Oral Health Needs Assessment* report (the report that formed the basis for the passage of bill AB733). To carry out the review, they turned to a Tennessee firm known as the SENES Oak Ridge Center for Risk Analysis. The SENES firm specializes in "energy, nuclear, and environmental sciences" with special expertise in "applications in human health and ecological assessment." They claim to have carried out consulting contracts for many government agencies, including the Centers for Disease Control, the Environmental Protection Agency, the U.S. National Park Service, and the U.S. Army Corps of Engineers. However, they were also known by the majority councilors to be firmly in the anti-fluoridation camp, and they were apparently selected for the review on the advice of Jeff Green of the California Citizens for Safe Drinking Water. The SENES researcher who carried out the review admitted to talking to two of the councilors and to Jeff Green before submitting her proposal. She has provided other supposedly independent reviews of fluoridation issues that have proven very useful to anti-fluoridation lobbyists. In the Escondido case, she pointed out in her review that the *California Oral Health Needs Assessment* was never published in a peer-reviewed journal (a rather peculiar charge given the long record of self-published, media-directed pamphlets common to the anti-fluoridation literature), and that the "conclusion reported ... does not necessarily follow from the data." (The review is full of careful wording such as "does not *necessarily* follow.") The covering letter that accompanied the review, which was widely quoted by the majority councilors, emphasized all these negative aspects of the review. The full review was much more temperate in tone, with many sentences that start with disclaimers of the type "This is not to say that fluoride is not beneficial, just that. ...," and the like.

On a more personal level, the SENES reviewer charged that R. Isman, one of the authors of the *California Oral Health Needs Assessment* (the second listed author in a nonalphabetical listing of six) was under indictment in Oregon for election code violations associated with an Oregon fluoridation ballot issue. This charge has some significance because Isman later became the California state dental director, and he helped lobby bill AB733 through the California state legislature.

Personalities also came to the fore in the Escondido city council itself. When the SENES proposal first came up for a vote, it turned out that no one other than the three majority councilors, Keith Beier, Marie Waldron, and Jerry Kaufman, had seen copies of the proposal.[27] There was no mention of the firm or its proposal in the council meeting agenda; the city clerk and city manager didn't have copies, nor did the other two council members.

When queried by a TV reporter, June Rady, one of the minority councilors answered that she had not seen the proposal, and that if Beier said she had, he was lying. The following week an agenda item was tabled by the majority councilors under the heading "discussion of council ethics." The purpose of this discussion was to censure Rady publicly for her comments to the press. A resolution to that effect was pushed through by the three majority councilors at the following week's council meeting. Perhaps all this has less to do with the fluoride issue than meets the eye; at the time of their discord, Beier and Rady were opposing candidates in the Republican primary for California's 74th Assembly District.

The final word on the whole Escondido fracas is reserved for the San Diego Taxpayers Association, a government watchdog group that highlights wasteful public spending. In May 2000 the association gave their Golden Fleece Award to the Escondido city council for their "bogus fluoride study."

REFERENCES

1. The information on Jackie Speier's political career comes from her website, which can be accessed through http://democrats.sen.ca.gov, and from articles in the press identified through a media search engine.

2. The information on Darlene Sherrell's life and all the quotes ascribed to her come from the wealth of autobiographical material posted by Stop Fluoridation, http://www.rvi.net/~fluoride, and from a biographical article by journalist Barry Newman that appeared in the *Wall Street Journal*, April 12, 2000.

3. I. R. Campbell, *The Role of Fluoride in Public Health: A Selected Bibliography*, Kettering Laboratory, University of Cincinnati, Cincinnati, OH, 1963.

4. E. Groth III, Two issues of science and public policy: air pollution control in the San Francisco Bay area, and fluoridation of community water supplies, Ph.D. dissertation, Stanford University, 1973.

5. K. Roholm, *Flourine Intoxication*, H.K. Lewis, London, 1937.

6. U.S. National Academy of Sciences Board on Environmental Studies and Toxicology, *Health Effects of Ingested Fluoride*, National Academics Press, Washington, DC, 1993.

7. World Health Organization, *Fluorides and Human Health*, Monograph 59, WHO, Geneva, Switzerland, 1970.

8. Newman, 2000, op. cit.

9. Newman, 2000, op. cit.

10. Speier website, http://democrats.sen.ca.gov, op. cit.

11. The information on events leading up to the Port Kaituma massacre, and to events at Jonestown on November 17–18, 1978, come from the following sources: G. Klineman, S. Butler, and D. Conn, *The Cult That Died: The Tragedy of Jim Jones*

and the People's Temple, G. P. Putnam Sons, New York, 1980; D. Layton, *Seductive Poison: A Jonestown Survivor's Story of Life and Death in the People's Temple* (including the Foreword by C. Krause), Doubleday Anchor Books, New York, 1998; M. M. Maaga, *Hearing the Voices of Jonestown*, Syracuse University Press, Syracuse, NY, 1998; R. Moore, *Alternative Considerations of Jonestown and People's Temple*, http://www-rohan.sdsu.edu/~remoore/jonestown/faq.html; F. Steel, *Jonestown Massacre: A Reason to Die*, http://www.crimelibrary.com/serial4/jonestown/index.html; U.S. Foreign Affairs Committee, *Report on Assassination of Representative Leo J. Ryan*, 1979.

12. Maaga, 1998, op. cit.

13. Ibid.

14. C. Krause, in Foreword to Layton, 1998, op. cit.

15. Klineman et al., 1980, op. cit.

16. Ibid.

17. Maaga, 1998, op. cit.

18. Speier website, http://democrats.sen.ca.gov, op. cit.

19. M. W. Easley, Organizational and legislative efforts on behalf of AB733: a lesson in civic and professional cooperation, presented at the 124th Annual Session, American Public Health Association, New York, November 20, 1996.

20. U.S. Department of Health, Office of the Surgeon General, *Healthy People, 2000*, U.S. DH, Washington, DC, 1991.

21. H. F. Pollick, R. Isman, J. I. Fine, J. Wellman, P. Kipris, and J. Ellison, *California Oral Health Needs Assessment, 1993–94*, California Dental Health Foundation, for the California Department of Health Sciences, Sacramento, CA, 1994.

22. As posted at http://www.slugwire.org/weekly/archives/97Nov6/fluoride.html.

23. J. Yiamouyiannis, We can and will stop fluoridation in California, as posted at http://trufax/fluoride/yiamou.html.

24. The description of the San Diego and Escondido fluoridation battles are taken from news articles gleaned from the *San Diego Union Tribune* during the period October 7, 1999–September 6, 2000.

25. S. Golding, Why San Diego should OK fluoridation, *San Diego Union Tribune*, April 11, 2000.

26. San Diego County Superior Court, Case gic749524, *Citizens for Safe Drinking Water v. Council for the City of San Diego*, September 1, 2000.

27. A nasty fluoridation scrap: zealots appear bent on shooting down opponents, *San Diego Union Tribune*, February 21, 2000.

CHAPTER 5

THE ROAD TO FLUORIDATION

The road to fluoridation began with mottled teeth. There is no getting around it. Anti-fluoridationists point to this fact as proof of an illegitimate birth. Pro-fluoridationists point to the serendipity of it: a cloud with a silver lining.

BEAUTIFUL WOMEN AND BLACK TEETH

To begin the tale, we must transport ourselves across an ocean and back in time to the dawn of the twentieth century: to Naples, Italy in 1901. It was a time of political stability in Europe, the upheavals of the midcentury forgotten. Germany had yet to flex her military muscle. Times were good, and in Italy national confidence was high. Many Italians had achieved fame and fortune through their prominent roles in the great technological achievements of the day. Guglielmo Marconi was the first to transmit human speech by radio in 1900; and it was the recordings of Enrico Caruso that popularized the phonograph around the world. However, whereas Milan and the other great commercial centers of northern Italy prospered, the good times faded dramatically as one headed south. From Rome to Naples, and on down into Sicily, the largely rural population eked out a hardscrabble existence from the rocky Italian landscape. As the population swelled, there was simply not enough land to go around. It is no wonder that dreams of leaving for the United States began to capture the souls of poor peasants living on the Neapolitan hillsides. The New World. A land of plenty. A melting pot where everyone could start anew and make their way no matter where they came from. It was the same across Europe. Between 1900 and 1914, over 70 million Europeans emigrated from their homelands to seek a new life in new lands.[1]

We have all read about the bittersweet arrival of the immigrants to the United States: packed like sardines into pitching freighters, the thrill of their first view of the Statue of Liberty, and then the thoughtless Anglicization of their unfamiliar Italian names on Ellis Island. One seldom thinks of the tribulations, back in Europe, that must have preceded the trip. There would have been application forms in triplicate, in a foreign language. Lineups, and screwups, and inquisitions from officious bureaucrats. One of the most anxiety-ridden steps in the procedure was undoubtedly the medical examination. What would be more ironic than to have one's hopes of a new life dashed on the rocks of some long-forgotten medical ailment. One can picture these prospective new Americans sitting in doctors' waiting rooms, cloth caps in hand, hoping for medical absolution. And improbably, it is here that the story of fluoridation begins.

The medical examination of prospective immigrants in the Naples area took place in a hospital run by the U.S. Marine Hospital Service. The Hospital Service established several U.S. military hospitals on foreign soil under the auspices of a congressional act that dated back to the presidency of John Adams in 1798. The original act, for the "relief of sick and disabled seamen," made provision for a tax of 20 cents per month to be taken out of the wages of all U.S. seamen to pay for these hospitals. The Marine Hospital Service was a precursor of today's Public Health Service. In fact, it was in the following year that President Teddy Roosevelt signed legislation that renamed and expanded the mission of the Marine Hospital Service into a full-fledged Public Health Service.[2]

One of the medical examiners in the Naples hospital in 1901was a 37-year-old American surgeon named John M. Eager.[3] He had joined the service in 1891 and was initially assigned to duty in Naples to help stem the tide of a local cholera epidemic. Now he found himself engaged in the more prosaic task of vetting the medical status of throngs of prospective U.S. immigrants. As the seemingly endless line of candidates began to pass beneath his professional gaze, he couldn't help but notice their teeth. An inordinate number of these subjects had a dark brown staining on their teeth. It was almost black in some cases. The locals referred to these black teeth as *denti neri*. Others had fine horizontal black lines across their teeth that resembled minute hieroglyphic inscriptions. These were known as *denti scritti*. Eager was sufficiently taken by this strange dental disorder that he wrote up his observations in a brief communication which he sent to Walter Wyman, the Surgeon General of the Marine Hospital Service in the United States. The following year, Eager's article was published by the newly established Public Health Service (PHS). It was the first dental article ever published by the PHS and the first scientific document in the long and contentious history of stained and mottled teeth.[4]

In his paper, Eager described the blackened teeth as "quite unlike any other dental disease or other maladies of the teeth" that he had ever observed.

He referred to the condition as *denti di Chiaie*, apparently in honor of a Professor Chiaie, who had first described the disorder. Later dental historians have questioned this connection, suggesting it is more likely that the name derives from La Villa Chiaia, a town on the Neapolitan Riviera where blackened teeth were particularly common. In his article, Eager drew attention to the fact that those who exhibited *denti di Chiaie* tended to come from particular villages in the Neapolitan region, and he made the observation that many of these towns were situated on volcanic terrain. He made the remarkable conjecture that the condition might have something to do with the spring-fed drinking-water systems common in these communities, which he thought might be "charged under pressure with volcanic fumes".

While Eager was the first to provide scientific documentation of the *denti di Chiaie*, he was certainly not the first to comment on it. In a review of the Neapolitan arts published in 1892, the philosopher and critic Benedetto Croce lamented the tragedy of "the beautiful women with black teeth" in La Villa Chiaia.[5] And centuries earlier, the Roman poet Martialis provided a different explanation in describing the teeth of Thais, a mistress of Alexander the Great: "Thais has black teeth. Laecania has snow-white ones. Why? The latter's teeth were bought, the former has her own."[6]

FREDERICK McKAY AND THE MYSTERY OF THE COLORADO STAIN

In the same year that John Eager sent his dispatch from Naples, a young dentist named Frederick McKay set up practice in Colorado Springs, Colorado. Here, thousands of miles and an ocean away from La Villa Chiaia, McKay found that many of his patients also suffered from stained teeth. He called the condition *Colorado stain*. Unaware of Eager's article, he began to investigate the question of stained and mottled teeth, and unlike Eager, who apparently dropped the topic after his article was published, once McKay got the bit between his teeth, he would not let go. He began a quest to find an explanation and a cure for this peculiar affliction. It would be three decades before he met success.[7]

Photographs of McKay taken in the early years of the new century show a tall, slender, young man dressed in the finery of the day: double-breasted suit, tight starched collar, and string tie. Colleagues described him as having a dynamic, persistent, and inquisitive personality. He was a lover of music who became the president of the Colorado Springs Symphony Orchestra in later life. He arrived in Colorado Springs in 1901, at the age of 26, just a year after he graduated from the University of Pennsylvania dental school. In Colorado Springs he found a booming frontier town joyously cashing in on the prosperity of the nearby Cripple Creek goldfields. The town advertised itself as a scenic wonderland and health resort. It claimed to be the wealthiest city per capita in the United States.

As he began his practice, McKay was repeatedly taken aback by the number of patients, rich and poor alike, who showed up in his dental chair with stained and pitted teeth. He began to keep records. With the help of another local dentist he carried out a systematic examination of almost 3000 schoolchildren in Colorado Springs. He was astonished to find that over 80% had defects in tooth enamel. Despite these alarming statistics, McKay found it difficult to arouse the interest of the local dental community or of the small cadre of nationally recognized dental researchers, most of whom held their chairs at faraway eastern universities. He even exhibited one of his severely affected patients at a meeting of the Colorado State Dental Society, to little notice. The lack of interest seemed all the more peculiar as he learned that many other Colorado communities also experienced this mysterious condition. He visited most of these towns, examined the afflicted, and built up his files. He persisted in his lonely campaign, writing up his findings and waiting for the rest of the dental community to catch up with him.[8]

It was over 15 years before his persistence finally paid off. In 1915, he managed to attract the interest of G. V. Black, dean of the Dental School at Northwestern University in Chicago. Black came to Colorado and worked with McKay, and together they published a series of five papers in the respected journal *Dental Cosmos*.[9] They described browned and yellowed teeth with "ghastly chalky white patches." They revealed a human touch by confiding how the disfigured teeth "materially injure the countenance of the individual" and create "intense self-consciousness and a bitter attitude." They presented evidence to support their claim that the damage is apparently done in youth, during tooth development, thus identifying Colorado stain as a childhood disease worthy of societal attention. Thanks to Black's reputation and his colorful writing style, the dental community finally took notice. Reports began to come in of other cases around the country: in Arizona, Washington, Virginia, Idaho, Texas, and South Dakota.

In 1905, McKay had moved to St. Louis for three years, where he never saw a single case of stained teeth. On moving back to Colorado Springs, he was struck again by the pervasive reality of the disease there. Some cities were damned, it seemed, whereas others got off scot-free. As he studied the reports coming in from around the country, he noticed that in almost every case, certain communities were affected, whereas others nearby were not. McKay began to suspect an environmental driver, and he zeroed in on the drinking water in the endemic communities. He requested water samples and had them analyzed, but nothing out of the ordinary ever showed up.

The mystery now caught the attention of other dental experts, each of whom had their own pet theories. It was a nutritional issue. It was a calcium deficiency. Too much iron. Radioactivity. Heredity. One researcher even claimed to have found a connection between mottled teeth and freckles.[10]

McKay was not impressed. "Colorado stain," he wrote, "disregards nationality, social status, and every condition of physical health."[11] As the years went by, he systematically eliminated every possible cause except the drinking water. This hypothesis was strengthened further when he learned that stained teeth had appeared in the children of Britton, South Dakota only after that small community had changed its water supply from one well to another.[12] Then in 1927, on a trip to Italy, he discovered in John Eager's old stamping ground that the children in the Neapolitan suburb of Pozzuoli no longer suffered from the stained teeth that were endemic to their parents. A brief investigation uncovered the fact that this community had also recently changed the source of its water supply.[13] Sometimes a change in drinking water created the problem, and sometimes it resolved it, but one way or another, McKay knew that he was homing in on a solution.

In 1925, despite his continued ignorance as to the specific constituent of drinking water that was responsible for stained teeth, McKay helped persuade the citizens of the small town of Oakley, Idaho to change their water supply for the sole purpose of eradicating this dental affliction. The Oakley Women's Civic League was campaigning for a $35,000 bond issue to change the town water, and McKay went to Oakley to speak on their behalf. The night before the election the townsfolk filled the local theater to hear the expert from Colorado tell his tale. Flashing before-and-after lantern slides from Britton, South Dakota onto the movie screen, he drew the parallels between these two small western towns. The bond issue passed, and McKay recommended that the nearby Carpenter Spring be used as the new water supply, because rural children who had been raised on this water showed no ill effects. Seven years later, "with a good deal of trepidation," McKay returned to Oakley to examine the teeth of the 24 children born in the community since the change in water supply. To his immense pleasure, none of these children exhibited even a hint of Colorado stain.[14]

So: "It's the water!" as the beer ads are wont to exclaim. But what exactly was it *in the water* that does the damage? There was the rub for Fred McKay in 1928. Hundreds of water analyses from endemic areas had revealed nothing. In retrospect, it is clear that the problems lay in the types of analyses that were carried out and in the equipment that was used to do so. Chemical labs were simply not equipped to measure anything other than the few primary chemical constituents that are commonly found in all waters: calcium, sodium, magnesium, chloride, sulfate, and carbonate. They were not capable of assaying trace constituents, and those labs that were capable of such measurements could not guarantee sufficient accuracy with the primitive measurement methods then available.

The breakthrough finally came in 1931. The town of Bauxite, Arkansas, about 25 miles southwest of Little Rock, was a company town owned by a mining subsidiary of the Aluminum Company of America (Alcoa). The town got its drinking water from two deep wells, and all the children in town suffered from stained teeth. The children in the town of Benton, only 5 miles away, which took its water supply from the Saline River, exhibited normal teeth. Grover Kempf, the director of the child hygiene group at the Public Health Service, who had been made aware of the situation in Bauxite, called in Fred McKay to help study the problem. Once again, careful water analyses provided no special clues. McKay and Kempf suggested closing the wells anyway, and recommended a pipeline to the Saline River. They wrote up their findings for publication and went home.[15]

Back at Alcoa headquarters in Pittsburgh, H. V. Churchill, Alcoa's chief chemist, watched the events unfolding at Bauxite with concern. His superiors worried that stories about pitted teeth in an Alcoa company town might harm the company image, and they wanted Churchill to solve the problem and absolve Alcoa from all potential blame. Churchill put his lab technicians to work testing the waters from the Bauxite deep wells, but this time he demanded that they test not just for the standard constituents but for all identifiable trace constituents as well. When the results came back, an unusual anomaly leaped off the page. The Bauxite well waters contained fluoride at 13.7 ppm. Normal fluoride concentrations in well and spring waters are usually less than half a part per million. Churchill then asked for samples from Oakley and other endemic communities. The Oakley spring came down at 6 ppm fluoride. Some samples from deep wells in South Dakota had 12 ppm. Surprisingly, samples from Colorado Springs, where it all started, turned up concentrations of only 2 ppm, higher than normal but not excessively so. Churchill wrote up his results for publication, emphasizing his discovery of "hitherto unsuspected constituents" in the endemic waters.[16] In his paper, Churchill was exceedingly careful, noting that "no precise correlation" had been established between the fluoride content of the water and mottled teeth, and warning the reader that fluoride determinations in water are "fraught with difficulty."

No matter. The culprit was identified. And so it has remained to this day. The relation has become so clear that the disease that causes stained and mottled teeth is now known as *dental fluorosis*. Back in 1931, however, it remained to make the connection causal rather than just correlative. Unbeknown to Fred McKay, the research that would cement this relationship was already under way. A husband-and-wife team of research chemists, Margaret Cammack Smith and her husband Howard Smith, working at the University of Arizona Agricultural Experiment Station, were alarmed by the prevalence of mottled teeth in the nearby town of St. Davids, Arizona, where the well water used by the town water supply ran up to 7 ppm fluoride. They fed controlled concentrations of highly fluoridated water to white rats and observed the formation of defects in the rats' teeth that were "similar if not identical to the mottling seen in human teeth." They concluded that their studies advanced definitive proof that mottled enamel "is caused by the destructive action of fluorine present in the water supply of afflicted communities."[17] It had taken 30 years, but Fred McKay finally had his answer.

H. TRENDLEY DEAN AND THE TOWNS WITHOUT TOOTHACHES

So, you may be dying to ask: What has all this got to do with cavities and fluoridation? Well, Fred McKay may have been obsessed with mottled teeth, but he was certainly not averse to recording other aspects of his patients' dental health. As early as 1916, he observed that the mottled condition itself, "contrary to what may be expected ... does not seem to increase the susceptibility of the teeth to decay."[18] Again, in a 1925 article, he asked: "How do we explain the comparatively high immunity to decay of mottled enamel when its structural elements lie wrecked and disorganized?"[19] Then in a 1928 article entitled "The Relation of Mottled Teeth to Caries," McKay laid it on the line. He stated for the first time that teeth with mottled enamel are not just the equivalent of their unmottled cousins when it comes to dental caries; they are superior. They show "a singular absence of decay."[20]

Yet, despite proffering these provocative harbingers of the future, McKay did not carry these ideas forward. The search for a solution to the problem of mottled teeth consumed him, and he was not the type of person to be sidetracked by peripheral issues along the way. Moreover, McKay had finally convinced the Public Health Service, which had rebuffed his many requests for support during the 1920s, to take up the cudgels in support of mottled-teeth research. Ironically, it would be these late bloomers in government service who would preside over the impending paradigm shift.

The catalyzing action was the transformation in 1930 of the old Hygienic Laboratory of the Public Health Service into a new and expanded National Institute of Health (NIH) in Bethesda, Maryland, and the appointment of a 38-year-old career dental officer named H. Trendley Dean to form a team within NIH to pursue full-time research on mottled teeth. Dean, who obtained his dental degree from the St. Louis University Dental School in 1916, served in the Army Dental Corps in World War I and joined the Public Health Service in 1921.[21] He worked in U.S. Marine hospitals in Boston, New York, and San Francisco, generating a steady stream of clinical research papers as he went along. It was this record of scholarly production that impressed his superiors and led to his appointment to the NIH position. Pictures of Dean hunched over his desk at NIH reveal a short, stocky man with glasses and a brushcut. He was a cautious and conservative man, given to homely midwestern aphorisms and malapropisms that led to much sniggering behind his back. Yet, despite his "gee, shucks" facade, he had the ability to design and carry out an effective program and to garner unquestioned loyalty from his colleagues. He was quickly anointed as chief scientist of the Dental Research Section of NIH. When Congress established the National Institute of Dental Research in 1948, Trendley Dean was appointed its first director. But all that was in the future. In 1931, his assignment was clearly put to him. He was asked to determine, first, whether fluoride was the sole cause of mottled teeth; second, whether there was a threshold concentration of fluoride in the water below which mottling is not observed, and above which defects in tooth enamel first become apparent; and third, whether fluoride could be removed from water, and at what cost. This last item seems especially ironic in light of later developments.

Dean took as his initial task the development of a classification system for the diagnosis of mottled teeth. He formulated a rigorous set of criteria that could be used by dental examiners to distinguish objectively between normal teeth and very mild, mild, moderate, and severe cases of fluorosis.[22] Under Dean's classification, *normal* teeth are "translucent, … smooth, glossy, and usually a pale creamy white color." Very *mild* fluorosis involves "small, opaque, paper-white areas scattered irregularly over the tooth, but not involving as much as 25% of the tooth surface." *Mild* fluorosis exhibits the same flaws but involving up to 50% of the tooth surface. *Moderate* fluorosis involves all tooth surfaces and includes "disfiguring brown stain." *Severe* fluorosis is indicated by "widespread staining," "a corroded appearance," and "discrete or confluent pitting."

With this classification system in place, he initiated a series of demographic studies to further clarify the scope of the problem. He sent out questionnaires to dental societies, county health officers, and local dentists and physicians around the country. Once this information was in hand, he made confirmatory visits to afflicted areas, examining children's teeth, collecting water samples, and conferring with local health officers. He described these investigations as "a lot of shoe leather, a ball of string, and a pencil," giving rise to his team's pride in their "shoe-leather epidemiology." He also began a lifelong friendship with Fred McKay, who was by then practicing dentistry in New York City, often inviting him to his home to discuss the latest developments. Ultimately, he and McKay published a paper identifying 375 known endemic areas of dental fluorosis in 26 states.[23]

Over the years, Dean added three new colleagues to the team that would ultimately play an important role in the birth of the fluoridation movement. Elias Elvove, a rotund, balding native of the Soviet Union, had research expertise in both pharmacy and chemistry and a reputation for meticulous accuracy in his work. He developed a quicker and more accurate method for the analysis of fluoride concentrations in water. In later years, he patented a technology for removing fluoride from high-fluoride waters. Frank McClure was a toxicologist who had published several papers on fluoride metabolism. He was asked to further investigate how fluoride intake affected the human body. Francis Arnold, a protégé of a friend of Dean's, was brought onto the team as an additional pair of hands. Known quaintly to his friends as "Pokey," he had dreamed of a career in dental research ever since his days as a teenage dental assistant in Oroville, Ohio.

Using Elvove's improved fluoride-assay procedures, Dean measured fluoride concentrations in drinking water supplies across the nation. By 1936 he had built up a sufficiently large file of data to produce the figure shown here as Figure 5.1.[24] It exposes the clear relationship between the prevalence of mottled enamel in a given water district and the concentration of fluoride in the water supply of that district. *Normal* teeth are associated with low fluoride content; *mottled* teeth (including the very mild, mild, moderate, and severe types) are associated with higher fluoride contents. (The *questionable* cases included with the *normal* in Figure 5.1 are those cases where a *normal* classification is not justified due to "slight aberrations" in the translucency

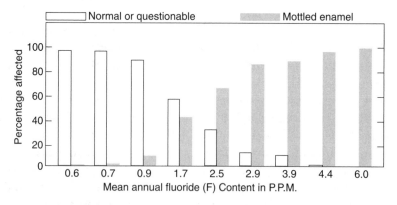

FIGURE 5.1 Prevalence of mottled enamel in areas with differing concentrations of natural fluoride in the water supply. (*Source:* H. T. Dean, Chronic endemic dental fluorosis, *J. Am. Med. Assoc.*, 107, 1269–1272, 1936. Copyright © 1936 American Medical Association. All rights reserved.)

of the enamel, but a definite diagnosis of the mildest form of fluorosis is not warranted.) Dean concluded on the basis of these data that a concentration of 1.0 ppm fluoride was the minimal threshold that he had been asked to determine: the level at which fluoride begins to blemish teeth. At this concentration, only 10% of the population exhibits any evidence of mottling, and this only in its very mildest form (a level that Dean felt was not even of cosmetic significance). In time, the data that appear in this figure, the 1.0 ppm value in particular, would take on additional significance.

Unlike McKay, Dean was intensely interested in the observation that mottled teeth might be cavity-resistant. Starting with his earliest field studies, he always ensured that observations of patients with stained and pitted teeth also included a record of their history of dental caries. As early as his first annual report in 1932, he noted that people in endemic areas of fluorosis often show a lower incidence of dental caries than those in nearby nonendemic areas. Consequently, he argued, "the study of mottled enamel may disclose some lead applicable to the vastly more important problem of dental caries."[25]

By the mid-1930s, Dean was not alone in his observation that higher fluoride levels in drinking water seemed to presage a reduced prevalence of dental caries. New articles were appearing in the dental literature every month attesting to the fidelity of the correlation.[26] A well-documented case study based on data from a number of Indian reservations in the American West appeared. Others came from Minnesota, England, Argentina, and Japan. All of these studies concurred that, like mottling, the effects of fluoride on cavity reduction were dominated by fluoride exposure in childhood, during the years of tooth eruption and development. By 1937, the focus of Dean's studies had switched completely from the role of fluoride in mottling to the role of fluoride in caries prevention. Dean's team carried out confirmatory studies of ever-widening scope[27]: a study based on the records of 236 nine-year-old children already on file in 1938; a study of 885 twelve-to-fourteen-year-old children in four Illinois cities (Galesburg, Quincy, Monmouth, and Macomb) in 1939; and finally, a study of 7257 twelve-to-fourte-year-old children in 21 cities in four states (Illinois, Ohio, Indiana, and Colorado) in 1942. The results were consistent with earlier observations and with one another. In Quincy, Illinois, with less than 0.2 ppm fluoride in the water supply, only 14% of the children were free of dental caries, whereas in Galesburg, with 1.6 ppm fluoride, almost 35% of the children had no decay. In the 21-city study, the team found that children in cities with fluoride content in the water of less than 0.5 ppm had nearly three times as many cavities as did those in cities with an excess of 1.4 ppm fluoride in the water supply. The relation is illustrated in Figure 5.2.[28] The acronym DMF in the figure refers to decayed, missing, and filled teeth, an overall measure of dental caries.

Number of cities studied	Number of children examined	Number of DMF teeth per 100 examinees 0 100 200 300 400 500 600 700	Fluoride content of water (ppm)
11	3867		<0.5
3	1140		0.5–0.9
4	1403		1.0–1.4
3	847		>1.4

FIGURE 5.2 Data from 21-city survey grouped according to the fluoride content of water. (*Source: Fluorides and Human Health*, World Health Organization, Geneva, Switzerland, 1970).

It is unlikely that the public would have learned much of these arcane goings-on in the dental research community were it not for an article that appeared in the December 19, 1942, issue of *Collier's* magazine, at that time one of the leading weekly magazines in the United States. The article was written by a journalist named J. D. Ratcliff and had the provocative title, "The Town Without a Toothache."[29] It told readers about the miraculous absence of cavities in Hereford, Texas, and the role of a 3-ppm fluoride concentration in the water supply in creating this happy situation. These were the darkest days of World War II, and the public was ready for good news. Excerpts from the article appeared in many newspapers, and it was reprinted in the February 1943 issue of *Reader's Digest*. Press releases on fluoride issues from Dean's team at NIH that had always been relegated to the back pages of the newspaper suddenly warranted front-page coverage. The relationship between fluoride and the reduced incidence of tooth decay was firmly cemented in the public's mind. In point of fact, the fluoride concentrations in the Hereford water were well above Dean's threshhold value of 1 ppm, but neither the *Collier's* article nor the press releases mentioned the existence of childhood fluorosis, which was also endemic in the Hereford area.

LATHERED UP TO GO

If fluoride in drinking water prevents cavities, and by the late 1930s this fact seemed well established, it is not much of a stretch to suggest that fluoride could be added to those water supplies that do not have enough of it. Surely there must have been considerable discussion of this possibility within the dental community, and probably many could lay claim to being the first to suggest it. The official credit (or blame, depending on from which pulpit you are preaching) is usually given to Gerald J. Cox, a biochemist from the Dental School at the University of Pittsburgh, who was also active in the Mellon Institute of Industrial Research at that university. He was apparently the first to specifically recommend the treatment of water supplies with fluoride in a published article. He argued that the addition of fluoride to prevent cavities ought to be no more controversial than the addition of chloride to prevent bacteriological and viral diseases. He felt that such a program would be the "most practical means of approaching the goal of sound teeth for all children."[30]

Dean, ever cautious, was aghast. He felt that such a proposal was grossly premature: that there was need for more confirmatory studies, more examination of other potential health impacts of fluoride, and more consideration of the logistic and engineering complexities. He was beginning to think about the possibility of a 10- to 15-year clinical trial, but in his opinion, even that undertaking would be premature without more study. He pleaded for more groundwork, a 10- to 15-year study, and *then*, all things remaining copacetic, it would be time to consider action. Only after a successful long-term clinical trial would he be willing to climb onto his own bandwagon.

Surprisingly, in light of their later strong support, the American Dental Association was also nervous. Even as late as October 1944, an editorial in the *Journal of the American Dental Association* warned that although the potential benefits of fluoride as a therapeutic procedure to prevent dental caries "may appear speculatively attractive, in the light of our present knowledge (or lack of knowledge) of the chemistry of the subject, the potentialities for harm far outweigh those for good." Some ADA members were displeased with this discouraging statement and told the editor so. The December issue of the journal carried a semiretraction in which the editor stated that he had "not intended to present an alarmist attitude." However, he did not back down from the association position that more research was needed before fluoridation of water supplies could be considered as an acceptable public health measure.[31]

Despite these warnings, or perhaps because of them, the director of the National Institutes of Health convened a conference of government health mandarins in 1942 to discuss the possibility of introducing fluoride into drinking water as a public health measure.[32] Heeding Dean's pleas, they developed both a short- and a long-term plan to investigate the effect of fluoride on the general health of the population. The short-term plan would be carried out as a comparative health survey in two Texas towns, Bartlett and Cameron, one that had a high natural fluoride content in its drinking water and one that did not. Investigators would check the medical histories of the residents of the two towns and set up a program of regular physical exams, dental exams, x-rays, blood sampling, and urine sampling. They would record the comparative incidence of a variety of potential health problems over a 10-year period, including arthritis, osteoporosis, high blood pressure, cataracts, thyroid difficulties, cardiovascular problems, hearing loss, tumors, fractures, gallstones, urinary problems, and dental fluorosis.[33] Dean and his team were instructed to begin planning a large-scale clinical trial of artificial fluoridation, which would go forward if the Texas study provided suitable solace.

One issue that had to be settled was the concentration of fluoride that would be introduced into the water supply in the trial city. Dean argued successfully that the target concentration should be the maximum fluoride level that does not lead to dental fluorosis. This, of course, was the 1.0 ppm threshold that he had identified in his earlier studies. A few years later, a fluorine chemist named Harold Hodge (the same Harold Hodge who made the dosage error identified by Darlene Sherrell in Chapter 4, and who will figure further in our story in due course) published a paper entitled "The Concentration of Fluoride in Drinking Water to Give the Point of Minimum Caries with Maximum Safety."[34] In his article, Hodge presented the figure shown here as Figure 5.3,

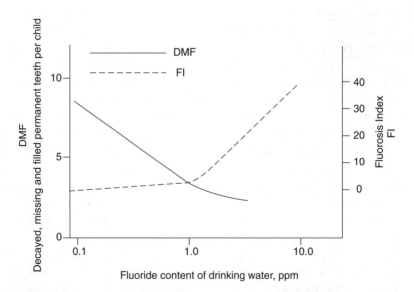

FIGURE 5.3 Relationship between the fluoride content of drinking water, caries occurrence, and dental fluorosis. (*Source*: H. C. Hodge, The concentration of fluorides in drinking water to give the point of minimum caries with maximum safety, *J. Am. Dent. Assoc.*, 40, 436–439, 1950. Copyright © 1950 American Dental Association. All rights reserved. Adapted 2008 with permission of the American Dental Association.)

which superimposes the decreasing trend in dental caries with increasing
fluoride content (the solid line) and the increasing occurrence of dental fluorosis at fluoride content greater than 1.0 ppm (the dashed line). Hodge's analysis
further confirmed Dean's argument for an optimal concentration of 1.0 ppm,
and that value has been considered appropriate by fluoridation proponents
ever since.

Dean envisaged a 15-year study of artificial fluoridation in a representative U.S. city, with one or more unfluoridated cities acting as a control.
Together with W. J. Pelton of the Public Health Service, Dean and Arnold
began the search for a suitable pair of cities to carry out the fluoridation
trial. They zeroed in on the midwestern states, where Dean's database
from earlier studies was most complete. The state of Michigan came naturally to the fore. Arnold had ties with state dental health authorities there,
and the University of Michigan was preeminent in caries research. There
would be no legal obstacles in Michigan because the state department of
health was already empowered by state law to carry out all necessary
water supply treatment. Furthermore, Arnold already had an offer on
file from C. R. Taylor of the Michigan Bureau of Public Health Dentistry
urging such a study in Michigan and offering their support. The letter
began "Dear Pokey" and stated that everybody in Michigan was "lathered
up" to go.[35]

In the end, Dean and Arnold selected Grand Rapids, Michigan, as the
fluoridation city and nearby Muskegon as the control. Both cities used
Lake Michigan water from areas not too far apart, and they shared a
similar cultural demography. A third city, Aurora, Illinois, was added as a
different kind of control. The water supply in Aurora was naturally fluoridated at a level close to the optimal value, so a comparison of these two
cities would test the hypothesis that there was no difference in response
to natural or added fluoride. Grand Rapids seemed an ideal choice for
the trial city. It had a large school population, a stable demography,
and a history of having used the same fluoride-free water supply since
1912.

Together with their Michigan supporters, Dean and Arnold began the
process of getting civic approval of the project. They emphasized the benefits
that would accrue to Grand Rapids children and the recognition that the city
would receive for its leadership role in this public health breakthrough. They
provided assurances against any negative health impacts, using as a basis for
this claim Dean's studies across the land, recent studies by Frank McClure
on a large number of armed forces inductees, and the positive findings that
were coming in from the Bartlett–Cameron study in Texas. The final step was
a vote by mayor George Welsh and the city commission on July 31, 1944, to
approve the fluoride study.[36]

Strategic planning for the Grand Rapids study took about a year and a half. Arrangements had to be made with the Michigan Department of Health, the University of Michigan School of Dentistry, the Grand Rapids City Commission, the Grand Rapids School Department, and the Grand Rapids Waterworks. Decisions had to be reached about examiners, recorders, examination protocols, statistical analyses, office space, laboratory facilities, fluoride supplies, parental consent forms, transportation, lodging, and more. By the fall of 1944, the project was geared up and almost ready to roll. The first step would be a full-scale pre-fluoridation dental examination of all the children in the three cities, a monumental task in itself.

Although Trendley Dean may have harbored some doubts going into the Grand Rapids study, the same could not be said for Pokey Arnold. In 1943 he predicted that artificial fluoridation would bring about a 60% reduction in caries and a sixfold increase in the number of caries-free children by the time of their high-school graduation.[37] As it turned out, these predictions may have been a bit optimistic, but they weren't that far off.

LITTLE GIRLS IN GINGHAM DRESSES

So we arrive once again at Grand Rapids. Our story started in Naples, Italy, but since then it has been an odyssey across the hinterlands of the United States. It has taken us to the gold-fueled frontier town of Colorado Springs; to tiny western hamlets such as Britton, South Dakota, St. Davids, Arizona, and Oakley, Idaho; and to turn-of-the-century mining towns such as Bauxite, Arkansas. It has taken us to Bartlett, Cameron, and Hereford on the Texas Great Plains; and to midwestern "our-towns" such as Quincy and Galesburg, Illinois. Along the way the idea survived depression, drought, and two world wars.

Grand Rapids in 1944 was a city of immigrants, many of them originally drawn to America's "Furniture City" to work in the cabinetmaking trade. Of course, in 1944, most of the men were off in the war, and many of the women worked on "war work" in the refurbished old furniture factories. In the backyards of their working-class homes, families tended their "victory gardens," and each night, mothers and children gathered around their radios and listened to the news. It was through the disembodied voices of the newscasters that they learned to hate Hitler. That fall they cheered the Allies through the battle of Normandy and the liberation of Paris.[38]

The other topic on everybody's lips was the November election. Franklin Delano Roosevelt had been nominated yet again, and in the blue-collar cities of southern Michigan this was viewed as a good thing. His Republican opponent, Governor Thomas E. Dewey of New York, was seen as a bit of a silk stocking who would not understand the problems of working people. Most Grand Rapids mothers felt that if FDR were elected, the men would soon be home.

In early September, the kids returned to school to start classes. They soon received the obligatory start-of-the-school-year swatch of mimeographed notices to take home to their parents. Most of them were the usual boring messages about gym outfits, renting a clarinet for band, and working with 2H pencils with a soft eraser. However, there was one notice that was definitely different. It seemed that the students of the Grand Rapids school district had been selected to take part in a scientific experiment that would keep people from getting cavities in their teeth. If their parents signed the form, each child would get a free dental checkup at school. Not only that, but the notice also said that those taking part in the trial would get to spit into a plastic cup, and that sounded like fun. Some of the boys were already practicing.

While the parents of Grand Rapids pondered this unusual request, David Scott, a postdoctoral student in the University of Rochester School of Medicine and Dentistry in Rochester, New York, was packing his bag in response to what he viewed as an equally unusual request. In the summer of 1944, as a part of the strategic planning for the start of the fluoridation trial in Grand Rapids, Trendley Dean and his colleagues had recruited four dental examiners to carry out the first examinations of Grand Rapids schoolchildren. Three of them came from within the NIH; the fourth was David Scott. The four arranged lodgings around town and set up shop in office space made available to them by the Grand Rapids School Department in their building on Bostwick Street. From there, Scott and his colleagues made the rounds of the local schools, one after the other, carrying out dental examinations and collecting saliva samples from almost 32,000 students in Grand Rapids (and in the control towns of Muskegon and Aurora) during the 1944–1945 school year.[39]

As it turned out, and as Dean had envisaged, the trial went on for 15 years, with dental examiners returning every year to look into the mouths of the 10,000 or so students chosen to be included in the study from the three cities. All in all, about 150,000 examinations were made. Pictures survive of these examinations.[40] They took place in the back of schoolrooms with simple tools and primitive lighting. The children sat in a straight-backed chair while the young white-smocked examiners leaned over and asked for them to "open wide." The next few students watched as they waited in line, the little girls in gingham dresses and saddle shoes, the young boys in Hawaiian shirts and crisply ironed pants. A dental assistant took notes at a desk just off to the side.

There were many changes in personnel over the years, but David Scott managed to return every year. In later years, Scott was asked how he survived the grind of examining student mouths day after day, week after week, month after month. In answer, he gives credit to the people of Grand Rapids, who welcomed the research team into their community with open arms. School principals and teachers cheerfully helped keep things running smoothly. City leaders and local newspapers gave their unqualified support. Scott was an amateur thespian and he found a second home with the Grand Rapids Civic Theater as an actor and stage manager. Years later he still remembered his role in the Grand Rapids fluoridation trial as one of the great experiences of his life. He speaks of the "thrill that came some six years into the program when ... [we saw the] ... huge increase in the numbers of young children entering school caries-free. Witnessing firsthand a success like that, with all its implications, is a privilege accorded to but a few people."[41]

One of the issues that Dean and his colleagues had investigated in the planning stages of the project was the question of engineering feasibility. On this front, they were encouraged by the confidence of H. W. Streeter, chief engineer of the Public Health Service in Cincinnati, Ohio, who assured them in October 1942 that no engineering difficulties need be anticipated in the process of controlled fluoridation. Once Grand Rapids was selected as the trial city, W. L. Harris, chief chemist of the city waterworks, who would be responsible for the maintenance of the desired fluoride content, expressed these same views. The fluoride concentrations in the incoming water from Lake Michigan ran about 0.05 ppm, and Harris calculated that 400 pounds of a suitable fluoride compound would have to be added to the water supply each day to bring it up to the optimal concentration of 1.0 ppm. For the additive, he recommended the use of sodium fluoride, which was commercially available in the form of a soluble granular powder. He and his engineers designed a system of basins, hoppers, filters, and tanks that would produce the desired concentration of 1.0 ppm fluoride in the water, and would offer strong protection against any overdosage.[42]

On the morning of Thursday, January 25, a three-month supply of sodium fluoride was in place at the Grand Rapids waterworks. That afternoon the first barrel of sodium fluoride went into the system hopper. A few minutes later, artificially fluoridated water began coursing through the pipes of the Grand Rapids' water distribution system. Harris notified the NIH team by cable with a single understated sentence: "Sodium fluoride application to the local water supply started 4:00 P.M., Thursday, January 25."[43]

The citizens of Grand Rapids learned about the fluoridation experiment in their city through articles in the *Grand Rapids Herald*, the *Detroit Free Press*, and local radio. The coverage was universally positive, from the first intimations that Grand Rapids was under consideration as a trial site, right through the early years of the trial. The public was informed that the project had the support of mayor Welsh, the local dental community, the University of Michigan, and all state and federal health agencies. They were given little cause for concern, and the matter never became a serious political issue.

Hints of future conflicts over fluoridation were there if you searched hard enough. One local doctor wrote several letters to the editor of the *Grand Rapids Herald* opposing the experimental program, but his letters didn't generate much debate. Perhaps even more prescient of future concerns over the health effects of fluoridation were the calls that began coming in to city offices from people complaining of sore gums and peeling tooth enamel. One woman even claimed that all her teeth had fallen out. These calls arrived in *early* January, when some press reports had stated that fluoridation would begin but some weeks *before* the actual advent of fluoridation on January 25.[44]

With fluoridated water now trickling regularly from the taps in Grand Rapids, the months went by and the world continued to turn on its axis. Franklin Delano Roosevelt had been reelected in November 1944, but he died suddenly from a cerebral hemorrhage on April 12, 1945, and Harry S Truman became President. Adolf Hitler committed suicide on April 30 in Berlin. On August 6 the *Enola Gay* dropped the atomic bomb on the Japanese city of Hiroshima and changed the way we think about war.

In 1948, President Truman approved the creation of the National Institute of Dental Research. The NIDR became the third independent institute in the National Institutes of Health. The strong public visibility of the Grand Rapids fluoridation trial is widely cited as the driver that led to the elevation of the federal dental research program to full Institute status. Trendley Dean was the first NIDR director, and both Francis Arnold and David Scott went on to become director in later years.

Mayor Welsh did not garner much political credit for his support of the fluoridation trial in Grand Rapids. Four years later, a grassroots organization known as Citizen's Action, with a charismatic leader named Dorothy Judd, called for the removal from office of mayor Welsh and several of the city commissioners. Supporters of Citizen's Action hung brooms on their homes to indicate their desire to clean up city government.[45]

Fifty years later, on September 15, 1995, a Fluoridation Commemorative Monument was unveiled in the courtyard of the Van Andel Public

Museum in Grand Rapids to celebrate the fiftieth anniversary of fluoridation. It is a stylish set of engraved stone tablets arranged in a semicircle, with text that pays homage to the pioneering researchers and to the schoolchildren of Grand Rapids. In the lead article from a scientific symposium that accompanied the celebrations, fluoridation is described as "the single most important clinical event in the history of dentistry, an event of such profound impact that the pandemic of dental decay has ended." No longer do senior citizens "expect to lose all their teeth." No longer do youngsters have to "experience the excruciating pain of a toothache." The author concludes that thanks to fluoride, "we in dentistry are now in control of our clinical destiny."[46]

The strategic plan of NIDR (now called the National Institute of Dental and Craniofacial Research) also venerates Grand Rapids: "We dedicate this plan to the men and women scientists who had the vision to conduct the first trial of a unique public health measure of water fluoridation in Grand Rapids, Michigan, in 1945, and to the mothers, fathers and schoolchildren who made that vision a reality. They and the generations of research scientists and clinical volunteers who follow them continue to demonstrate the intellectual curiosity, the courage and commitment to the principles of science that have enabled oral health research to achieve unprecedented progress in the last half of the 20th century. Following in their footsteps, we face the dawn of a new millennium with the prospect of even more dramatic advances in the conquest of disease and the preservation of long and healthier lives for all Americans."

These ringing resolutions take us back to the heady euphoria of 1945, when the war to end all wars was ended, when science was king, and when citizens still gave their full trust to government and all its agencies. For better or for worse, times have changed. When the medical and political establishment gathered around the new Fluoridation Monument at the Grand Rapids public museum in September 15, 1995, to celebrate the fiftieth anniversary of fluoridation, a small band of anti-fluoridation activists stood on the other side of the street with their signs, their slogans, and their anger. They were members of the National Health Federation, the New York State Coalition Opposed to Fluoridation, and the Grand Rapids Citizens Opposed to Fluoridation. They were committed enough to their cause to give up a day at the ballpark to spoil the party. Their flyers accused the dental agencies of covering up the true results of the early fluoridation trials of 1945. They gave interviews claiming that the trials were flawed. They warned against the adverse side effects of artificial water fluoridation and decried the loss of freedom of choice. And to the chagrin of the organizers of the celebration, their protests garnered equal time on the six o'clock news. The TV lead-in featured

protesters plodding up and down the sidewalk carrying placards that proclaimed "Only You Know What's Best for Your Body."

FLUORIDE ON TRIAL

In late 1944 and early 1945, as we now know, Robert Oppenheimer and his
team of scientists at Los Alamos were putting the finishing touches on the
bomb that would end the war. On the other side of the country, teams of
scientists of a different stripe had thoughts only of fluoride. Dean and Arnold
were not the only team of dental researchers who were putting together plans
for a trial run with a fluoridated water supply. David B. Ast had taken time
off from his post with the dental bureau of the New York State Department
of Health to finish up a master's degree in public health at the University of
Michigan. His thesis, a version of which was published in the open literature in 1943,[47] outlined a plan for adding fluoride to public water supplies
to reduce decay. In 1944, back in New York, he began to put his plan into
action. He gained the consent of two cities on the upper Hudson River to participate in a trial. Newburgh would be the fluoridated city, and Kingston the
unfluoridated control. The Newburgh–Kingston trial started on May 2, 1945,
only a few months after the Grand Rapids–Muskegon trial began. At about
the same time, a Canadian team instigated a fluoridation trial in three small
cities in southern Ontario. Brantford was the fluoridated city, with Sarnia
acting as the nonfluoridated control and Stratford as a naturally fluoridated
comparison. A year or so later, a very detailed trial began at Evanston,
Illinois, with nearby Oak Park as the control, under the auspices of the
Zoller Memorial Dental Clinic of the University of Chicago.

In the years that followed there were fluoridation trials in many countries
of the world, most notably perhaps the Hastings trial in New Zealand, and
the Tiel–Culemborg trial in the Netherlands.[48] In fact, the American Dental
Association reports in *Fluoridation Facts* that by 1993 there had been 113
studies on the effectiveness of controlled fluoridation in 23 different
countries.[49] In Chapter 7 we look in more detail at the outcome of these
studies (by way of the many reviews of this body of work that have been prepared by various reasonably objective groups and agencies over the years).
In the present chapter we limit ourselves to the four pioneering studies in
Grand Rapids, Newburgh, Brantford, and Evanston. These were the trials
that had historical impact. It was the favorable results reported from these
trials that drove the fluoridation movement forward.

One should note the careful use of the word *trial*. In using this term for
these studies, we are following the historical lead of the proponents, who
avoided the word *experiment* as if it were blasphemous. It was their general

belief that the studies carried out by Dean and other workers in the 1930s and early 1940s, comparing the dental-caries experiences of communities that were naturally high and low in fluoride, had already provided the experimental proof of the efficacy of fluoride in the reduction of dental caries. They did not anticipate any chemical or biological differences in the impact of fluoride on teeth, regardless of whether the fluoride content was artificially enhanced or naturally occurring. They viewed the trials not as experiments but as "demonstration projects" that would provide politicians and bureaucrats with the necessary evidence to approve community fluoridation projects in due course. Even Dean and Ast, both of whom wanted to see their trials proceed for many years before addressing the policy issues, stuck to the accepted pro-fluoridation terminology. Their inclination to postpone widespread fluoridation of public water supplies was based on a desire to give medical scientists more time to investigate the broader health impacts. It was not based on any real concern that the trials would not prove successful.

In the first two or three years of the Grand Rapids trial, no significant improvement was noted in the dental health of Grand Rapids schoolchildren. This was not unexpected, as those children receiving fluoridated water since birth were not yet in the school system. What *was unexpected* was the flood of positive results that began to emerge from the several trials as early as 1949. The dental examinations carried out in the schools of Grand Rapids for that year showed a marked reduction in caries. Similar results were coming in from the other trials: a 32% reduction in caries from Newburgh, and a 40% reduction from Brantford. The research teams were ecstatic. David Scott recalls sitting around the old Pantlind Hotel in Grand Rapids with Trendley Dean, who had come to town on an inspection trip. They were discussing the improvements in the children's teeth that were just then coming to light. Dean, eyes bright, summed things up in his inimitable style. "Those children are just as neat and clean as little bird dogs," he said.[50]

During this period the Public Health Service and the American Dental Association both faced tremendous pressure from fluoridation proponents who wanted to see an early endorsement of the practice from these national groups. Proponents sensed that they needed such government and professional support before their proposed fluoridation programs would have any chance of gaining local political approval. They felt that the initial results coming from the trials were proof enough; they did not want to wait another 10 years. Pressure was especially intense from the Wisconsin Fluorine Study Committee, and especially its leaders, Frank Bull of the Wisconsin State Board of Health and John Frisch of the state dental society. They accused Dean of "fogging the issue," "stalling," and "playing safe." But Dean continued to use his influence within the PHS to have the agency maintain its publicly stated position that mass fluoridation could not be recommended until such time as all the results were in hand from the Grand Rapids trial. The ADA trotted along behind, using the PHS position as a shield.

Frisch was a particularly feisty gadfly, turning every scientific meeting he attended into an all-out battle over fluoridation. He spoke of "oiling up the old shotgun for fun in Atlantic City," and then was all but kicked out of the meeting. At another meeting he engaged in a heated exchange, finally threatening to take his opponent and "sock him in the nose."[51] Considering the all-out war that they were soon to face with the anti-fluoridationists, it is hard not to take guilty pleasure from the apparent farce of these heated internecine scraps within the fluoridation movement.

In June 1950, the pressure from Wisconsin finally paid off. After a meeting called by Bruce Forsyth, Assistant Surgeon General and chief dental officer of the Public Health Service, and attended by Dean, Arnold, and many state dental directors, including Bull, the PHS announced its support for community fluoridation. The decision was based on the encouraging results coming in from Grand Rapids and Newburgh. The Surgeon General, Leonard Scheele, went on record saying that communities wishing to fluoridate their water supplies should be "strongly encouraged" to do so. The American Dental Association, whose position had been so closely tied to that of the PHS, quickly added their name to the list of advocates. In New York State, the Department of Health, acting against David Ast's wishes, recommended that all communities that could fluoridate their water supplies under adequate control measures should do so now. Dean and Ast and the rest of the cautious trialmasters had essentially been hung out to dry.

That is not to say that they did not continue to administer the fluoridation trials with care and deliberation. They did, with summary articles coming out every two or three years to report the latest results. And year after year, in trial after trial, the results supported the clear-cut conclusion that children who drank fluoridated water in their formative years had significantly less dental decay than those who did not. Table 5.1 summarizes the reduction in dental caries that occurred over the life of the trials in the fluoridated cities in the four pioneering fluoridation trials.[52] The measure is the DMF/child (where the DMF score is the number of decayed, missing, and filled teeth in each child's mouth). Reductions in DMF on the order of 35 to 55% are indicated in the four cases.

One might note in Table 5.1 that the age groups of the children differ from study to study. This is because the results are posted for the oldest group of children that had experienced fluoridation for their full life, at the stage indicated for each trial. It is not an important point because by the end of the trials, results were similar for all age groups under study in each trial.

TABLE 5.1 Reduction in Dental Caries in Fluoridated Cities During Fluoridation Trials

City	Period	No. of Years	Age Group	DMF/Child Start	DMF/Child End	Percent Reduction
Grand Rapids, MI	1945–1959	15	12–14	9.58	4.26	55.5
Newburgh, NY	1945–1955	10	13	7.40	4.80	35.1
Brantford, ON, Canada	1945–1959	15	12–14	7.01[a]	3.23	53.9
Evanston, IL	1946–1960	14	14	11.66	5.95	48.9

[a]Back-calculated from the values reported in the two rightmost columns.

TABLE 5.2 Difference in Dental Caries between Fluoridated and Control Cities at the End of the Fluoridation Trials

Fluoridated City	Control City	Date	No. of Years	Age Group	DMF/Child Control City	DMF/Child Fluoridated City	Percent Difference
Grand Rapids, MI	*Muskegon, MI*	1951	6[a]	12–14	9.52	7.52	20.0
Newburgh, NY	*Kingston, NY*	1955	10	10–12	8.40	4.80	42.9
Brantford, ON, Canada	*Sarnia, ON, Canada*	1959	15	12–14	7.46	3.23	56.7
Evanston, IL	*Oak Park, IL*	1956	10[b]	14	—[b]	—[b]	57.0[b]

[a]Muskegon became fluoridated in 1951. Data in the four rightmost columns are for the period 1945–1951.
[b]No measurements in Oak Park after 1956. The value in the rightmost column is for the period 1946–1956. It comes from the sources listed in note 52. The authors were not able to locate the detailed DMF values for 1956.

An outcome similar to that found in Table 5.1 can be gleaned from Table 5.2, which summarizes the difference in dental caries experience between fluoridated cities and control cities. Differences greater than 42% are indicated for three of the four studies. The smaller difference indicated for the Grand Rapids–Muskegon trial is based on only six years of record rather than the 10 to 15 years of record in the other three cases. It is not possible to look at a longer record for the Grand Rapids trial, because in 1951,

TABLE 5.3   Percent Caries-free Children in Fluoridated and Control Cities at the End of the Fluoridation Trials

					Percent Caries-free	
Fluoridated City	Control City	Date	No. of Years	Age Group	Control City	Fluoridated City
Grand Rapids, MI	**Muskegon, MI**	1955	10[a]	12–14	2.0	9.9
Brantford, ON, Canada	**Sarnia, ON, Canada**	1962	18	16–18	0.4	11.8

[a]In the final three years of this 10-year period, the water supply was fluoridated in both cities.

the citizens of Muskegon, not wanting to be deprived of this new health benefit, fluoridated their water supply. From that date on, Muskegon was lost to the experiment as a control city, and the Grand Rapids trial continued as a single-city retrospective analysis without a control. Similarly, DMF measurements are not available for Oak Park, Illinois after 1956, and the reported difference of 57% between Evanston and Oak Park applies to the 10-year period 1946–1956 rather than the full 14-year period of the Evanston study.

Table 5.3 provides another comparison between fluoridated and non-fluoridated cities in two of the trials. This table presents data on the number of caries-free children at the end of the trial period. It documents the very large increase observed in the percentage of caries-free children in the fluoridated cities relative to the control cities.

We have noted some of the inconsistencies in the periods of study that are recorded for the various trials cited in Tables 5.1, 5.2, and 5.3. The premature end of the Muskegon and Oak Park data are noted above. In the Brantford–Sarnia study, DMF data are most complete through 1959, whereas caries-free data continue through 1962. Furthermore, for those who might choose to examine the source we have referenced, beware the many different age groups that are reported in the various publications. There are a lot of numbers out there. Where our figures differ from those you first find, it is probably because the age groups are not the same. In any case, these imperfections in the comparative record are of no import. The conclusions of these studies are so transparent that no amount of jockeying with the data could possibly point in any other direction.

In fact, the results of the four pioneering trials are so startlingly clear that is hard to imagine how anyone could possibly find fault. One would assume that by the end of the trials in 1960, every one would be on the same page. But of course they weren't. The attack dogs were ready to be unleashed.

BLIND EXAMINERS AND CONFOUNDING FACTORS

First off the mark was Philip R. N. Sutton, a senior research fellow in the Department of Oral Medicine and Surgery at the University of Melbourne, Australia. In 1957, Sutton was asked by Sir Arthur Amies, dean of the university's dental science faculty, to check out the data and methods in the papers from the North American fluoridation trials, which were by then flooding the dental literature. The result was an aggressive attack on the trials in a monograph entitled *Fluoridation: Errors and Omissions in Experimental Trials*, published by the University of Melbourne Press in 1959. Sutton claimed that the trials had major shortcomings, including data limitations, inconsistencies and errors in sampling, inadequate control populations, inappropriate weighting of results, and misleading presentations and discussion. The monograph provoked a passionate response from the United States, and several hostile reviews of the Sutton monograph were published in the Australian dental literature. Sutton then brought out a second edition of his book, which included the hostile reviews in full, together with his responses to their arguments.[53] Because of his standing as a reputable dental researcher and the credibility of his publisher, Sutton's critique had considerable impact. Forty years later, it is still the most widely quoted source on the shortcomings of the trials. Its arguments are dogma to the more reputable, quasiscientific wing of the anti-fluoridation movement. Sutton himself was largely ostracized by the dental community following publication of his monograph, but he never wavered in his views, holding an anti-fluoridation position until his death in 1995.[54]

Sutton accused the organizers of the trials of failing to check the composition of the waters in the comparison cities for factors other than fluoride, of ignoring differences in the standard of dental care between the cities, and of forgetting to take population migrations into account. Perhaps Sutton's most telling arguments revolved around the consistency and objectivity of the dental examiners. He pointed out that there is no standard definition of what constitutes a cavity. In the Brantford study, for example, the lowest limit for a carious lesion that would be counted was defined as one in which "the point of a No. 5 Clev-dent explorer would stick and resist direct withdrawal, or in which softness could be felt."[55] Other definitions are possible, and all of them are quite subjective. Over the years, in the various trials, hundreds of examiners took part, and Sutton questioned whether a sufficient level of standardization could be achieved.

More important, he drew attention to the fact that examiners knew which city their subjects represented, and he felt that this could easily introduce bias. In his opinion, it left the studies open to criticism that examiners might unconsciously see what they wanted to see. He argued that the studies should have been done using proper "blind" procedures, with the children from each city, both fluoridated and unfluoridated, brought to a central location where examiners would not know which child came from which city.

Those who supported the results of the trials pointed to the reduction in caries that was observed in the individual fluoridated cities irrespective of any comparisons with the control cities. But Sutton and his cohorts argued that these results could also be biased, representing nothing more than wish fulfillment on the part of the examiners. On the question of examiner consistency, at least one city had an answer. In Brantford, the same dentist, B. W. Linscott, carried out all the examinations over 12 annual dental surveys, a total of 56,347 examinations in all.[56]

It is perhaps not surprising that an aggressive attack on the validity of the original trials is part of the lexicon in the anti-fluoridationist camp. It comes as more of a surprise to find that the current dental research community also finds much to fault with the original trial methodologies. B. A. Burt and S. A. Eklund, in their widely used textbook *Dentistry, Dental Practice, and the Community*, state that by present-day standards, the original trials were "crude and unrefined." A recent review of the benefits and risks of water fluoridation commissioned by the Ontario Ministry of Health in Canada concluded that research connected with the original trials is only "of historical interest; it is no longer relevant to an assessment of the current benefits of water fluoridation." In Britain, a systematic review of public water fluoridation carried out for the National Health Service judged the overall quality of evidence in the original trials as "poor."[57]

However, the issues raised in these forums are not questions of motivation or bias on the part of examiners. Rather, they deal with the lack of appropriate controls for *confounding factors*, and the crudeness of the statistical methodologies. Confounding factors are the many other possible environmental conditions, other than fluoride, that might conceivably have been responsible for the reductions observed in dental caries, among them, changes in the socioeconomic status of the children's families, changes in demography in the comparison cities, and improved diet or improved dental hygiene on the part of the subjects. There is no evidence in most of the studies that any record of these details was ever kept. (The counterexample is the Evanston study,[58] which presented findings by age group, by race, by type of infant feeding, by public school versus parochial school upbringing, and with respect to several other dental health indicators. Even with all these factors attended to, the primary influence on dental caries reduction over the trial period remained the presence of fluoride in the water supply.)

One possible confounding factor that *did not escape* the attention of the study teams at the time of the trials was the growing popularity of topical applications of fluoride in the form of fluoride rinses and mouthwashes, often administered by dentists in their offices. Given the euphoria of the times with respect to the power of fluoride, it is not surprising that some parents in the unfluoridated control cities felt that their children were getting the short end of the stick and demanded the best that the dental profession had to offer their children. In Muskegon, Dean and his colleagues considered the possibility of trying to convince local dentists to hold back on the procedure until the trials were complete, but eventually, they decided that such an approach would be an unacceptable withholding of a beneficial medical practice, and hence immoral. In any case, it seemed that the number of affected children was small, and no influence on the results was ever detected. Of course, after 1951, when Muskegon fluoridated its water supply, the question became mute. In the antifluoridation camp, the issue of topical fluoride as a confounding factor had little resonance, because bringing it up would imply that some types of fluoride did some good, and any such admission has always been anathema in the anti world.

On the statistical front, Sutton found fault with "percentage reduction" statistics such as those presented on Table 5.1. He pointed out that depending on the number of teeth in a child's mouth, fairly large percentage reductions may reflect a difference of only one or two affected teeth. Other critics draw attention to the lack of statistical rigor in the presentation of results for the original trials. All of the conclusions are based on statistical means of the measures observed, but no formal estimates of variance are associated with the means. No hypothesis tests are applied. No confidence intervals are calculated. It is not really possible for an informed reader to determine the statistical significance of the results reported.

Apparently, the statistical naivete of the fluoridation trials was sufficiently well known that discussion of it became a staple offering in a course on "statistical fraud" offered by Hubert Arnold on the Davis campus of the University of California. Arnold (presumably no relation to Francis Arnold, Trendley Dean's right-hand man) found the published papers "rich in fallacies, improper design, ... and just plain muddleheadedness and hebetude." He claimed that "many of the blunders were so glaring that I gave them to my beginning freshman classes in statistics at the very first meeting.

The students see through them straightway, and are afforded great amusement." All this would make a better tale were it not for the obvious anti-fluoridation bias that Arnold exhibits in the letter that is the source of these quotes.[59]

One of the other early critics of the fluoridation trials was the irascible Albert Schatz. Schatz is a brilliant agricultural microbiologist who at the age of 23 was credited with the discovery of the antibiotic streptomycin. The value of streptomycin in vanquishing tuberculosis led Schatz to receive hundreds of awards, medals, and honorary degrees from the scientific and medical establishment. However, much like Linus Pauling, in his later years Schatz became somewhat of a professional curmudgeon, happily ruffling the feathers of his former colleagues and benefactors, and espousing unpopular causes. One of these causes was the anti-fluoridation movement, and Schatz has been an active participant over many decades. His method of attack tends to be tongue-in-cheek, and in one memorable contribution[60] he made his point with some statistics of his own. Writing about one of the British trial summaries, he had this to say: "The official report repeats in one way or another no less than 89 times that fluoride protects against caries. This is an average of 10.7 times per page, and 1.8 times per paragraph. It uses the word 'benefit' as a verb, noun, and adjective 30 times. ... The preface of the report has seven paragraphs and tells us 13 times that fluoridation protects against caries. ... [It] extols the alleged benefits of fluoridation an average of once every four of its 52 lines." Point taken.

So where does all this leave us? Is the edifice of fluoridation built on a house of cards? Should we view the results of the original trials as invalid under the weight of charges of methodological malfeasance? Well, apparently not. After raising all these flags and throwing a jolt of doubt into every fluoridation proponent who is still willing to harbor them, the authors of the Ontario Ministry of Health study have this to say: "Because the historical trials were conducted when the prevalence of childhood caries was high, it is likely that the magnitude of the effect of fluoride on dental decay was large relative to the bias introduced into the studies by methodological flaws." Burt and Eklund are even more straightforward: "Despite the flaws, it is difficult for an objective observer to reject the conclusion that fluoridation was effective."[61]

The fact is that the original fluoridation trials have been under review for almost 40 years, and although many methodological shortcomings have been identified, the fundamental conclusions remained robust. There should be no doubt in any reasonable person's mind that enhancing the fluoride content of the water supplies in the trial cities to a concentration of approximately 1 ppm led to a reduction in the number of cavities suffered by the children in those communities. It is undoubtedly true that were fluoridation being proposed now, it would undergo more rigorous scrutiny as a potential health hazard than it received in the 1950s when government agencies first gave the practice a green light, but that is another question, and we save its consideration for another chapter.

THE MAVERICKS EMERGE

As the postwar boom took hold in the United States in the early 1950s, fluoridation proponents had every reason to believe that success was theirs. The triumph of the fluoridation trials in Grand Rapids, Newburgh, and Evanston had been widely publicized in the popular press. The Public Health Service and most other state and federal health and dental agencies were on board. This band of visionaries could see the road ahead clearly: Fluoridate the country's water supplies, let our children enjoy the benefits of better dental health, and stand ready to exploit the next great medical breakthrough, whatever it might be and whenever it might make itself known. Unfortunately, they couldn't see into the hearts and minds of those members of society who don't jump on bandwagons. And even if they could, they would never have dreamed that this ragtag band of doubters would be able to rally enough popular support to put fluoridation into that select group of issues that never get solved. They certainly didn't envisage 60 years (and counting) of manning the trenches against what they perceived as an illiterate, antiscientific, paranoid opposition.

As early as 1950 the battle was joined. In the small town of Stevens Point, Wisconsin, right in the heartland of the fiercest fluoridation proponents, a few gadflies began to question the wisdom of tampering with the town's water supply. They argued that such decisions should go to the people rather than being decided by city councils, health agencies, or waterworks departments, as was being done in other towns and cities around the country. The town council acceded to this demand and placed the fluoridation question on the ballot. During the campaign there was much talk of rat poison and communist plots, but even sophisticated voters who were not likely to be swayed by these crude arguments were disturbed by the idea that the government was pushing fluoridation down their throats before all the results were in. The people of Stevens Point did not want to be guinea pigs. They defeated the fluoridation measure, thus becoming the first of many cities that would reject fluoridation by referendum in the ensuing years.

Given the scientific backgrounds of most of the early fluoridation proponents, it is likely that they were caught by surprise by the politicization of their pet issue. They were used to logical discourse and rational debate. They were not prepared for the hurly-burly, emotional street fights that arose in the cities and towns of the nation. But no matter what they may have thought about those developments, there is no doubt that they were caught even further offguard by yet another development. It turned out that some of their own weren't toeing the line. A group of maverick scientists emerged around the country who began to report the results of laboratory experiments that seemed to implicate fluoride in a variety of health concerns. Most of these researchers were of dubious reputation, and investigation of their claims usually led more reputable researchers to discount their findings. However, because these investigators tended to report directly to the public rather than through the time-consuming and threatening process of peer review in scientific journals, the seeds of doubt that they sowed were often difficult to eradicate from the public's mind.

The first such case involved a University of Texas biochemist named Alfred Taylor, who claimed that cancer-prone laboratory mice that drank water containing 1 ppm fluoride exhibited accelerated development of their cancerous tumors. A team of reviewers from the National Cancer Institute visited Taylor's laboratory and found many fatal flaws in his procedures.[62] Despite the refutation of his results, Taylor continued to press them on all who would listen. He became a regular on the anti-fluoridation circuit, the first of many ostracized scientists who would play this role.

In 1952, fluoridation made it to Congress. New York Congressman James J. Delaney included consideration of the fluoridation question in his hearings on chemicals in food and cosmetics.[63] The committee confined testimony to that of "expert" witnesses. The list included Trendley Dean and several of his NIH colleagues, but it also included Alfred Taylor and other maverick scientists whose work had been denigrated by the medical establishment. More harmful yet to the fluoridation cause was the testimony of Margaret Cammack Smith, the very reputable Arizona scientist whose research back in 1931 had provided the clinching argument that implicated fluoride as the cause of Colorado stain. In the intervening years, she had come down on the side of the anti-fluoridationists, largely because of her concern that adding fluoride to water supplies would create an unacceptable increase in the prevalence of mottled teeth. Two years later she would reverse her stand and endorse the value of fluoride, but her reversal garnered far less attention than her earlier congressional testimony. At the 1952 hearings, several of the congressmen on the committee were quite receptive to the anti-fluoridation arguments and they grilled Dean and his team in an adversarial courtroom style that the scientists were not expecting. Although nothing much came of the Delaney hearings, anti-fluoridationists had found a pulpit from which they could preach their gospel to much public attention. It was a strategy that they would use to their advantage many times in future years.

By 1955, George Waldbott, the Detroit allergist, had instituted his bimonthly anti-fluoridation newsletter *The National Fluoridation News*. In 1952, Seattle rejected fluoridation in a hotly contested referendum, the largest city yet to turn its back on fluoride. So, what just a few years earlier had looked like a slam-dunk had become a down-to-the-wire finish in city after city. Some of the early proponents simply shook their heads in dismay and went back to their laboratories. Others continued to fight the good fight.

They tried to keep the controversy on rational ground. Fluoridation reduces tooth decay, they argued, and it doesn't cause cancer. Case closed. When the opposition talked communist plots or government cover-ups, they simply refused to play. Heaven knows what they would have thought about the truly paranoid ideas that were beginning to take hold of the extreme wings of the anti-fluoridation movement; or that such ideas would continue to have appeal into the new millenium. Read on, dear reader, and enter the strange but alluring world of fluoridation conspiracy theory.

REFERENCES

1. *The World Almanac*, World Almanac Books, New York, 1999.
2. R. C. Williams, *The United States Public Health Service, 1798–1950*, U.S. PHS, Washington, DC, 1951.
3. The story of John Eager in Naples is based on accounts from R. R. Harris, *Dental Science in a New Age: A History of the National Institute of Dental Research*, Montrose Press, Rockville, MD, 1989; and F. J. McClure, *Water Fluoridation: The Search and the Victory*, National Institute of Dental Research, Bethesda, MD, 1970.
4. J. M. Eager, Denti di Chiaie (Chiaie teeth), *Publ. Health Rep.*, 16, 2, 1901. Abstract reprinted in *Dent. Cosmos*, 44, 300–301, 1902.
5. McClure, 1970, op. cit.
6. G. L. Waldbott, A. W. Burgstahler, and H. L. McKinney, *Fluoridation: The Great Dilemma*, Coronado Press, Lawrence, KS, 1978.
7. The story of Frederick McKay's long campaign to solve the mystery of mottled teeth is based on accounts from Harris, 1989, op. cit.; McClure, 1970, op. cit.; D. R. McNeil, *The Fight for Fluoridation*, Oxford University Press, New York, 1957; and J. J. Murray, A. J. Rugg-Gunn, and G. N. Jenkins, *Fluorides in Caries Prevention*, 3rd ed., Butterworth-Heinemann Publishers, Boston, MA, 1991.
8. F. S. McKay, Investigation of mottled enamel and brown stain, *J. Natl. Dent. Assoc.*, 4, 273–278, 1917; F. S. McKay, Mottled enamel: a fundamental problem in

dentistry, *Dent. Cosmos*, 67, 847–860, 1925; F. S. McKay, Do water supplies cause defects in teeth enamel? *Water Works Eng.*, 79, 1321–1335, 1926.

9. F. S. McKay (in collaboration with G. V. Black), An investigation of mottled teeth, *Dent. Cosmos*, 58, (I) 477–484, (II) 627–644, (III) 781–792, (IV) 894–904, 1916; G. V. Black (in collaboration with F. S. McKay), Mottled teeth, *Dent. Cosmos*, 58, 129–156, 1916.

10. McNeil, 1957, op. cit.

11. Ibid.

12. F. S. McKay, Progress of the year in the investigation of mottled enamel with special reference to its association with artesian water, *J. Natl. Dent. Assoc.*, 5, 721–750, 1918.

13. McClure, 1970, op. cit.

14. F. S. McKay, Mottled enamel: the prevention of its further production through a change of water supply at Oakley, Idaho, *J. Am. Dent. Assoc.*, 20, 1137–1149, 1933.

15. G. A. Kempf and F. S. McKay, Mottled enamel in a segregated population, *Publ. Health Rep.*, 45, 2923–2940, 1930.

16. H. V. Churchill, Occurrence of fluorides in some waters of the United States, *J. Ind. Eng. Chem.*, 23, 996–998, 1931. See also *J. Am. Water Works Assoc.*, 23, 1399–1407, 1931.

17. M. C. Smith, E. M. Lantz, and H. V. Smith, The cause of mottled enamel, a defect of human teeth, *Univ. Ariz. Coll. Agric. Tech. Bull.*, 32, 253–282, 1931.

18. McKay, 1916, (I), op. cit.

19. McKay, 1925, op. cit.

20. F. S. McKay, The relation of mottled enamel to caries, *J. Am. Dent. Assoc.*, 15, 1435, 1928.

21. Information on H. Trendley Dean's career comes from Harris, 1989, op. cit.; Williams, 1951, op. cit.; and from Dean's obituary in the U.S. Public Health Service, Centers for Disease Control and Prevention, *MMWR*, 48(41), 935, 1999.

22. H. T. Dean, Classification of mottled enamel diagnosis, *J. Am. Dent. Assoc.*, 21, 1421–1426, 1934.

23. H. T. Dean and F. S. McKay, Production of mottled enamel halted by a change in common water supply, *Am. J. Publ. Health*, 29, 590–596, 1939.

24. H. T. Dean, Chronic endemic dental fluorosis, *J. Am. Med. Assoc.*, 107, 1269–1272, 1936; H. T. Dean, Some epidemiological aspects of chronic endemic dental fluorosis, *Am. J. Publ. Health*, 26, 567–575, 1936.

25. Harris, 1989, op. cit.

26. R. W. Bunting, M. Crowley, D. G. Hard, and M. Keller, Further studies of the relation of bacillus acidophilus to dental caries, *Dent. Cosmos*, 70, 1002, 1928; N. J. Ainsworth, Mottled teeth, *Br. Dent. J.*, 60, 233–250, 1933; W. D. Armstrong and P. J. Brekhus, Possible relationship between the fluoride content of enamel and resistance to dental caries, *J. Dent. Res.*, 16, 394, 1937; H. Klein and C. E. Palmer, Dental

caries in American Indian children, *Publ. Health Bull.*, 239, 37, 1937. For additional references, see McNeil, 1957, op. cit., Harrisand, 1989, op. cit.

27. H. T. Dean, Endemic fluorosis and its relation to dental caries, *Publ. Health Rep.*, 53, 1443–1452, 1938; H. T. Dean, Domestic water and dental caries, *J. Am. Water Works Assoc.*, 35, 1161–1186, 1943; H. T. Dean, Fluorine in the control of dental caries, *J. Am. Dent. Assoc.*, 52, 1, 1956.

28. This figure, based on Dean, 1956, op. cit., P. Adleris taken from, Fluorides and dental health, in *Fluorides and Human Health*, World Health Organization, Geneva, Switzerland, 1970.

29. J. D. Ratcliff, The town without a toothache, *Colliers*, December 19, 1942; reprinted in *Reader's Digest*, February 1943.

30. G. J. Cox, New knowledge of fluorine in relation to dental caries, *J. Am Water Works Assoc.*, 31, 1926–1930, 1939.

31. Editorial: Effect of fluorine on dental caries, *J. Am. Dent. Assoc.*, 31, 1360–1363, 1944; Clarification, *J. Am. Dent. Assoc.*, 31, 1660–1661, 1944.

32. McNeil, 1957, op. cit.

33. N. C. Leone, M. B. Shimkin, F. A. Arnold, Jr., C. A. Stevenson, E. R. Zimmerman, P. B. Geiser, and J. E. Lieberman, Medical aspects of excessive fluoride in a water supply: a ten-year study, *Publ. Health Rep.*, 69, 925–936, 1954; also in *Fluoridation as a Public Health Measure*, edited by J. H. Shaw, American Association for the Advancement of Science, Washington, DC, 1954, pp. 110–127.

34. H. C. Hodge, The concentration of fluorides in drinking water to give the point of minimum caries with maximum safety, *J. Am. Dent. Assoc.*, 40, 436–439, 1950.

35. McClure, 1970, op. cit.

36. McClure, 1970, op. cit.

37. F. A. Arnold, Jr., Role of fluorides in preventive dentistry, *J. Am. Dent. Assoc.*, 30, 499–508, 1943.

38. These vignettes of Grand Rapids during the war years are drawn from R. Harms, *Grand Rapids Goes to War: The 1940s Homefront*, Grand Rapids Historical Society, Grand Rapids, MI, 1993, and from a collection of annotated photographs that appear under the title A Grand Century: One Hundred Years of Photographs from 20th Century Grand Rapids, at http://www.grpl.org/coll/grandintro.html.

39. D. B. Scott, Evolution of the Grand Rapids water fluoridation project, *J. Publ. Health Dent.*, 49(1), 59–61, 1989; D. B. Scott, The dawn of a new era, *J. Publ. Health Dent.*, 56(5), 235–241, 1996; Harris, 1989, op. cit.

40. Harris, 1989, op. cit.

41. Scott, 1989, op. cit.

42. Harris, 1989, op. cit.

43. McClure, 1970, op. cit.

44. *Grand Rapids Herald*, February 3, 1945, as reported in Scott, 1996, op. cit.

45. *A Grand Century*, op. cit.

46. W. Loesche, The 50th anniversary of water fluoridation in Grand Rapids, Michigan, *J. Publ. Health Dent.*, 56(5), 233–234, 1996.

47. D. B. Ast, A program of treatment of public water supply to correct fluoride deficiency, *J. Am. Water Works Assoc.*, 35, 1191, 1943.

48. T. G. Ludwig, The Hastings fluoridation project, *N. Z. Dent. J.*, 67, 155–160, 1971; G. W. Kwant, B. Houwink, O. Backer-Dirks, A. Groeneveld, and T. J. Pot, Artificial fluoridation of drinking water in the Netherlands: results of the Tiel–Culemborg experiment after 16–1/2 years, *Neth. Dent. J.*, 80, Suppl., 9, 6–27, 1973.

49. American Dental Association, Fluoridation Facts, http://www.ada.org.

50. Scott, 1996, op. cit.

51. The anecdotes and quotes in this paragraph come from McNeil, 1957, op. cit.

52. The data in Tables 5.1, 5.2 and 5.3 are taken from articles that present the final results of the original trials, as listed below, and from B. A. Burt and S. A. Eklund, *Dentistry, Dental Practice, and the Community*, W.B. Saunders, Philadelphia, 1999; Adler, 1970, op. cit.; and J. J. Murray, A. J. Rugg-Gunn, and G. N. Jenkins, *Fluorides in Caries Prevention*, 3rd ed., Butterworth-Heinemann Publishers, Boston, MA, 1991.

Grand Rapids: F. A. Arnold, Jr., H. T. Dean, P. Jay, and J. W. Knutson, Effect of fluoridated public water supplies on dental caries prevalence: tenth year of the Grand Rapids–Muskegon study, *Publ. Health Rep.*, 71, 652–658, 1956; F. A. Arnold, Jr., R. C. Likens, A. L. Russell, and D. B. Scott, Fifteenth year of the Grand Rapids fluoridation study, *J. Am. Dent. Assoc.*, 65, 780–785, 1962.

Newburgh: D. B. Ast, D. J. Smith, B. Wacks, and K. T. Cantwell, Newburgh–Kingston caries fluorine study: XIV. Combined clinical and roentgenographic dental findings after ten years of fluoride experience, *J. Am. Dent. Assoc.*, 52, 314–325, 1956; D. B. Ast and B. Fitzgerald, Effectiveness of water fluoridation, *J. Am. Dent. Assoc.*, 65, 581–587, 1962; J. V. Kumar, E. L. Green, W. Wallace, and T. Carnahan, Trends in dental fluorosis and dental caries prevalences in Newburgh and Kingston, NY, *Am. J. Publ. Health*, 79(5), 565–569, 1989.

Brantford: W. L. Hutton, B. W. Linscott, and D. B. Williams, Final report of local studies on water fluoridation in Brantford, Canada, *Can. J. Publ. Health*, 47, 89, 1956; H. K. Brown and M. Poplove, Brantford–Sarnia–Stratford, fluoridation caries study: final survey, 1963, *J. Can. Dent. Assoc.*, 31, 505–511, 1965.

Evanston: J. R. Blaney and I. N. Hill, Fluorine and dental caries, *J. Am. Dent. Assoc.*, 74, 233, 1967.

53. P. R. N. Sutton, *Fluoridation: Errors and Omissions in Experimental Trials*, 2nd ed., Melbourne University Press, Melbourne, Australia, 1960.

54. Obituary and editorial on Philip R. N. Sutton, *Fluoride*, 28(3), 1995.

55. McClure, 1970, op. cit.

56. McClure, 1970, op. cit.

57. Burt and Eklund, 1999, op. cit.; D. Locker, *Benefits and Risks of Water Fluoridation*, Ontario Ministry of Health, Toronto, Ontario, Canada, 1999; M. McDonagh, P.

Whiting, M. Bradley, J. Cooper, A. Sutton, I. Chestnutt, K. Misso, P. Wilson, E. Treasure, and J. Kleijnen, A Systematic Review of Public Water Fluoridation, NHS Centre for Reviews and Dissemination, University of York (UK), 2000.

58. McClure, 1970, op. cit.; Blaney and Hill, 1967, op. cit.

59. Letter from Hubert A. Arnold to Ernest Newbrun, May 28, 1980, as posted at http://www.fluoridealert.org.

60. As quoted in A. L. Gotzsche, *The Fluoride Question: Panacea or Poison?* Stein and Day, New York, NY, 1975.

61. Burt and Eklund, 1999, op. cit.; Locker, 1999, op. cit.

62. Harris, 1989, op. cit.

63. Ibid.

CHAPTER 6

FLUOROPHOBIA

Those on the far side of the anti-fluoridation movement have never traveled down the same road to fluoridation as the rest of us. They do not accept the smooth ride offered in Chapter 5. They choose to cruise a bumpier set of roads, using a different route, a different map, perhaps an entirely different atlas.[1]

On the Stop Fluoridation website there is a year-by-year chronology of events put together by Philip Heggen under the title *How We Got Fluoridated*. It is 26 pages long, yet it contains not a word about Frederick McKay, John Eager, or any of the other early dental researchers. Trendley Dean is scarcely mentioned, certainly not as the "father of fluoridation." He appears only on the eighth page of the chronology, and then only to judge his shoe-leather surveys as "worthless." The famous trials receive only passing mention; they are seen as a fraud and a hoax. The entry for 1945 makes no mention of the first fluoridation in Grand Rapids; the items singled out for that year highlight two publications, one in which "fluoride was found to have marked adverse effects to the central nervous system," and one which claims that "22% to 84% of American children are afflicted with dental fluorosis."[2]

The Stop Fluoridation anti-history begins long before John Eager's encounter with *denti scritti* in Naples. It begins with an entry for the year 1855, which is the date when the smelting industry in Freiburg, Germany, first paid damages to their neighbors for the poisoning of livestock by emissions from their smelters (emissions, it is claimed, that contained fluoride gases). Eighty-six items later, there is an entry for the year 1999, which quotes a news release urging cities and municipalities to disconnect their water-fluoridation equipment during the Y2K (year 2000) rollover to prevent possible fluoride fatalities. The intervening entries highlight the dates of alleged fluoride poisoning events, the year of publication of influential anti-fluoridation articles and books, the dates of anti-fluoridationist exposure of secret agendas at industrial laboratories, and the periods of alleged collusion between government agencies and industrial corporations.

The advent of fluoridation is seen not as a path toward the light, but as a spider's web of conspiracy and deceit. Evil motives are ascribed to individuals, organizations, companies, and government agencies. Allegations are made against a cabal of conspirators that includes such disparate entities as the Mellon Institute, the University of Cincinnati, the Public Health Service, and even the Manhattan Project. However, these agencies are just the supporting cast. The lead role in this evil empire is saved unreservedly for the Aluminum Company of America. The thread of perceived Alcoa malfeasance runs through this alternative history like blood across a Civil War battlefield.

In the first five sections of this chapter we let the conspiranoians have their say. We summarize their arguments more or less as they are presented in the underground literature of the anti-fluoridation movement. We highlight the points of fact on which their arguments are based, and the sometimes-convoluted interpretations of these facts that lead them to their conspiratorial viewpoint. We do not present the counter-arguments to each strand of their tale as it is presented, because we believe that this approach would destroy the strange allure of their tangled web. After allowing readers to immerse themselves in this esoteric world, without commercial interruption so to speak, we bring us all back to Earth in the final section of the chapter. There we turn a critical eye on these tales, presenting the counter-arguments and providing the large dose of skepticism that many readers may have felt was missing earlier.

SATAN'S METAL

One event that plays a prominent role in the historical chronologies of *both* pro- and anti-fluoridation camps is the research carried out in 1931 in the Aluminum Company of America labs in Pittsburgh, Pennsylvania, that led to the identification of fluoride as the mysterious constituent of drinking water that is responsible for the development of mottled teeth. The role of Alcoa chemist H. V. Churchill is featured in both versions, but the motivation for his research is seen through different eyes. In the pro-fluoridation version, he is a dedicated scientist who solves this long-standing riddle through careful research and publishes his results to the betterment of humankind. In the anti-fluoridation version, he is a tool of his evil employers, who hijack his results for selfish, nefarious motives, thus starting us down the long road of collusion and cover-up that eventually leads to the fluoridation of public water supplies.

To see how this tale of conspiracy could find any resonance in the public mind, we have to take ourselves back to the scientifically less-sophisticated era of the early twentieth century and the strange campaign that arose in opposition to the new wonder metal, aluminum.

Aluminum is the most abundant metal in the Earth's crust. It is a common element in many rock-forming minerals, including the feldspars, which are the predominant minerals in granitic rocks. It is a commonly measured constituent in water, soil, and air. Unlike other metals, aluminum never occurs in nature in its pure metallic form as do gold and silver, nor even in minerals that have a metallic appearance, such as iron pyrite or the lead ore, galena. Although known to the ancients in the form of alumina (an oxide of the metal), the metal itself was not isolated until 1827, and it was not until 1866 that a commercial method of separation was devised.[3]

Aluminum ore occurs as bauxite, a weathering product of granite that takes the form of an easily mined, claylike, reddish, earthy material. Bauxite is a hydrated aluminum oxide which must first be dehydrated in a refinery to form alumina. The pure metal is then separated from the alumina at high temperature through an electrolytic process using a molten electrolyte of sodium and calcium fluoride salts. The original process used molten cryolite (a naturally occurring fluoride mineral mined in Greenland) as the electrolyte, but this approach soon gave way to the less expensive alternative of using electrolytes made up of synthetically produced fluoride salts. The smelting of aluminum thus provided impetus for growth in the production of fluorine-based chemicals, and also created a manufacturing process that produced large amounts of fluoride-rich wastes. The nexus of aluminum and fluoride that runs through this conspiratorial version of history rests on these connections. A fluorophobic movement is very likely to be aluminophobic as well.

On the face of it, aversion to aluminum seems foolish: at best, quixotic. Pure aluminum is a silvery white metal with a wonderful set of properties, quite different from all other metals. It is light, malleable, ductile, corrosion-resistant, nonmagnetic, and an excellent conductor of heat and electricity. It is easily machined and cast, and becomes hard and strong when alloyed with minor amounts of copper, magnesium, manganese, or zinc. These favorable properties have led to its widespread use in the manufacture of automobiles, aircraft, munitions, high-tension cable, and thousands of other applications that enrich our daily life. By the early twentieth century, aluminum was already big business.

In 1922, the aluminum industry decided to test a new market. It was in that year that Alcoa introduced a line of aluminum cooking ware. New advertising campaigns appeared in popular magazines with housewives as the target audience rather than industrial buyers. The new aluminum kitchen utensils were feted for their lightness, their ease of use, and their soft silvery appearance. Consumers were impressed, and aluminum cookware became the norm in many well-off suburban homes. Who would have imagined that this new marketing strategy would set off storms of protest over the purported dangers of cooking food in pots made from "Satan's metal?"[4]

The leaders of this peculiar crusade were two men who dedicated their lives to an obsessive quest for public acceptance of their anti-aluminum viewpoint. Despite questionable credentials and a long gestation period of bitter rejection, they were eventually successful in finding outlets for their views and became a significant thorn in the side of the budding aluminum industry. As an echo to Darlene Sherrell's story from Chapter 4, both men first developed their antipathy to aluminum as a result of a self-diagnosis of their own health problems. In later life, both men found a second home in the anti-fluoridation movement.

Leo Spira was an Austrian doctor, a graduate of the University of Vienna Medical School, who moved to London in 1922 and then to New York in 1951. During his early years in London he became sickly, developing a set of symptoms that included constipation, numbness in the fingers, boils, rashes, peeling skin between the toes, thinning hair, brittle nails, and blisters in the mouth. He noticed similar symptoms in many of his patients. After carrying out unspecified investigations, he concluded that his troubles, and those of his patients, resulted from the "poisons" that were released upon heating the recently introduced lines of aluminum cookware.

The medical establishment did not accept his findings. His submissions to medical journals were rejected and his requests to speak at medical conferences turned down. He developed strong feelings of persecution by the establishment. He joined the British Army and during World War II carried out unofficial studies of his fellow soldiers, adding to his database of aluminum poisoning. After the war, and after many rejections, he was accepted as a doctoral student in physiology at the Middlesex Hospital Medical School of the University of London. With fluorides now in the news, he turned his attention in that direction, suggesting that the poisons released by aluminum cooking ware might be generated by the fluorides that are used in the production of aluminum. At Middlesex he carried out a set of experiments that documented the demise of rats under high doses of fluoride. He was awarded a Ph.D. for this work in 1950.[5]

With his new degree in hand, Spira came to the United States. He now suspected a link between aluminum, fluoride, and cancer. He proposed to supervise a set of controlled experiments on inoperable cancer patients in which he would attempt to cure them by placing the patients on a fluoride-free diet while eliminating the use of aluminum cookware in the preparation of their food. His proposal was rejected by all the granting agencies he approached, including the Rockefeller Foundation, the Public Health Service, and the American Cancer Society. He had come to the United States seeking a more open research climate, but found himself once again thwarted by the medical establishment. His feelings of persecution were fanned, and his anti-establishment proclivities sharpened. Like many before him, when rejected by the ruling class, he turned elsewhere for approval. He found a home in the anti-fluoridation movement, which was by then just heating up. He was finally able to get his anti-aluminum and anti-fluoride writings disseminated through their underground network. Rather than being mocked, he was now feted for his double-doctoral credentials and pushed forward as an expert. He enthusiastically jumped into the fray. In 1953, he published a book that was part autobiographical potboiler and part polemic against fluoride. He called it *The Drama of Fluorine: Arch Enemy of Mankind*.

One of the people that Spira contacted on his arrival in the United States was Charles T. Betts, the North American guru of the anti-aluminum movement. Betts was a Toledo dentist who had been turning out pamphlets and books attacking aluminum cookware since the 1920s. He was the author of a 1928 book entitled *Aluminum Poisoning*.[6] In time, Betts placed himself in opposition not only to aluminum, but also to vaccination, immunization, pasteurization, and fluoridation. More obscurely, he also opposed the use of aspirin, holding that most of the problems that lead people to take aspirin are caused by aluminum poisoning. His dental beliefs were also offbeat. He recommended that children under 15 years of age should not brush their teeth. He argued that brushing causes many diseases of the mouth. This viewpoint was based in part on the observation that cats and dogs do not brush their teeth, yet they suffer little from such diseases.[7]

Betts claimed that in 1913, at the age of 34, he was told by three doctors that he only had months to live. Shortly thereafter, while visiting a mineral spring in the hopes that it would improve his health, he had a life-altering experience. He noticed that when he poured springwater into an aluminum cup, it effervesced, whereas in a glass cup it did not. He associated the effervescence with the aluminum, and the aluminum with his illness. He went home, discontinued his use of aluminum cookware, and was cured.

If Betts's writings on aluminum had been limited to self-published pamphlets, it is unlikely that they would have had much impact on the public at large. However in 1928, Betts found a willing outlet for his work. His anti-establishment viewpoint found communion with the tenets of the Watchtower Society of the Jehovah's Witness religion. In 1928, despite the fact that Betts was a lifelong Presbyterian, the Watchtower magazine *The Golden Age* accepted one of his articles for publication.[8] It was the beginning of a half-century crusade by the Watchtower Society against aluminum cooking utensils. Unbelievably, *The Golden Age* published over 130 articles railing against aluminum cookware between 1925 and 1969, many by Betts, but many more in the form of news items by the magazine's long-time editor, Clayton J. Woodworth. Among the titles of the articles are "Death in the Aluminum Bucket," "Coffee Poisoning by Aluminum," and "Disease and an Early Grave Via the Modern Kitchen."[9] Almost all of the articles are case histories of food poisoning of one kind or another, some of them fatal, all ostensibly due to the use of aluminum cooking pots. Many are first-person stories of readers who cured themselves from a variety of ailments through the elimination of aluminum cookware. In one issue, the editor asks: "How many fathers and mothers will be made ill; how many babies slain before the government takes a hand in this thing and prevents this unnecessary slaughter?" In another issue, a cartoon shows a *Leave-It-to-Beaver* family sitting down to dinner: mother, father, and young teenage son. Floating ominously in the air above their heads are ghostly images of "the unseen guests at the aluminum dinner table": food poisoning, cancer, and death.[10]

Interestingly, Betts and Spira never made any claims with respect to geriatric senility, which is the one disease that modern medical researchers suspect may be affected by aluminum intake. Of course, all this happened in the distant past. Alzheimer's disease didn't even have a name yet. From our current perspective, it is hard to believe that their unsophisticated attacks could have had much impact. But they did. Anti-aluminum thinking was so prevalent, and ran so counter to the accepted scientific thinking of the day, that the respected journal *Scientific American* felt the need to publish a long article in their March 1929 issue defending the use of aluminum and trying to assuage the fears of the populace.[11] In the same year, the editors of *The Golden Age* fanned the flames further, clarifying the conspiracy that they saw at work. They concluded that the reason the government had not banned aluminum cookware was "because the principal officers and stockholders in the aluminum trusts are such an important part of the government itself and have such power to control its activities" that action is impossible.[12] Statements like this were widely quoted in the popular press.

This, then, was the climate of opinion when the news arrived at Alcoa headquarters in 1931 that the children of Bauxite, Arkansas, an Alcoa company town, were all suffering from mottled and pitted teeth. If one has a conspiratorial mind, one sees a situation that is ripe for deceit and cover-up. If one believes that the aluminum industry was purposely poisoning the population in the name of profit through its marketing of aluminum cookware, mottled teeth just look like further evidence of aluminum's sins. One is not likely to believe any explanation that might be extended by the guilty party. Although there is no published record that describes the reaction of the anti-aluminum lobby to the announcement by H. V. Churchill that the source of the problem lay in the fluoride content of the town water supply, one must assume that they were incredulous, suspecting a cover-up under pressure from the Alcoa hierarchy. To this group at this time, long before fluoride had any public visibility, the attempt to transfer the blame from the hated aluminum atom to some johnny-come-lately like fluoride must have seemed almost laughable.

The response of the anti-fluoridation lobby is a post facto one, because in 1931 there *was* no anti-fluoridation lobby, the entire issue still being some 10 years in the future. Retrospectively, however, in their conspiratorial history of fluoridation, they too suspect that Churchill's findings were made under duress from above in the self-interest of the aluminum industry. The current leaders of the anti-fluoridation movement have long since abandoned the cooking-ware issue in the light of public skepticism, but they have a different conspiratorial twist to put on the affair. It is a twist that first requires a short review of the aluminum industry's long-standing problems with air pollution.

ALCOAnoia

As already noted, the production of aluminum involves the electrolysis of dehydrated bauxite in a molten fluoride bath. One of the less desirable outcomes of this process is the venting of hydrogen fluoride gas to the atmosphere. Although sulfur dioxide is usually considered the most serious industrial air pollutant, fluoride emissions are serious in their own right. Excessive hydrogen fluoride emissions are known to cause agricultural damage to forage crops and fruit orchards. It is also accepted that such emissions can produce lameness in domestic animals, especially cattle. The well-documented releases of hydrogen fluoride gas from the Rocky Mountain Phosphate Company plant in Garrison, Montana, had a severe impact on livestock. It was the sad image of crippled cows crawling across pastures on their knees near Garrison that led Montana state legislators to toughen up their air pollution standards.[13]

During the early 1950s, aluminum companies experienced a spate of lawsuits claiming damages from farmers and ranchers who lived in the shadow of aluminum smelters. Four such cases in Washington and Oregon alone are documented by George Waldbott in his influential anti-fluoridation book.[14] Most of these cases claimed loss of cropland. Several involved crippled livestock. At least one of them involved a claim of human health impact. The potential growth in the number of such lawsuits posed a threat to the aluminum industry, and it is the view of those in the anti-fluoridation movement with a conspiratorial turn of mind that this fear of regulation and litigation led the industry, and Alcoa in particular, to take covert action.

In this light, at least according to Philip Heggen in his chronological time-line of *How We Got Fluoridated*, H. V. Churchill's exposure of fluoride as the causative agent of mottled teeth is suspect, but not for the reasons put forth by anti-aluminum gurus like Leo Spira and Charles Betts. In Heggen's eyes, it is the claim of *water-based fluoride* rather than *air-based fluoride* that is suspect. It is Heggen's hypothesis that mottled teeth were a common occurrence in the vicinity of aluminum smelters due to the hydrogen fluoride emissions that poured forth from their smokestacks. This was especially true in Pitts-burgh, Heggen claims, where Churchill worked, and where Alcoa smelters were sure to come under suspicion. In this scenario, the primary motivation behind Churchill's announcement was to get people to believe that water was the chief source of fluoride, not air pollution, and thus stem the tide of legal damage claims against the company.[15]

Once the public was convinced that the only source of fluoride in their lives came from the water they drink, the next step in Alcoa strat-egy becomes crystal clear to those with paranoid leanings. The next step was to convince the public that fluoride in the water supply was a good thing. It is a widely held belief in the anti-fluoridation camp that scientists, lawyers, and bureaucrats with Alcoa connections purposefully infiltrated the relevant government agencies and prodded them down the road to fluoridation. In 1948, for example, when the Public Health Service sampled hydrogen fluoride concentrations over 27 major cities as part of a nation-wide air pollution probe, 12 of the cities were found to have serious fluo-ride exceedances (Pittsburgh, Baltimore, Chicago, Cleveland, Milwaukee, St. Louis, Philadelphia, San Francisco, Buffalo, Denver, Oklahoma City, and Indianapolis). In the collaborationist scenario, the Public Health Service then embarked on a strategy to fluoridate the water supplies of these cities as soon as possible in order to camouflage their toxic air pollution problems. In this script, the premature announcement of support for fluori-dation by the PHS in 1950, after only five years of the proposed 15-year study at Grand Rapids, was not a result of public pressure, but rather a calculated ploy by the PHS and their Alcoa henchmen for quick and effi-cient pursuit of their hidden agenda of deception with respect to fluoride air pollution.

Collusion on this scale between Alcoa and the Public Health Service would not have been possible without people in high places, and the conspiracy theorists think they know who these people were. Pick any book from the anti-fluoridation bookshelf, read any one of a hundred articles, or bring up any anti-fluoride webpage at random; it will not be long before you encounter one of the four *bête noires* of the anti-fluoridation movement: Andrew Mellon, Gerald Cox, Oscar Ewing, or Edward Bernays.[16] So here follows, in somewhat abbreviated form, their tangled tale. Most readers will probably find the alleged kinship between these men a bit thin, but if you have a suspicious turn of mind, you may find it seductive.

The earliest villain in the alleged rogue's gallery is Andrew W. Mellon, one of the founders of Alcoa and a major stockholder in the company, who in 1925 became Secretary of the Treasury in the federal cabinet. At that time, the Public Health Service fell under Treasury jurisdiction, and it is one of the tenets of anti-fluoridation lore that Mellon influenced the direction of the emerging dental research program and pointed it down the road to fluoridation, to the greater benefit of the aluminum industry. It is also during this period that Andrew and Richard Mellon established the Mellon Institute, an applied science laboratory that was heavily funded by industry and purportedly catered to their needs.[17] Some of the most influential pro-fluoride research was carried out at the Mellon Institute.

Gerald J. Cox was a biochemist who worked at the Mellon Institute, where some of his research was allegedly funded by Alcoa. He was one of the first scientists to carry out experiments on rats that proved the efficacy of fluoride in reducing dental caries.[18] He became a strong supporter of the fluoridation movement, and prepared several pro-fluoridation research summaries for both state and federal government review boards. It was Cox who is generally given credit (or blame) for first proposing the systematic fluoridation of public water supplies.[19] Anti-fluoridationists find it significant that this first proposal came from Cox, who was "not a doctor, not a dentist, but an industry scientist working for a company threatened by fluoride damage claims."[20]

The Mellon Institute is not the only industrial laboratory that is censured in anti-fluoridation literature. The Kettering Laboratory, located at the University of Cincinnati, also raises their ire. This laboratory was established in 1930 to carry out contract research on chemical hazards that arise in industrial operations. Anti-fluoridationists charge that it is little more than a lobby group for industry. Considerable research was carried out in the early years at Kettering on the toxicology of fluoride, and most of it minimized the possibility of health impacts. It was the Kettering Laboratory that was responsible for the alleged sanitization of abstracts uncovered by Darlene Sherrell, as described in Chapter 4. The sanitized document, which Sherrell claims downplayed the toxicological dangers of fluoride, was widely distributed to health care professionals across the nation.

When it comes to alleged villainy, the anger trained on Mellon and Cox is strictly small change compared to the animosity that is directed at Oscar R. Ewing. Ewing was a lawyer who took the post of administrator of the Federal Security Agency (a forerunner of the Department of Health, Education, and Welfare) between 1947 and 1953. The Public Health Service fell under his jurisdiction. It was under Ewing's watch that the final steps toward public water fluoridation were taken. The 27-city air-pollution study was carried out in 1948, and the "premature" endorsement of community water fluoridation was made in 1950. If the two were connected, as fluoride foes claim, the connection was consummated under Ewing's leadership. In 1951, Ewing allocated $2 million to promote fluoride nationwide.

Anti-fluoridationists see skullduggery at every turn. They claim that Alcoa was a major client of Ewing's law firm and that prior to his acceptance of the position with the Federal Security Agency, Alcoa paid a large sum of money to Ewing's firm to buttress the loss of salary that Ewing would suffer by going into government service, and to buy his support for industry aims in the coming fluoridation battles.[21]

The final rider of the four horsemen of the anti-fluoridationist apocalypse was Edward L. Bernays. In the early years of the twentieth century, Bernays played a leading role in the development of the new discipline of public relations. His impact on advertising techniques, which he called "the engineering of consent," earned him a place on *Life* magazine's listing of the 100 most influential Americans of the twentieth century. He was widely quoted as an icon of the booming American consumer culture.[22]

Anti-fluoridationists claim that Bernays was Oscar Ewing's public relations strategist for the water fluoridation campaign that followed the PHS endorsement of the practice.[23] They note pointedly that one of Bernay's best-selling books was titled *Propaganda*. They see significance in the fact that Bernays was a nephew of Sigmund Freud. (In fact, he was a double nephew; his mother was Freud's sister, his father was Freud's wife's brother.) They accuse Bernays of applying his uncle's subversive theories to government propaganda in support of fluoridation. In their view, it was under the onslaught of this tax-supported propaganda machine that the image of fluoride changed from that of rat poison to that of gleaming smiles. Fluoride opponents were engraved on the public mind as crackpots and loonies. Newspapers influenced by industry advertisers became key dispensers of this propaganda. Whenever the anti-fluoridation camp is accused of one-sidedness and lack of balance in their literature, they point to Bernays, and say, "He started it!"

TOXIC COUP?

Camouflage of their air pollution sins is not the only scurrilous motivation ascribed to the aluminum industry by the anti-fluoridation camp. Large amounts of fluoride waste are generated from the electrolytic process used to produce aluminum, and anti-fluoridationists contend that the aluminum industry supported fluoridation to create a market for these waste streams. Indeed, there was a period between 1957 and 1968 when Alcoa sold sodium fluoride to cities for the fluoridation of their water supplies. Many anti-fluoridation books reproduce one or another of the Alcoa advertisements that appeared in the *Journal of the American Waterworks Association* during this period. In the one shown in Waldbott's book, a large hand holds a glass of clear water, with the invitation to "Fluoridate Your Water with Confidence" by using "High Purity Alcoa Sodium Fluoride." The accompanying text states that "Alcoa sodium fluoride is particularly suitable for the fluorida- tion of water supplies. If your community is fluoridating its water supply, or is considering doing so, let us show you how Alcoa sodium fluoride can do the job for you. Write to the Aluminum Company of America."[24]

The aluminum industry was not the only industry trying to recoup some of their production expenses by selling fluoride by-products from their waste stream. The phosphate fertilizer industry was also able to break into the new market. Phosphates for use in fertilizer production are separated from phosphate-rich rock by dissolving the rock in sulfuric acid. The phosphate-bearing mineral in the rock is apatite, which also contains calcium and fluorine. Steam and fluorine gas are produced by the process, but the fluorine is easily removed from smokestacks through the use of scrubbers. The gas is then mixed with water to produce fluosilicic acid, which is particu- larly well suited to the fluoridation of water supplies. In fact, it was the entry of this source of fluoride into the marketplace that priced Alcoa out of the fluoride market in 1968. Since then, most fluoride that is used for community water fluoridation has come as a by-product from the fertilizer industry.

Of all the issues that make the anti-fluoridation movement see red, it is this "toxic coup"—that is the sorest point of all.[25] To their mind, the thought that anybody could support what they perceive as the dumping of toxic industrial effluent into our drinking water passes all understanding. This is the issue that they push hardest in every fluoridation campaign. It is beyond their ken how a voter who learns where fluoride comes from could still support the fluoridation of community water supplies. Not only that, but they argue that these by-products of aluminum and fertilizer production are impure, nowhere near the pharmaceutical-quality fluoride used in drugs or the food-grade quality used in toothpaste. They warn (albeit without any convincing evidence) that these waste fluorides might well be laced with heavy metals such as arsenic, lead, and chromium, or other proven carcinogens.[26] They charge that if the fluoride doesn't get you, the impurities will.

In most cases, citizens who feel that they are being poisoned by industrial chemicals would turn to their government for investigation and recompense. Anti-fluoridationists, of course, cannot make this turn because they believe that their governments are in collusion with the guilty parties. As Joel Griffiths puts it in his article *Fluorine: Industry's Toxic Coup*, "whenever new scientific evidence threatens fluoride's protected pollutant status, the government appoints a commission, typically composed of veteran fluoride defenders and no opponents. These commissions dismiss the new evidence and reaffirm the status quo."[27] Philip Heggen has written that the Public Health Service and the Environmental Protection Agency have "become clearly identified with the motivations of industry" and that through their support for fluoridation, they have "abandoned their charge to promote human and environmental health."[28]

If at this point we pause to summarize the anti-fluoridationist case against industry (especially the aluminum industry, and more specifically, Alcoa), it would appear that their argument has three facets. It is their contention that industry supported the fluoridation movement (and indeed, took covert action to achieve their goals), first, to deflect blame for fluoride air pollution that they had caused; second, to provide a profitable market for waste fluorides from their production sites; and third, to avoid litigation and compensation for parties affected by their waste disposal practices.

Each of these charges comes with its own special lore. Anecdotal stories that support the charges are cycled and recycled through the incestuous maze of pamphlets, books, and websites until the messages become almost biblical in their clarity. The air pollution claim, for example, is based on a real-life tragedy that occurred in Donora, Pennsylvania, in 1948, but it rests almost totally on the interpretation of this event by an investigator named Philip Sadtler, obscure and unknown to most of us, but held up as a visionary hero by those who oppose fluoridation.

THE DONORA DEATH FOG

There was no Halloween on October 31, 1948, in Donora, Pennsylvania. For the four days and nights before Halloween, the town of Donora and the neighboring community of Webster suffered the worst recorded industrial air pollution incident in United States history. The town of Donora sits on the inside of a sharp horseshoe bend in the Monongahela River in a narrow valley 30 miles south of Pittsburgh. The valley is highly industrialized, and in 1948, Donora's townscape was dominated by two huge smelters that extended for almost 3 miles along the banks of the Monongahela. There was a steel plant and a zinc plant, jointly known to the citizens of the area as the Donora Zinc Works. During the deadly smog, gaseous emissions from the smelters of the Donora Zinc Works became trapped in the valley under the influence of a temperature inversion. The smog was so thick that even natives of the area became easily lost, and streamers of carbon appeared to hang motionless in the air. Over half the citizens in the town of 14,000 were sickened in the incident. Hundreds of residents were evacuated and hospitalized. Many suffered permanent respiratory damage. By the fifth day, when rain showers finally dispersed the smog, 20 people were dead. A local doctor estimated that if the smog had lasted another night, "the casualty list would've been 1000 instead of 20."[29]

In the months following those deadly nights in Donora, at least three official investigations were carried out to look into the disaster: one by the Kettering Laboratory of the University of Cincinnati, one by the state of Pennsylvania, and one by the U.S. Public Health Service. The Kettering study was commissioned by the American Steel and Wire Company, a subsidiary of U.S. Steel, which owned the Donora Zinc Works. It was an attempt to get friendly scientific support for the mill owners, who publicly denied responsibility for the incident, describing it as an "act of God." The state's study was rather cursory, being one of the first to be carried out by the newly formed Division of Industrial Air Pollution. The U.S. Public Health Service initially declined involvement but eventually succumbed under the communal entreaties of the Pennsylvania Department of Health, the United Steelworkers Union, and the Donora borough council. There was much nervousness on the part of the borough council, in that Donora was basically a single-employer town with a strong economic dependency on the Zinc Works. The Public Health Service was happy not to rock the boat, being a politically cautious agency with no mandate to carry out forensic studies designed to assign blame. They limited their studies to air sampling, weather modeling, and epidemiological surveys.

When published in 1949, their results sidestepped any comments that might offend American Steel and Wire, and blamed the disaster on the temperature inversion, the topography, fumes from a variety of sources, and preexisting respiratory and cardiovascular conditions in the victims. The report recognized the presence in the smelter emissions of sulfur dioxide, carbon monoxide, nitrous oxides, and "heavy metal dust," but it concluded that "no single substance" was responsible for the toxic impact. Because of the inadequacies of the data available, the investigating team was unable to document the levels of pollution that occurred during the event. The report recommended that a warning system tied to weather forecasts be designed and installed, and that a more comprehensive air sampling program be put in place.[30]

Anti-fluoridationists strongly believe that there *was* a single substance responsible for the death and illness at Donora. They believe that the guilty substance was hydrogen fluoride gas. They see the hand of the Kettering Lab once again muddying the waters. They regard the Public Health Service Bulletin as a whitewash that failed to report the strong evidence of acute fluoride poisoning. They see the report as yet another example of collusion between government and corporate America. They are not surprised at this perceived cover-up, because once again all this took place during the Washington tenure of Oscar Ewing.

For support, anti-fluoridationists point to the work of Philip Sadtler, a consulting forensic chemist who investigated the Donora tragedy on behalf of some of the victims. His results were reported in a brief news item in the December 13, 1948, issue of *Chemical and Engineering News,* a highly regarded technical journal published by the American Chemical Society. Sadtler apparently undertook a fluoride-sampling program in the days following the tragedy. He claimed that his measurements uncovered high fluoride levels in vegetation and homes in the area. He also found that the fluoride concentrations in the blood of dead and hospitalized victims were 12 to 25 times the normal level. In his opinion, the symptoms reported by the victims before their death, and by hospitalized survivors, were consistent with fluoride poisoning.[31]

Even more in line with anti-fluoridationist thinking, Sadtler believed that there was a cover-up at Donora. In an interview with an investigative reporter, Chris Bryson, shortly before Sadtler's death in 1996, Sadtler charged that the Public Health Service helped U.S. Steel escape its liability for the Donora tragedy. He claims that a PHS chemist told him at the time, "I know you're right, but I am not allowed to say so." Furthermore, he claims that the editor of *Chemical and Engineering News,* the journal that publicized his results, told him that they would not be able to accept any more submissions from him because of pressures that were brought to bear on the leadership of the American Chemical Society from their colleagues at the Mellon Institute.[32]

The Donora event spawned many lawsuits. A class-action suit against U.S. Steel by the families of Donora victims was settled out of court. The tragedy also garnered national attention when the syndicated columnist

Walter Winchell covered the incident in his national radio show. Before Donora, there had not been much concern over air pollution among the public, or even among public health professionals, but the notoriety of the Donora disaster led to the first national legislation to protect the public from air pollution in 1955, ultimately culminating in the Clean Air Act of 1963.

In an historical context, there is no controversy over the scope of the Donora tragedy, the widespread illness, the number of deaths, or even the culpability of the industrial air pollution emanating from the corporate smelters. The point of contention between mainstream scientific observers and anti-fluoridation conspiracy theorists revolves around the relative importance of hydrogen fluoride in the tragedy. While fluoride gases are known to be a primary toxin from aluminum smelters and phosphate fertilizer plants, the question as to whether they can be singled out for blame in air pollution events that emanate from steel and zinc smelters is unclear. The anti-fluoride camp points to the fact that the most noted retrospective study of one of the world's first documented steel mill–generated pollution events, in the Meuse Valley of Belgium in 1933, placed the blame for the loss of human life primarily on fluoride emissions.[33] On the other hand, EPA analysis of a killer smog that arose from steel mill pollution in April 1971 in Birmingham, Alabama blamed the toxic impacts primarily on particulates, and implied that fluoride gases were not implicated.

Perhaps the last word in this section should go to one of the survivors of the Donora tragedy. A resident of the area directed folklorist Dan G. Hoffman to a ballad entitled *Death in Donora*. It begins with the following quatrain:

"I have felt the fog in my throat,
The misty hand of Death caress my face;
I have wrestled with a frightful foe,
Who strangled me with wisps of grey fog-lace.[34]

PROJECT F

Four years before the Donora tragedy, and not all that far away, another air-pollution incident has led historical sleuths from the anti-fluoridation movement to broach yet another alleged conspiracy, this one suggesting a sinister role for the Manhattan Project in the early development of pro-fluoridation government policy. The tale is set out in a classic underground exposé entitled *Fluoride, Teeth, and the Atomic Bomb*.[35] It was written by Joel Griffiths and Chris Bryson, two investigative reporters who have written many articles that tweak the complacency of mainstream science and medicine. Their story is based on recently declassified government documents that they obtained under the Freedom of Information Act. The story was originally commissioned by the *Christian Science Monitor*, but it never appeared there. The authors claim that at least a dozen mainstream media outlets subsequently expressed strong interest in their story, but all later declined. Ultimately, they found a home for their article in the obscure journal *Waste Not*, an environmental periodical put out by well-known anti-fluoride activists Paul and Eileen Connett. Griffiths and Bryson state that their facts are not in question and have been known to many insiders for years. "The fluoride story," they say, "is a hangover from the Cold War, when the U.S. media would not abrogate 'national security.'" It is worth noting that their 1997 article was selected by the Censored Project of the journalism faculty at Sonoma State University (in northern California) in their annual listing of the 25 most important, undercovered news stories of the year.[36]

The air pollution incident in question was a hydrogen fluoride release that occurred in 1944 from the E. I. du Pont de Nemours chemical plant in Deepwater, New Jersey, just across the Delaware River from Wilmington, Delaware. Farmers in Gloucester and Salem counties claimed that their fruit and vegetable crops were blighted, and their poultry and livestock sickened, by the du Pont emissions. They brought in Philip Sadtler, later of Donora fame, to investigate their claims, and they instigated legal action against du Pont.

During World War II, du Pont was a prime contractor for the Manhattan Project. Although it was not widely known in the community at the time, the Deepwater plant had largely been converted to the production of fluorine. Large supplies of fluorine were needed by the Manhattan Project for the separation of uranium isotopes in the construction of the atomic bomb. In nature, uranium occurs with two atomic structures, known to physicists as U-238, and U-235. It is the U-235 isotope that is needed for atomic fuel. Manhattan Project scientists had decided that the best way to separate U-235 from U-238 was to convert the uranium into a gaseous compound, and then separate the uranium isotopes by gaseous diffusion. The gas they selected to use was uranium hexafluoride (popularly known as "hex" in the project), hence the need for a fluorine supply to use in the gasification reaction. In the gaseous-diffusion separation process, gases diffuse through porous materials at rates that are determined by their molecular weight, with lighter gases diffusing faster than heavier gases. The separation equipment consists of a cascade of tubes, each filled with metal foil punctured with millions of microscopic holes. As the hex diffuses through the tubes, it is selectively enriched in the lighter isotope, U-235. Because the enrichment is so slight with each pass, many thousands of passes are needed. With enough passes, almost 100% enrichment can be achieved. The du Pont plant at Deepwater, New Jersey, delivered thousands of tons of fluorine to the separation facility at

Oak Ridge, Tennessee, in the final years of the war and in the immediate postwar years.[37]

During the war, the farmers' grievances over their crop and livestock losses were deflected on the grounds of national security, but in 1946, with the war over and du Pont's emissions still unchecked, the farmers reopened their lawsuit, and things came to a head. The Food and Drug Administration was sufficiently worried about the fluorine levels in the food and vegetable crops that they were considering an embargo on produce from Salem and Gloucester counties. The results of Sadtler's investigations were about to become public knowledge, indicating high fluoride levels not only in the produce and livestock, but also in the bloodstream of "human individuals residing in the area."[38]

These developments alarmed the military. They were more cognizant than the general public of the escalating tensions between the United States and the Soviet Union, and it was their intention to flaunt the U.S. monopoly on the bomb as a stratagem of deterrence in the Cold War. Their plan to produce a sufficiently fearsome arsenal of atomic bombs required continued production of large quantities of fluorine. The specter of a rash of lawsuits against the Manhattan project and its contractors raised grave apprehensions. According to the files uncovered by Griffiths and Bryson, these worries led to a spate of meetings in the spring of 1946 organized under the personal direction of Manhattan Project chief, Major General Leslie R. Groves. As a result of these meetings, the U.S. Army Chemical Warfare Service was brought in to carry out a new fluoride-testing program in New Jersey, the Food and Drug Administration was dissuaded from their embargo, and the Department of Justice settled the lawsuits out of court.

The Manhattan Project was not unaware of the dangers associated with their fluorine production activities. They had already created a special medical section of the project at the University of Rochester in upstate New York to study the health effects of radiation. Once the role of fluorine became clear, they added a fluoride toxicology program at Rochester, under the leadership of Harold C. Hodge, to investigate the impact of fluoride exposures on the human body. The research program there was the largest such program in the United States, and much of the information on the toxicity of fluoride that later emerged during the fluoridation battles came from Hodge and his co-workers. It is the contention of the anti-fluoridation camp that this work is tainted by the fact that its original purpose was to protect the Manhattan project from politically inconvenient litigation. They also question the sincerity of Hodge's later activity in support of water fluoridation, pointing to a declassified memo from Hodge to his superior officer, Colonel Stafford L.Warren, chief of the Manhattan Project Medical Section, in which he asks:

"Would there be any use in making attempts to counteract the local fear of fluoride on the part of residents of Salem and Gloucester counties through lectures on fluoride toxicology and perhaps the usefulness of fluoride in tooth health?"[39]

Some of the other internal memos between Hodge and Warren that came to light in Griffith and Bryson's Freedom of Information foray show that Hodge suspected that acute fluoride exposure could have deleterious effects on the central nervous system (CNS), perhaps causing mental confusion, drowsiness, and lassitude. He even proposed a program of animal research on CNS effects, but it was apparently never funded. Anti-fluoridationists wonder why he never raised these concerns in any of his later articles on fluoridation or on any of the many government fluoridation panels on which he sat over the years.

The final link in the chain that ties the Manhattan project to the pro-fluoridation movement lies in the involvement of Harold Hodge and his University of Rochester toxicology team in the Newburgh–Kingston fluor-idation trial. When the New York State Department of Health decided to follow up on David Ast's proposal to carry out the Newburgh demonstra-tion project, they appointed a committee to assess the feasibility of such a study. Harold Hodge was asked to preside over that committee as chairman. Anti-fluoridationists see this appointment as grossly inappropriate, and they see sinister motivations in allowing a Manhattan Project scientist to "shape and guide" the Newburgh studies.[40] Griffiths and Bryson claim that Hodge's military connections were never revealed to the public. They further charge that Hodge misused his position by convincing Ast to allow blood samples to be taken from Newburgh children for use in his Manhattan project studies at the University of Rochester (more accurately, his Atomic Energy Com-mission (AEC) studies, the Manhattan Project having been closed down and replaced by the new AEC). They claim that during the first 10 years of the trial, blood samples were duly collected by health department personnel and shipped to Rochester.

According to Griffiths and Bryson the purpose of the Rochester fluoride studies was not healthy teeth, it was "to furnish scientific ammunition which the government and its nuclear contractors could use to defeat lawsuits." The studies were code-named Program F. They were directed by Hodge, funded by AEC, and carried out at Strong Memorial Hospital in Rochester. It was during this same time frame and at the same hospital that the medical section of the Manhattan Project carried out its infamous program of pluto-nium injections on unsuspecting patients, as outlined by Eileen Welsome in her Pulitzer Prize–winning book *The Plutonium Files: America's Secret Medical Experiments in the Cold War.*[41] The plutonium studies were carried out behind closed doors, under Army guard. They were exposed by a 1995 investigation, prodded by Welsome's investigative reporting, which ultimately led to a multimillion-dollar settlement for the families of the victims. Anti-fluoridationists feel that all studies that were carried out in this milieu are tainted. They see the forced consumption of fluoridated water by Newburgh schoolchildren as crossing the same unethical line as the secret injection of plutonium on the Rochester patients.

The results of Project F were not included in the final report of the Newburgh–Kingston fluoridation trial, nor is there any mention of blood samples being taken from the Newburgh schoolchildren.[42] The authors conclude that the low concentrations of fluoride proposed for use in water fluoridation programs pose no health risk to participating citizens. Griffiths and Bryson are suspicious because they claim that Project F documents uncovered under the Freedom of Information Act reveal evidence of AEC censorship. They claim that conclusions on public health impacts in the published versions of Project F studies were often softened from those appearing in earlier drafts. In one case, comparison of draft and final versions of a paper that appeared in the *Journal of the American Dental Association*[43] indicated significant differences in the results of a study on dental health impacts on workers at a wartime chemical production plant (possibly Deepwater). They claim that the draft version highlighted many health problems experienced by the workers, whereas the published version describes the workers as "unusually healthy." Conspiracy mavens suspect that the Rochester contributions to the Newburgh studies may have been excised from the final report by AEC censors; however a comparison of draft and published versions of the Newburgh fluoridation study is not possible, because no draft versions of the paper were found in the declassified AEC files. Anti-fluoridationists find the absence of this file even more damning than anything that might be contained within it.

THE FAR SIDE

If you can give credence to stories of malicious collusion between atomic scientists and the leaders of the early fluoridation trials, you may be ready for the final step in the fluorophobian chain. Conspiracy lovers on the outside edges of the anti-fluoridation movement suspect that the fluoridation of public water supplies is nothing more or less than an attempt by the government to control the minds of the populace. They note that many mood-altering drugs, such as Prozac and Rohypnol (the "date-rape" drug) are composed of fluorinated compounds. They have read the fluoride toxicology literature. They are aware that those who suffer *acute* exposure to hydrogen fluoride gas, the kind of exposure experienced by laboratory workers who inadvertently lean into the wrong fume hood, may exhibit "mental confusion, drowsiness, and lassitude." It is their contention that if such effects are known to occur in response to short-term, high-dose, *acute* exposure, perhaps they also occur in response to long-term, low-dose, *chronic* exposure, such as would occur from the ingestion of fluoridated drinking water.

Of course, there is always an anecdote to back up every paranoid suspicion, and mind control through fluoridation is no exception. In his book *Conspiranoia*, author Devon Jackson takes the reader on a skeptical tour of the far side, telling us about the Illuminati, the Rosicrucians, and the Freemasons; charting the unrecognized links between the international Zionist conspiracy, the military–industrial complex, and the Human Genome Project; and spelling out the sinister connections between Howard Hunt, Marilyn Monroe, and the Teletubbies (we exaggerate, but not much).[44] In his section on fluoride, Jackson tells the oft-told tale (or at least, oft-told in the conspiracy netherworld) of Charles Elliott Perkins, a prominent scientist sent to Germany at the end of World War II to take over control of the I. G. Farben chemical plants. These are the plants that manufactured the Zyklon-B gas used in the Auschwitz gas chambers, a fact that has no bearing on our tale, but which never escapes mention. Perkins claims that he was told by Farben engineers that near war's end the Third Reich had approved a scheme for mind control of the German population through mass medication of drinking water using sodium fluoride. Nazi medical researchers supposedly told the Gestapo that fluoridated citizens would be "more docile towards authority."[45]

According to Anne-Lise Gotzsche in her anti-fluoride book *The Fluoride Question: Panacea or Poison?*, fluoride is not the only supplement that has come under consideration as an additive to public water supplies.[46] She sees fluoridation as the thin edge of the wedge. If we allow one, she argues, why not others? She worries about tranquilizers and other mind-control drugs, such as lithium. She alleges that a former president of France once suggested adding Antabuse to drinking water to cure the French of alcoholism. She claims that some groups have promoted adding contraceptive drugs to check the population explosion. Anti-government suspicion runs very deep in the world of conspiranoia.

LET THERE BE LIGHT: AN ASSESSMENT OF ANTI-FLUORIDATION CONSPIRACY CLAIMS

It is our opinion that these dark tales of toxic coups, death fogs, and secret projects represent an unduly paranoid view of the history of the fluoridation movement. These anti-fluoridation stories are larded with unfair interpretation. Normal interactions between scientists from different agencies are termed secret trysts. Cooperative steps between government and industry are termed collusion. Meetings that took place openly and publicly are called secret. Ordinary business strategies are identified as hidden agendas. The complexities that underlie massive interdisciplinary and interagency undertakings like the Manhattan Project or the fluoridation trials are given devious meaning. People who left high-paying jobs in industry to serve their country in times of depression and war are given sinister motives. Nobody escapes obsessive suspicion, whether they make their home in science, industry, business, government, or the military. Anybody who favors rather than opposes fluoridation is considered suspect, malicious, and dangerous. No credence is given to the possibility that honest persons can be in honest disagreement over a controversial undertaking. In our opinion, this dark side of the anti-fluoridation movement is demonstrably obsessive and unfair.

We will try to defend this strong position by assessing each of the questions raised in the foregoing sections of this chapter and summarized in Table 6.1. The questions reflect historical anti-fluoridation concerns about aluminum cookware, Alcoa motivations, industrial laboratories, air pollution events, the Manhattan Project, and mind control. Perusal of the short

TABLE 6.1 An Assessment of Anti-fluoridation Conspiracy Claims

Issues	Questions	Short Answers
Aluminum cookware	Does aluminum cookware release poisons into food that threaten health?	No.
Alcoa motivation	Is H.V. Churchill's finding that waterborne fluoride is the cause of mottled teeth open to any question?	No.
	Are by-products from the waste streams of the aluminum and fertilizer industries used as a source of fluoride for public water fluoridation?	Yes.
	Is this tantamount to dumping industrial effluent into drinking water?	No.
	Did these industries lobby on behalf of fluoridation in order to see these markets develop?	Possibly.
	Are there any health concerns associated with impurities in the fluoride from these sources?	No.
	Did Oscar Ewing promote fluoridation while in government service?	Yes.
	Did he purposely enter government service to promote fluoridation?	Unlikely.
	Did he promote fluoridation to camouflage the fluoride air pollution problems of the aluminum industry?	Very far-fetched.

TABLE 6.1 (*Continued*)

Issues	Questions	Short Answers
Industrial labs	Did the Mellon Institute and the Kettering Laboratory cater to industrial needs?	Yes.
	Did scientists at these institutes rig their research results in favor of fluoridation to please industrial sponsors?	Very unlikely.
	Did they promote their favorable fluoride results on government panels and committees?	Yes.
Air pollution	Were atmospheric effluents from the Zinc Works responsible for the Donora air pollution disaster?	Yes.
	Was the USPHS report of the Donora incident a purposeful cover-up of Zinc Works complicity?	Yes and no.
	Were the health impacts at Donora due to hydrogen fluoride gas as claimed by Sadtler or to a mix of effluent gases as claimed by the USPHS?	Unclear. More likely a mix.
	Is hydrogen fluoride gas from industrial plants a significant air pollutant in the United States?	Significant but secondary.
Manhattan project	Is there any reason to doubt the reliability of Project F fluoride toxicology studies?	No.
	Were published versions of Project F papers censored under Manhattan Project security concerns?	Probably.
	Was there anything inappropriate about Hodge's involvement in the Newburgh fluoridation trial?	Not really.
	Is there any reason to question Hodge's motivations in supporting fluoridation?	Not really.
	Are Hodge's concerns about the impacts of acute fluoride poisoning on the central nervous system germane to the fluoridation discussion?	Only marginally.
Mind control	Is there any evidence that fluoridation could be used for mind control?	No.
	Would it be possible for government to add mind-controlling substances to water supplies without public knowledge?	No.

answers that I have provided on Table 6.1 clarifies the debating strategy. Conspiracy buffs like to start with historical facts that nobody can deny (e.g., Did Oscar Ewing work for the government? Yes!), then build a beguiling house of cards based on the underlying fact, but leavened with supposition and interpretation. It is sometimes difficult to see where the facts end and the supposition begins. Whatever truths may underlie the stories, the interpretation given to these truths is always malign.

Over the years these obsessive stories have taken on the stuff of legend in anti-fluoridation circles. It is time to heed the difference between legend and myth.

Aluminum Cookware

The charge that the use of aluminum cookware might release poisons into food probably requires little refutation. The claims of Spira and Betts have long since been discredited, and even anti-fluoridation conspiracy theorists don't push this one anymore. Although it is true that material from cooking pots does enter the food we cook in them, the amounts released are only a miniscule percentage of the safe daily intakes. Furthermore, most aluminum pots sold nowadays are anodized, which reduces the amount of leachate even more. Like other metals, large intakes of aluminum can do harm to human health, but the extremely small concentrations released during the heating of aluminum cookware, anodized or not, are benign. There is no credible evidence that there is any danger in using aluminum pots and pans in the kitchen.

Having said this, readers may be surprised to learn that the issue was still alive as late as 1987. In that year, an article appeared in the prestigious scientific journal, *Nature,* claiming that fluoridated water boiled in aluminum pots leached a greater concentration of aluminum into the water than did unfluoridated water. The concentrations were miniscule in both cases and unlikely to have any significance on human health, but the reference was picked up nevertheless and highlighted in anti-fluoridation literature. Unfortunately for the authors of the *Nature* article (and the writers of anti-fluoridation literature), the methodology and results of this research were discredited a few months later in the same journal, and a few months after that the authors were forced to publish a retraction.[47]

Alcoa Motivations

Anti-fluoridationists have long questioned the motivation behind H. V. Churchill's 1931 finding of fluoride, waterborne fluoride in particular, as the cause of mottled teeth. They suggest that he or his superiors may have been trying to deflect suspicion from *airborne* fluorides emanating from Alcoa smelters. However, it is highly unlikely that Churchill or his superiors knew about the possible dangers associated with fluoride emissions at that time (or perhaps even that hydrogen fluoride was one of the gases belching from their smokestacks). Public concern over air pollution had not developed by that date, and did not really do so until the Donora incident 17 years later.

Furthermore, it was not until six years later, in 1937, that Roholm published his studies in Europe suggesting a toxic role for fluoride emissions
in the Meuse Valley air pollution deaths.[48] If by chance Churchill knew of
this budding work, I suppose it is possible that he was led to measure fluoride contents in the water from Bauxite, Arkansas (and the waters from the
other areas where mottled teeth had been observed) because of his suspicion that airborne fluorides had done similar damage elsewhere, but it is
hard to ascribe venal motives to such a master stroke, if such it was. On the
contrary, it seems that Churchill's fluoride finding was more likely to draw
attention *to* Alcoa's airborne fluoride emissions than *away from* them. In any
case, Churchill's forensic chemistry has stood the test of time. It is now an
accepted scientific fact that fluoride (both airborne and waterborne) is the
cause of mottled teeth, so clear that the disease is now known as *dental fluorosis*. One must conclude that Churchill's work was solid science carried out in
good conscience.

The next four questions under the Alcoa heading on Table 6.1 arise from
the fact that by-products from the waste streams of the aluminum industry
were originally used as a source of fluoride for public water fluoridation.
Indeed, by-products from the waste streams of the fertilizer industry are still
used widely for this purpose. The question is *not* whether fluoride from such
sources is in use, but whether there is any significance to the charge that
such use is a danger to human health. Many anti-fluoridationists argue that
using these sources of fluoride is tantamount to dumping industrial effluent into drinking water. The pro-fluoride camp finds this charge patently
ridiculous, and it is hard not to side with this viewpoint. There is absolutely
nothing sinister in a company reclaiming by-products that are marketable.
Shareholders and consumers alike benefit from the economic efficiency of
such a business strategy. Environmentalists should appreciate the virtue of
this recovery of waste product for beneficial use and the spirit of recycling
that such an approach represents. Recycling of fluoride compounds lessens
industrial fluoride emissions to land and air, and lessens the need for mining
and smelting of fluorine-bearing minerals.

Anti-fluoridationists worry that fluoride from these sources will
somehow be less pure, and more likely to harm human health, than that generated synthetically by chemical companies or pharmaceutical firms. This
concern is unwarranted. Fluorides utilized in municipal water fluoridation
must meet strict standards of purity regardless of their source. The American Water Works Association has published lengthy requirements for each
of the three fluoride compounds that are commonly used in the fluoridation
process.[49] Any suppliers that do not meet these requirements will quickly
lose their share of the market. Furthermore, the processing that is necessary

to meet the standards is similar in all cases, regardless of whether the initial feed is mined fluoride ore, a synthetic chemical compound, or a by-product recovered from an industrial process. The chemical products division of an aluminum company is no more likely to produce fluoride that does not meet standards than is a chemical company or a pharmaceutical firm. In any case, we can find no anecdotal records of health problems arising from impurities in the fluoride feed from any of the common sources. It appears that health concerns associated with possible impurities in fluoride feed for municipal fluoridation are unfounded.

The last question in this regard is whether the aluminum and fertilizer industries carried out inappropriate lobbying activities on behalf of fluoridation in order to see the fluoride market open up for them. It is certainly possible that they did so, but once again, it is difficult to see anything very sinister in such a business strategy. Perhaps the real question is: Would they have done so even if they thought that fluoridation was an evil and dangerous gamble? We will never know the answer to this question, because at the time in question, fluoridation had the more-or-less unanimous support of all responsible health agencies. The fluoride-producing industries probably perceived a win–win situation: a chance to profit while playing a visible role in a widely championed new public health measure.

Regardless of motives, it is a matter of record that fluoride recovery and resale has never been a particularly large or profitable market for either the aluminum or fertilizer industries. An Alcoa spokesman interviewed in 1972 displayed open frustration at the anti-fluoridation attacks. He claimed that fluorides were never more than an "infinitesimal part" of Alcoa operations. "We are in business primarily to make and sell aluminum," he stated. "The future prosperity of the thousands of employees and shareholders who make up Alcoa depends principally upon how well we make aluminum, not on whether ... communities fluoridate their water."[50]

In fact, as pointed out by Martin in his book *Scientific Knowledge in Controversy: The Social Dynamics of the Fluoridation Debate*, the U.S. aluminum industry is a major purchaser of fluosilicic acid, the chemical that is now most often used in water fluoridation. The aluminum industry and municipal water supply authorities are thus in competition for supplies of this chemical. To whatever degree such competition may have affected prices or availability of fluosilicic acid over the years, it could be argued that the fluoridation movement has been a bane rather than a boon to the aluminum industry. On this topic Martin concludes that "the view that aluminum companies gained financially from sales of fluoride wastes has never had much basis." Similar conclusions can be drawn with respect to the fertilizer industry. It seems that at best they have been "passive beneficiaries."[51]

All of this leads naturally to the peculiar anti-fluoridationist obsession with Oscar Ewing. It is implied whenever his name surfaces in anti-fluoride literature that without his support and connivance, public acceptance of fluoridation would never have come to pass. There is no question that Oscar Ewing promoted fluoridation while in government service, but so did hundreds of other well-meaning government scientists and bureaucrats who accepted the dental health claims of the pro-fluoridation movement at face value. It seems far-fetched in the extreme to suggest that Ewing entered government service solely (or even primarily) to promote fluoridation. In his role as administrator of the Federal Security Agency (FSA), Ewing oversaw a vast array of postwar government health and welfare programs. The Public Health Service was only one of the many agencies that fell under his jurisdiction, and the fluoridation program only one of the many programs that were under way in that agency. It is unlikely that Ewing, or any other single government administrator, no matter what his rank, would have had sufficient influence to ensure the success or failure of any particular program.

Fluoride foes point to the $2 million budget approved by Congress in 1951 for support of community water fluoridation as proof of Ewing's cunning. However, they don't mention the $1 million budget approved in 1948 for a nationwide demonstration of the efficacy of *topical* fluoride applications (fluoride applications applied to tooth surfaces by dentists in dental offices).[52] This allocation also came under Ewing's tenure, and had it been successful in convincing the public to support voluntary topical fluoridation as the only method of delivery, there would have been less call for the involuntary fluoridation of public water supplies that the anti-fluoridation camp so despises.

None of the many detailed histories that have been written about the Public Health Service, or the fluoridation program per se, give Ewing any particular credit for the progress of the program. We might look, for example, at the "premature" decision by the Public Health Service to support community water fluoridation, well before the results of the fluoridation trials were completed, an event that holds a position of particular infamy in anti-fluoridationist annals. The steps leading up to this decision have been particularly well documented in the historical literature, especially in light of Trendley Dean's fierce opposition.[53] Despite the fact that this decision took place under Ewing's tenure as FSA chief, there is no evidence in the historical record of Ewing's direct or indirect involvement in the many meetings and negotiations that transpired at that time.

Ruth Roy Harris, in her history of the National Institute of Dental Research, looked rather carefully into the charges that Oscar Ewing was paid off to represent Alcoa interests while at the FSA.[54] Both Ewing and Alcoa formally denied the charges, of course, but even careful investigation doesn't reveal much of a smoking gun. Alcoa was just one of many clients served by Ewing's law firm prior to his government service. The only evidence presented by the anti-fluoridation camp (at congressional hearings in 1954)[55] consisted of records of fees paid to Ewing's law firm by Alcoa, which were large but probably not out of line for legal services to a large corporation by a large law firm. Filed affidavits show that Ewing divested himself of financial interest in his firm before joining FSA. One can never be absolutely certain regarding the sometimes-murky financial dealings of wealthy men, but the weight of evidence seems to suggest that Ewing took on his government post with public service in mind. Of course, Ewing may well have held to the conservative ethic of the day that *What's Good for General Bullmoose Is Good for the USA*, but whether this is true or not, the anti-fluoridation camp has not advanced any credible evidence that he was pandering to his severed aluminum connections in his support for fluoridation. If the charges are false, which they appear to be, anti-fluoridation activists are guilty of shameful character assassination of Oscar Ewing.

Industrial Labs

The first question under the heading of *Industrial Labs* on Table 6.1 dangles a straw man in our face and challenges us to knock him down. We are asked: "Did the Mellon Institute and the Kettering Laboratory cater to industrial needs?" Well, yes; during the period in question, in fact they did. So does it follow that scientists at these institutes would rig their research results in favor of fluoridation to please their industrial sponsors? Well, no; it doesn't. A "yes" answer to this second question shows a naive ignorance of how science works, and represents a grievous slur on two world-famous scientific centers that have played important roles in improving the health and welfare of the nation.

The Kettering Laboratory of Applied Physiology was created at the University of Cincinnati in 1930 under the leadership of Robert E. Kehoe.[56] Kehoe was the first research leader to assemble a multidisciplinary team of physicians, analytical chemists, toxicologists, industrial hygienists, and engineers to work in the newly emerging field of occupational and environmental health. His first studies, carried out under the aegis of General Motors Corporation, identified the health dangers of tetraethyllead, which would hardly seem to be climbing into the sponsor's pocket. As time passed, other corporate sponsors came to the Kettering Lab with health and safety concerns of their own. Anti-fluoridationists see this as a pact with the devil, ripe for collusion and cover-up. The contrary view, which I believe is more defensible, is that the corporations should be given some credit for their sponsorship of research designed to identify and mitigate health concerns associated with their workplace and their products. Certainly, one cannot be so naive as to believe that sponsorship did not buy them some favorable consideration, but the suggestion that Kettering scientists were in the pocket of corporate interests is an insult to those scientists. Sponsorship may have obligated them to soften the blow of bad news in public announcements, but there is little evidence that health and safety concerns uncovered by Kettering scientists were swept under the table.

As an example, we might look at the 1961 textbook *Fluorosis: The Health Aspects of Fluorine*, authored by Kettering scientist E. J. Largent.[57] Anti-fluoridationists are full of disdain for this book because of a statement that appeared on the dust jacket claiming that the book will "aid industry in lawsuits arising from fluoride claims." They charge that the book is an industry apologia. I suspect that most of those making this charge have never looked inside the pages of the book. If they did, they would find that it contains lengthy discussions of many of the aspects of acute fluorine poisoning that are so near and dear to anti-fluoridationist hearts, including skeletal fluorosis, dental fluorosis, animal intoxication, damage to plants, and occupational dangers. It is not exactly the stuff of apologia. It is true that there is a short chapter, "Fluorides and Claims of Damage" (only four pages out of 150), and the tenor there is perhaps a bit condescending. However, the claim on the dust jacket that so infuriates anti-fluoridationists really doesn't reflect the contents of the book. It was probably written by the book's publisher (an academic house with no connection to the Kettering Lab) rather than the author.

The Mellon Institute of Industrial Research has roots similar to those of the Kettering Lab.[58] It dates back to 1911, when the Mellon Brothers, Andrew and Richard, established a research institute at the University of Pittsburgh that they hoped would create a new kind of partnership between science and industry in order to create new and better consumer products. It is true that in the early years the Institute was organized on a contractual basis with all results obtained by institute scientists becoming the property of the contracting firm. By 1937, however, the Institute had evolved into a more conventional university research center. At Mellon, as at Kettering, most of the staff scientists held joint appointments in the associated university departments. Gerald Cox, for example, the man reviled in anti-fluoride literature for being the first to suggest community water fluoridation, and always identified as a Mellon Institute scientist, listed his primary affiliation in his published papers as the School of Dentistry at the University of Pittsburgh.

In fact, most Mellon and Kettering scientists had appointments on the faculty of the University of Pittsburgh or the University of Cincinnati. These appointments made them subject to the usual academic checks and balances that guarantee distinguished and unbiased scientific research. Like other faculty, they had to pass the tenure hurdle, and to do so, they had to present a satisfactory record of academic publication to their promotion committees. "Publish or perish" is not just a media catchphrase. A satisfactory publication record requires the acceptance of many articles by high-quality academic journals. Such journals are usually published by reputable scientific societies, and the articles in such journals must pass muster by an editorial board of research leaders in the authors' fields. It is highly unlikely that Mellon or Kettering scientists could gain access to these journals if their papers were biased or fudged to meet the goals of industrial sponsors. For that matter, the sponsors themselves would have little to gain, either publicly or privately, if their funded research did not have the credibility of the academic peer-review system. One must conclude that the fluoride toxicology studies carried out at the Mellon and Kettering labs, and the leadership role played by scientists at these institutes in the early years, represents good science carried out in good faith.

It would be tragic if those who have been influenced by anti-fluoridation literature formed their opinions of these two institutes from that source alone. Both institutions have a long history and have contributed much to science in the United States. Their early contributions to the fluoridation literature represent only a miniscule percentage of their total scientific output. The Kettering Lab no longer exists under that name. In 1965 it became part of the Department of Environmental Health in the College of Medicine at the University of Cincinnati. The department has a close and sustained linkage with the National Institute of Environmental Health Sciences, one of the National Institutes of Health. It is the largest research department at the University of Cincinnati, with a research budget over $20 million annually. It has a national ranking in the top 10% in its field. Faculty and doctoral graduates from the department are renowned for their many important contributions in such fields as molecular toxicology, statistical genetics, and lung cancer epidemiology. The Mellon Institute has also evolved. In 1967, the Institute merged with Carnegie Technical College to form Carnegie Mellon University, with its campus immediately adjacent to that of the University of Pittsburgh. The building for the original Mellon Institute, completed in 1937, is one of the great landmark university buildings in the country. It covers a city block, a huge Parthenon-like building of classical monumental grandeur. It now houses the Pittsburgh supercomputer center.

There is one anti-fluoridationist charge that does have some truth to it. Anti-fluoride forces have always claimed that the many government-sponsored review panels set up over the years to assess the costs and benefits of fluoridation were stacked in favor of fluoridation. A review of the membership of the various panels confirms this charge. The expert committees that put together reports by the American Association for the Advancement of Science in 1941, 1944, and 1954; the National Academy of Sciences in 1951, 1971, 1977, and 1993; the World Health Organization in 1958, and 1970; and the U.S. Public Health Service in 1991 are rife with the names of well-known medical and dental researchers who actively campaigned on behalf of fluoridation or whose research was held in high regard in the pro-fluoridation movement.[59] Membership was interlocking and incestuous. The names of many of the same scientists, Mellon and Kettering researchers among them, appear on the rolls of many of these studies. There is essentially no representation on any of the panels of reputable research scientists whose work found favor in the anti-fluoridation camp.

In the early years of the fluoridation movement, there may be mitigating circumstances that help explain the inherent bias in the makeup of the review boards. At that time, there was no well-established, credible scientific opposition to fluoridation. It would have been extremely difficult to find reputable medical or dental researchers to create balance on the panels. In later years, however, this explanation no longer holds. Opponents like Waldbott and Yiamouyiannis had research credentials similar to those chosen for service on the committees. The simple fact is that such opponents were considered quacks by the medical establishment, solely on the basis of their opposition to fluoridation. It was part of the shunning process, which is discussed later in this book, and which forced anti-fluoridation researchers to form their own organizations outside the medical mainstream.

One might ask the question: Would the fluoridation bandwagon have been derailed if these panels had included passionate opponents of the practice? Our opinion is that it would not. Even then, the clash of absolutes was in place. Pro-fluoridationists were in command, and they would have allowed no more than token opposition on the panels. Neither side would have suffered backsliders. The anti-fluoride panelists might have been able to append minority opinions to the majority reports, or perhaps they would have preferred to walk out in protest. Such actions might have had some influence on legislative decision makers, but we doubt it. We believe the saga would have run its course in much the same way, regardless of their actions. It might even be argued that the anti-fluoridation forces made their case more effectively by the very act of being excluded. To those of a conspiratorial turn of mind, exclusion is a powerful motivator.

Air Pollution

The Donora strand of the anti-fluoridationist argument asks us to accept a three-step reasoning process: first, that the tragic deaths in the Donora air pollution incident were caused by hydrogen fluoride gas in the smelter emissions; second, that on this evidence we should regard hydrogen fluoride as one of the primary toxic air pollutants in the United States; and third, that if this is so, then adding low concentrations of fluoride to the drinking water supply is likely to be harmful to human health. Let us examine these points in turn.

Atmospheric effluents from the Donora Zinc Works were without doubt responsible for the Donora air pollution tragedy. Without the effluents, the meteorological inversion would have caused harmless fog rather than deadly smog. The report of the investigation carried out by the U.S. Public Health Service did not unequivocally state this fact, and in that sense, it was a purposeful cover-up of Zinc Works complicity. However, as is made clear by Lynne Page Snyder in her historical reassessment of the Donora tragedy,[60] one must place PHS actions in the proper historical context. The Donora study was the first comprehensive survey carried out by the PHS on the health effects of air pollution. From the beginning, they made it clear that they did not intend to carry out a forensic study for the purpose of assessing blame. In fact, as a federal agency, the Public Health Service had limited jurisdiction in the matter. They did not want to get tangled up in the politically volatile issue of state regulation of the metal smelting industry. Their study was solely health related, and solely for the purpose of input to federal health policy. Moreover, two of the groups that requested PHS involvement, the borough of Donora and state of Pennsylvania, urged the PHS to sidestep the issue of responsibility, for fear of destroying the economic health of this single-employer town. In this day and age, when corporate environmental performance is regularly held up to public scrutiny, it is difficult to imagine a federal agency operating with such political caution, but such was the tenor of the times. Everybody knew who the culprits were, but it wasn't in anybody's interest to say it too loudly.

Anti-fluoridationist interest in Donora rests on the belief that the health impacts at Donora were due primarily to gaseous hydrogen fluoride effluent from the Zinc Works. The source of this belief is a single consulting report prepared by Philip Sadtler, who had developed a particular interest in hydrogen fluoride pollution through his involvement at the Deepwater site, where this gas was definitively identified as the primary pollutant responsible for the environmental degradation observed there. His views on Donora reached the mainstream through a brief three-paragraph news item that appeared in the journal *Chemical and Engineering News*, probably submitted by Sadtler himself, not peer-reviewed as a full article would have been. It turns out, on investigation, that Sadtler's view was not held widely at the time, nor has it become an accepted interpretation of events at Donora. The report of the official investigation carried out by the Public Health Service unequivocally dismisses fluoride as the culprit. If the credibility of this source is doubted, one can turn to the textbooks. The Donora tragedy is discussed in every leading air pollution textbook used in American universities. It is almost always identified as the event that triggered public interest in industrial pollution. We examined 10 such textbooks and not one of them referenced Sadtler's work or even mentioned hydrogen fluoride pollution in their discussion of the Donora disaster.[61] All of them lay the blame primarily on sulfur dioxide, long known to be a major gaseous effluent from zinc smelting operations. Frederick Lipfert's lengthy coverage also refers to "sulfuric acid," "total sulfur," "particulate matter," and a "wide variety of industrial emissions, including acid mists and trace metals." The latter are identified as "zinc, cadmium and lead." Other than Sadtler's paper, none of the contemporaneous discussions of the Donora tragedy even mention fluoride gas,[62] nor is it mentioned in a follow-up study carried out 10 years after the event,[63] or in Snyder's historical review.[64]

Anti-fluoridationists also look for support to Kaj Roholm, a respected European toxicologist who published a paper in 1937 suggesting that the victims of the 1930 air pollution disaster in the Meuse Valley, Belgium, may have suffered acute intoxication by gaseous fluorine compounds.[65] Conditions in the Meuse Valley episode were very similar to those at Donora. Dense fog and a temperature inversion in a narrow valley trapped industrial emissions from several factories that produced coke, steel, glass, phosphate, sulfuric acid, and zinc. Over 60 deaths were reported, and more than 6000 people became ill. Roholm's full body of work on fluoride toxicology has become classic, but on the question of the Meuse Valley, his is a minority opinion just like Sadtler's in Donora. The official commission of investigation into the Meuse Valley disaster specifically considered the question of fluorine intoxication, but credited it with only "doubtful" and "at most secondary" importance. Like Donora, the investigators failed to implicate any specific substance or chemical compound as the absolute cause of the deaths, but they did offer the opinion that the disaster "in all probability" had been brought about by sulfur dioxide emissions.

Before moving on, we should perhaps make one thing clear. We have not introduced these stories of the Donora and Meuse Valley air pollution disasters in order to deny the culpability of hydrogen fluoride as a toxic air contaminant. The dangers of gaseous fluoride emissions from aluminum plants and phosphate fertilizer plants are well documented, as we have seen from the case histories from Deepwater, New Jersey and Garrison, Montana. Rather, these events have been raised to illustrate the penchant of the anti-fluoridation movement to latch onto minority opinions that suit their cause and present them to the public as if they were proven fact. We may never know whether fluoride gas played a role in the pollution deaths at Donora or in the Meuse Valley, because the measurements that would allow independent observers to reach such a conclusion were never made. Sadtler's and Roholm's arguments are not without merit, but they are far from gospel truth.

So where *do* fluoride emissions fit into the spectrum of air pollution concerns? To answer this question, we turn first to the federal air pollution regulations and then to the leading air pollution textbooks. The first federal Clean Air Act was passed in 1963. It was amended in 1970 as part of the genesis of the Environmental Protection Agency, then again in 1977, and finally, in 1990. Under the current regulations, air pollutants are grouped into two classifications: *criteria pollutants*, and *hazardous air pollutants* (sometimes called *air toxics*).[66] Criteria pollutants are substances that are ubiquitous in most urban atmospheres and are deemed to present a general risk to public health. To date, six compounds have been identified by EPA as criteria pollutants: sulfur dioxide, nitrogen dioxide, carbon monoxide, ozone, inhalable particulate matter, and lead. For each of these pollutants, a National Ambient Air Quality Standard has been issued, and five of the six (all but lead) are used to calculate the Air Quality Index, which informs the public whether air pollution levels in their city pose a health concern. There are no fluoride compounds on the list of criteria pollutants.

Hazardous air pollutants are substances that tend to be identified with specific industrial emissions and the workplace. They are gaseous compounds that may cause cancer or other serious health effects, such as reproductive effects or birth defects, or adverse environmental or ecological effects. There are 189 compounds on the hazardous air pollutant list, and hydrogen fluoride is one of those compounds. Health hazard information published by EPA and the Centers for Disease Control state that "acute (short-term) inhalation exposure to gaseous hydrogen fluoride can cause severe respiratory damage in humans, including severe irritation and pulmonary edema." Furthermore, "severe ocular irritation and dermal burns may occur following eye or skin exposure."[67] As we have already learned, high levels of hydrogen fluoride in the air are also known to cause lameness in farm livestock, especially cattle, and to damage fruit and forage crops.

Regulatory control of these pollutants is achieved by identifying specific facilities within specific industries that produce unacceptable emissions, and then enforcing a maximum achievable control technology (MACT) at each facility. Final air toxics rules for hydrogen fluoride emissions have been set for both primary aluminum reduction plants and phosphate fertilizer plants. The rules are based on a combination of control techniques that either prevent the escape of hydrogen fluoride into the atmosphere or capture the pollutants and recycle them back into the process. The rules were developed in partnership with state regulators and industry stakeholders. They contain an "emissions averaging procedure" that allows facilities to overcontrol some emissions points and undercontrol others. Facilities that consistently meet the MACT standards are allowed to reduce the frequency of their emissions testing. Under the Clean Air Act Amendments of 1990, EPA's Office of Air Quality Planning and Standards is required to specify a "hazard ranking" for each of the 189 air toxics. Hydrogen fluoride gas is considered to be a pollutant of "high concern" under this ranking system due to its "severe acute toxicity."

If we turn to the standard textbooks on air pollution, we find quite a wide variance in the treatment of hydrogen fluoride. Wark, Warner, and Davis in their book *Air Pollution: Its Origin and Control* list hydrogen fluoride as one of the seven "primary gaseous air pollutants."[68] Boubel and coauthors in their text *Fundamentals of Air Pollution* give considerable coverage to gaseous fluoride emissions from phosphate fertilizer and aluminum reduction plants, and their chapter on human health includes more-or-less equally weighted discussions of the carbon cycle, the sulfur cycle, and the fluoride cycle.[69] Godish's book *Air Quality* does not list hydrogen fluoride as one of the 12 main gaseous pollutants but it does treat the compound in a chapter entitled "Welfare Effects," which discusses the impact of gaseous pollutants on plants and animals.[70] Lipfert, in his book *Air Pollution and Community Health*, scarcely mentions fluoride, dismissing the problem in a single sentence. "In the 1950s," he writes, "there was concern about the effects of fluoride on human and animal health, but these concerns seem to have since abated." Godish makes a similar statement, concluding that "fluorosis of livestock from air contamination is no longer as serious a problem as it was in the 1950s and 1960s ... as a result of the stringent control requirements now imposed on fluoride sources."[71]

The conclusion we draw from all this is that gaseous emissions of hydrogen fluoride from industrial sources, particularly phosphate fertilizer plants and aluminum reduction facilities, have the potential to do significant harm to natural vegetation, agricultural crops, and farm livestock. Their impact on human health is more problematic but certainly includes the possibility of severe respiratory impact. The threat of such releases into communities that host the suspect industries is much reduced over that of earlier years, thanks in large part to the effectiveness of the Clean Air Act Amendments of 1990, which placed stringent emissions controls on these industries.

So where does this conclusion lead us? The very fact that we have put this much effort into clarifying the facts about industrial hydrogen fluoride emissions is proof of the degree to which we are held hostage by the anti-fluoridation agenda. In truth, this entire topic is pretty much a red herring. The real issue before us is not whether hydrogen fluoride air contamination is harmful to our health, but whether this fact has any relevance in reaching a decision about the wisdom of adding 1 ppm fluoride to drinking water supplies. In point of fact, the response of the human body to the inhalation of hydrogen fluoride gas at high concentrations under acute short-term exposure has little to tell us about its response to chronic long-term exposure produced by ingestion of low fluoride concentrations in water. Many chemical substances (e.g., iron) are toxic at high concentrations but beneficial at low concentrations. Chlorine is a poisonous gas at high concentrations, but added to water at low concentrations it kills disease-carrying pathogens and makes our water safe to drink. Arsenic and lead are deadly poisons at high concentrations, yet trace amounts of these elements in our drinking water do us no harm.

For most chemical compounds there is a threshold level below which the human health impact is benign. In Chapter 10 we examine the controversies engendered by trying to identify this threshold for fluoride. In Chapter 8 we examine in much more detail the claims of potential health impacts from drinking fluoridated water. The point to be made here is not whether drinking fluoridated water is safe or unsafe, but that the anti-fluoridation strategy of inciting fear of fluoride in drinking water through reference to the very real dangers associated with hydrogen fluoride air pollution is unworthy of an honorable and rational opposition.

Manhattan Project

The Medical Section of the Manhattan Project was established at the University of Rochester to assess the radiation dangers associated with uranium and plutonium compounds. It was a huge program involving hundreds of medical researchers. The research results produced by this team of scientists were of immense importance in furthering human understanding of the effects of radiation on the human body. There is no question that the plutonium experiments carried out on human subjects at Strong Memorial Hospital that came to light after the war, and brought to public attention by Eileen Welsome in her book *The Plutonium Files*, placed a dark stain on this record, but this stain should not deflect acknowledgment of the overall value of the program through its many contributions to medical health for the nuclear age.

Once it became clear to Manhattan Project scientists that uranium hexafluoride was going to play a large role in the bomb program, a fluorine toxicology study was added to the Medical Section activities in Rochester. However, fluorine safety was never a major concern of the Manhattan Project leadership. The Deepwater incident does not rate a mention in Richard Rhodes' 886-page book *The Making of the Atomic Bomb*, or the most widely quoted of the earlier Manhattan Project histories, *Day of Trinity*.[72] At Rochester, the fluorine toxicology program received adequate funding to carry out its mandate, but it was far from the highest priority. A two-volume report of Manhattan Project activities at Rochester was published after the war. It was entitled *Pharmacology and Toxicology of Uranium Compounds*, but there was a subheading in smaller print that announced a "Section on the Pharmacology and Toxicology of Fluorine and Hydrogen Fluoride." This section, which comprised only one chapter out of 17, was dedicated to the "toxicity following inhalation of fluorine and hydrogen fluoride."[73] The emphasis on "inhalation" makes it clear that attention was focused on occupational accidents and atmospheric emissions rather than waterborne fluorides.

We can see no reason to doubt the reliability of fluoride toxicology studies carried out at Rochester. There is no reason to believe that contemporaneous interest in water fluoridation played any role in the Rochester studies. Service to the bomb program would surely have outweighed any peripheral interest that Manhattan Project scientists might have had in the progress of fluoridation efforts. In any case, their studies were not directly applicable to water fluoridation, focused as they were on exposure through inhalation rather than ingestion.

Nor do we see anything inappropriate in David Ast's invitation to Harold Hodge to join the advisory committee on the Newburgh fluoridation trial. By 1944, when this invitation was tendered, Hodge had established himself as the leading fluorine toxicologist in the country. It would seem logical to include such an expert on the advisory team, especially as he was based nearby in Rochester. Rather than being the sinister move seen by anti-fluoride foes, we see Ast's invitation to Hodge as rather brave. It must have taken some resolve to bring in a toxicologist who was familiar with acute fluoride poisoning and who might raise public concerns about such issues. It suggests a sincere interest on Ast's part to uncover negative health impacts if any were to arise. Ast seems to have had a firm hold on the program and a clear idea of where he was going; it seems unlikely that Hodge had much room to "shape and guide" the program as anti-fluoridationists charge.

Rather than censure, we also believe that Hodge's later support of fluoridation ought to be given considerable weight. Given his familiarity with the toxicological issues and his experience in an ongoing fluoridation trial, there was probably no other scientist better placed to assess both the risks and benefits of fluoridation. It is beyond belief that a scientist of his stature would have supported fluoridation so enthusiastically if he had even a shadow of a doubt about its safety. He certainly would not have done so just to get the AEC off the hook on a few lawsuits in New Jersey. As for his documented concerns about the possible impacts of fluorine on the central nervous system, these concerns arose with respect to acute exposures to high dose rates such as might be experienced by plant workers in an industrial accident. He never expressed any concern over chronic exposure to low dose rates such as occurs with the ingestion of fluoridated water. Indeed, he was the author of the paper that is most widely quoted in support of the complete safety of the 1.0-ppm concentration recommended for water fluoridation.[74]

The anti-fluoride camp also takes Ast to task for taking "secret" blood samples from the Newburgh subjects for analysis at Rochester. The fact is, there was nothing secret about the sampling program or its purpose. This program simply provides further evidence of the more sophisticated level of toxicological scrutiny in the Newburgh trial relative to that in other contemporaneous trials.

The question of internal censorship of externally published Manhattan Project articles is more problematic. There is little doubt that security was a very high priority issue in the project, particularly in the years following the Soviet spy scandals. The results of most scientific research were not released at all until many years after their genesis. The fluoride toxicology papers from the Medical Section staff in Rochester were among the first to be published in the outside literature after the war. This fact is a further indication that this work was not regarded as particularly sensitive by the AEC brass. Nevertheless, given the AEC traditions, it is quite likely that even these papers suffered under the red pen of project editors. Griffiths and Bryson are respected journalists and we have no reason to doubt their word that editorial changes were made to at least one postwar fluoride toxicology paper, and that these changes were in a direction favorable to AEC interests.[75] It is likely that most papers emanating from the Rochester group, including Harold Hodge's contributions to the Newburgh fluoridation trials, were edited to some degree.

Having said this, we cannot get as exercised about it as anti-fluoridationists do. First, it is not uncommon for papers written by scientists in an institutional milieu to undergo editing. Although it is unfortunate but true that such editing often includes changes that toe the company line, it is rare for scientists to allow their papers to be scientifically emasculated without a vicious fight. It is unlikely that AEC scientists allowed their papers to go forward for external publication if they felt that their scientific results were at all compromised in the editing process. Second, it seems unlikely that the AEC would feel particularly vulnerable with respect to the Rochester contributions to the Newburgh fluoridation studies. Despite anti-fluoridationist claims to the contrary, the AEC really had no vested interest in the fluoridation issue. Hodge was drawn into the program solely on the basis of his expertise, and AEC leaders were probably pleased to see one of their scientists involved in a project which was seen at the time by all reputable parties as an enlightened step toward better public health. Lastly, the results themselves do not seem at all doubtful or contentious. It is difficult to conjure up a reason for censorship. In our mind, the weight of evidence points to the harmless involvement of a reputable scientist in an interesting project, with his results appearing appropriately in the final reports, possibly edited, but surely uncorrupted.

Mind Control

Let's face it. If you believe the mind-control arguments, you qualify as a true-blue, bona fide conspiracy lover. When it comes to this level of paranoia, you either have it or you don't. We have to be honest: We don't. We think the space program *really landed* on the moon. We don't think the army is hiding aliens in that hanger in Roswell. And we don't think the government is trying to control our minds by putting fluoride in the water.

THE PERILS OF OBSESSION

Throughout the history of the fluoridation movement, and despite the strong backing of the medical and scientific establishment, more fluoridation referenda have been lost than won. Over the years, it has been a popular exercise for social scientists, most of whom came from the pro-fluoridation ranks themselves, to try to figure this out. "Given the recognized public health benefits of fluoridation," they ask, "how can anybody be persuaded to vote against it?" Some of the ideas they have put forward in this regard—the "alienation hypothesis," the "confusion hypothesis," and others—were discussed in Chapter 3. However, readers may also recall the less judgmental explanation offered there, wherein a well-informed and rational electorate may vote "no" on the basis of a perceived risk trade-off. While they fully believe that fluoridation offers a high likelihood of benefits, they see these benefits as relatively small (a few less cavities for their children), and in their mind, such benefits are offset by the admittedly low risk of a rather large disbenefit (like cancer or some other debilitating disease). In this light, social scientists perhaps ought to have addressed a question that we doubt they ever did: "Given the serious health and safety concerns that surface in every fluoridation battle," they might ask, "how can anybody be persuaded to vote for it?"

We believe that the answer to this second question often rests on who the voters most want to climb into bed with. On the one hand, they can align themselves with doctors and dentists and community leaders who appear to be making a rational case based on scientific evidence. On the other hand, they can join the shrill voices of apocalypse. Although some of the anti-fluoridation arguments about the health and safety of fluoridation may be worrisome, many voters balk at jumping into bed with a bunch of loose cannons who are blathering on about aluminum conspiracies and mind control. I suspect that these gaudy claims from the extreme fringe of the anti-fluoridation movement lost many more votes than they gained. One wonders if fluoridation would ever have taken hold without the benefit of these counterproductive activists. To the extent that fluoridation has established itself as a successful public health policy, the anti-fluoridation camp may well be a victim of its own shrill rhetoric, or at least that of its most extreme adherents.

REFERENCES

1. The term *fluorophobia* that appears in the title of this chapter has been appropriated from the National Center for Fluoridation Policy and Research, http://fluoride.oralhealth.org.

2. P. Heggen, *How We Got Fluoridated*, as posted by Stop Fluoridation USA, http://www.rvi.net/~fluoride/, 1999.

3. R. C. Weast, editor-in-chief, *Handbook of Chemistry and Physics*, 53rd ed. CRC Press, Boca Raton, FL, 1972, p. B-5.

4. The term *Satan's Metal* and much of the material in this section come from J. Bergman, *Aluminum: Satan's Metal and Killer of Millions? The Watchtower's Incredible Crusade Against Aluminum*, as posted at http://www.premier1.net. This website hosts the e-journal *JW Research: Research and Opinions on Jehovah Witnesses*. The articles in this journal, many by Bergman, are well researched and well written

but are far from unbiased. All reflect unfavorably on Jehovah Witness doctrine, in particular those aspects of doctrine that are seen to involve the occult, pseudo-science, and medical quackery.

5. Most of the biographical material on Leo Spira and Charles T. Betts included in this Section comes from D. R. McNeil, *The Fight for Fluoridation*, Oxford University Press, New York, 1957. Much of McNeil's Information on Spira Comes From Spira's autobiographical polemic *The Drama of Fluorine: Arch Enemy of Mankind*, Lee Foundation For Nutritional Research, San Diego, CA, 1953.

6. C. T. Betts, *Aluminum Poisoning*, Research Publishing, Toledo, OH, 1928. Betts was also the author of a later anti-fluoridation tract, *Dangers of Fluorine in Our Water Supply*, Research Publishing, Toledo, OH, 1953.

7. McNeil, 1957, op. cit.

8. C. T. Betts, An opinion upon aluminum kitchen utensils, *The Golden Age*, pp. 710–713, August 8, 1928.

9. Bergman, *Aluminum*, op. cit.

10. *The Golden Age*, p. 803, September 23, 1936.

11. A. A. Hopkins, Aluminum on trial, *Sci. Am.* 140(3), 246–248, March 1929.

12. *The Golden Age*, p. 275, January 23, 1929.

13. A. L. Gotzsche, *The Fluoride Question: Panacea or Poison*, Davis-Poynter, London, 1975. See also B. Merson, The town that refused to die, *Good Housekeeping*, January 1969.

14. G. L. Waldbott, A. W. Burgstahler, and H. L. McKinney, *Fluoridation: The Great Dilemma*, Coronado Press, Lawrence, KS, 1978.

15. Heggen, 1999, op. cit.

16. A clear exposition of the conspiracy can be found in an article by J. Griffiths, Fluoride: industry's toxic coup, *Covert Action Q.*, 42, pp. 26–30, 63, 66, Fall 1992 (reprinted in *Earth Island J.*, *Spring* 1998.) Among the anti-fluoridation books that cover this material are Waldbott et al., 1978, op. cit.; Gotzsche, 1975, op. cit.; and G. Caldwell and P. E. Zanfagna, *Fluoridation and Truth Decay*, Top Ecology Press, Reseda, CA, 1974. See also http://www.rvi.net/~fluoride/ and http://www.nofluoride.com.

17. *Life*, p. 38, May 9, 1938.

18. G. J. Cox, M. C. Matuschak, S. F. Dixon, M. L. Dodds, and W. E. Walker, Experimental dental caries: IV. Fluorine and its relation to dental caries, *J. Dent. Res.*, 18, 481, 1939.

19. G. J. Cox, New knowledge of fluorine in relation to dental caries, *J. Am Water Works Assoc.*, 31, 1926–1930, 1939.

20. Griffiths, 1992, op. cit.

21. Waldbott et al., 1978, op. cit. The figure mentioned there is $750,000.

22. S. Ewan, *PR: A Social History of Spin*, Basic Books, New York, 1996.

23. Griffiths, 1992, op. cit.; Heggen, 1999, op. cit.

24. Waldbott et al., 1978. The advertisement displayed there comes from *J. Am. Water Works Assoc.*, 43, 45, 1951. See also Caldwell and Zanfagna, 1974, op. cit.

25. The term *toxic coup* appears in the title of the article by Griffiths, 1992, op. cit.

26. See, for example, California Citizens for Safe Drinking Water, http://www.nofluoride.com.

27. Griffiths, 1992, op. cit.

28. Heggen, 1999, op. cit.

29. Contemporaneous descriptions of the Donora smog disaster are provided by J. Shilen, The Donora disaster, *Indust. Med.*, 18(2), 72, 1949; and J. G. Townsend, Investigation of the smog incident in Donora, Pennsylvania and vicinity, *Am. J. Publ. Health*, 40, 185, 1950. Historical perspective is provided by L. P. Snyder, The death-dealing smog over Donora, Pennsylvania: industrial air pollution, public health policy, and the politics of expertise, *Environ. Hist. Rev.*, Spring 1994; and C. Bryson, The Donora fluoride fog: a secret history of America's worst air pollution disaster, *Earth Island J.*, Fall 1998.

30. H. H. Shrenk, H. Heimann, G. D. Clayton, W. M. Gafafer, and H. Wexler, *Air Pollution in Donora, Pennsylvania*, Bulletin 306, U.S. Public Health Service, Washington, DC, 1949.

31. *Chem. Eng. News*, December 13, 1948, "Industrial News" column, item entitled "Fluorine gases in atmosphere as industrial waste blamed for death and chronic poisoning of Donora and Webster, Pa., inhabitants," apparently based on information submitted by Philip Sadtler.

32. Bryson, 1998, op. cit.

33. K. Roholm, *Flourine Intoxication*, H.K. Lewis, London, 1937.

34. Bryson, 1998, op. cit.

35. J. Griffiths and C. Bryson, Fluoride, teeth, and the atomic bomb, *Waste Not*, No. 414, September 1997. The conspiracy case is also made at greater length in a recent book by one of the original authors: C. Bryson, *The Fluoride Deception*, Seven Stories Press, New York, 2004.

36. Sonoma State University, Project Censored, press release: *Censored 1999: The News That Didn't Make the News*, March 1999.

37. R. Rhodes, *The Making of the Atomic Bomb*, Simon & Schuster, New York, 1987.

38. Griffiths and Bryson, 1997, op. cit.

39. Ibid.

40. Heggen, 1999, op. cit.

41. E. Welsome, *The Plutonium Files: America's Secret Medical Experiments in the Cold War*, Dial Press, New York, 1999.

42. D. B. Ast, D. J. Smith, B. Wacks, and K. T. Cantwell, Newburgh–Kingston caries fluorine study: XIV. Combined clinical and roentgenographic dental findings after ten years of fluoride experience, *J. Am. Dent. Assoc.*, 52, 314–325, 1956.

43. P. P. Dale and H. B. McCauley, Dental conditions in workers chronically exposed to dilute and anhydrous hydrofluoric acid, *J. Am. Dent. Assoc.*, 37, 131–140, 1948.

44. D. Jackson, *Conspiranoia*, Plume Books, New York, 1999.

45. H. Moolenburgh, *Fluoride: The Freedom Fight*, Mainstream Publishing, Edinburgh, UK, 1987.

46. Gotzsche, 1975, op. cit.

47. Original paper: K. Tennakone and S. Wickramanayake, Aluminum leaching from cooking utensils, *Nature*, 325, 202, January 15, 1987. Refutation: J. Savory, J. R. Nicholson, and M. R. Willis, Is aluminum leaching enhanced by fluoride? *Nature*, 327, 107–108, May 14, 1987. Retraction: K. Tennakone and S. Wickramanayake, Aluminum and cooking, *Nature*, 329, 398, October 1, 1987. The episode is discussed in B. Martin, *Scientific Knowledge in Controversy: The Social Dynamics of the Fluoridation Debate*, State University of New York Press, Albany, NY, 1991.

48. Roholm, 1937, op. cit.

49. American Water Works Association, *Standards for Fluoridation Chemicals*: B701-99, Sodium Fluoride; B702-99, Sodium Silicofluoride; B703-00, Fluosilicic Acid; AWWA, Denver, CO.

50. Fluoridation Reporter, *Am. Dent. Assoc.*, 10(2), 1972 (as quoted in Caldwell and Zanfaga, 1974, op. cit.)

51. Martin, 1991, op. cit.

52. R. C. Williams, *The United States Public Health Service, 1798–1950*, U.S. PHS, Washington, DC, 1951.

53. Williams, 1951, op. cit.; McNeil, 1957, Op. Cit.; R. R. Harris, *Dental Science in a New Age: A History of the National Institute of Dental Research*, Montrose Press, Rockville, MD, 1989.

54. Harris, 1989, op. cit.

55. Waldbott et al., 1978, op. cit.

56. Historical information on the Kettering Laboratory comes from the University of Cincinnati Department of Environmental Health, http://www.eh.uc.edu.

57. E. J. Largent, *Fluorosis: The Health Aspects of Fluorine Compounds*, Ohio State University Press, Columbus, OH, 1961.

58. Historical information on the Mellon Institute comes from the Carnegie Mellon University, http://www.cmu.edu.

59. References for these reports can be found in the References for Chapters 7 and 8, where the results of these studies are presented and asessed.

60. Snyder, 1994, op. cit.

61. See for example, F. W. Lipfert, *Air Pollution and Community Health*, Van Nostrand Reinhold, New York, 1994; or R. W. Boubel, D. L. Fox, D. B. Turner, and A. C. Stern, *Fundamentals of Air Pollution*, 3rd ed., Academic Press, San Diego, CA, 1994.

62. Shilen, 1949, op. cit.; Townsend, 1950, op. cit.

63. A. Ciocco and D. J. Thompson, A follow-up of Donora ten years after: methodology and findings, *J. Publ. Health*, 51, 155–164, 1961.

64. Snyder, 1994, op. cit.

65. K. Roholm, The fog disaster in the Meuse Valley, 1930: a fluorine intoxication, *J. Ind. Hyg. Toxicol.*, 19(3), 126–137, 1937.

66. Lipfert, 1994, op. cit.; W. L. Cleland, Hazardous air pollutants, *Chapter 13 of Air Quality Control Handbook*, prepared by E. Roberts Alley and Associates, McGraw-Hill, New York, 1998.

67. *Toxicological Profile for Fluorides, Hydrogen Fluoride and Fluorine*, Agency For Toxic Substances and Disease Registry, U.S. Public Health Service, Washington, DC, 1993; *Health Issue Assessment: Summary Review of Health Effects Associated with Hydrogen Fluoride and Related Compounds*, U.S. Environmental Protection Agency, Washington, DC, 1989. A summary of the first document can be found at http://www.atsdr.cdc.gov/tfacts11.html, and of the second document at http://www.epa.gov/ttnatw01/hlthef/hydrogen.html.

68. K. Wark, C. F. Warner, and W. T. Davis, *Air Pollution: It's Origin and Control*, 3rd ed., Addison-Wesley, Reading, MA, 1998.

69. Boubel et al., 1994, op. cit.

70. T. Godish, *Air Quality*, 3rd ed., Lewis Publishing, Boca Raton, FL, 1997.

71. Lipfert, 1994, op. cit.; Godish 1997, op. cit.

72. L. Lamont, *Day of Trinity*, Atheneum, 1965; R. Rhodes, *The Making of the Atomic Bomb*, Simon & Schuster, New York, 1986.

73. C. Voegtlin and H. C. Hodge, *Pharmacology and Toxicology of Uranium Compounds, with a Section on the Pharmacology and Toxicology of Fluorine and Hydrogen Fluoride*, National Nuclear Energy Series, Manhattan Project Technical Section, 2 vols., McGraw-Hill, New York, 1949. The chapter on fluorine is Chapter 17 by H. E. Stokinger, "Toxicity Following Inhalation of Fluorine and Hydrogen Fluoride."

74. H. C. Hodge, The concentration of fluorides in drinking water to give the point of minimum caries with maximum safety, *J. Am. Dent. Assoc.*, 40, 436–439, 1950.

75. Dale and McCauley, 1948, op. cit.

CHAPTER 7

LOOK, MA. NO CAVITIES: FLUORIDE AND TEETH

Men and women have been getting toothaches since time immemorial. Early medical savants recognized that the pain was associated with rotted pits and cavities in the teeth, but they didn't know the cause of the rot. The anonymous authors of Chinese medical texts written 27 centuries before the birth of Christ may have been among the first to speculate. They suggested that tiny worms invade the mouth and carve out the painful pits. This "worm theory" of dental caries, which sounds so fanciful to the modern ear, had remarkable staying power. Four thousand years later, Pope John XXI's *Treasure of Health* (first published in the late thirteenth century but still in print in a third edition in 1556), recommended roasting henbane seeds over hot coals and sucking the smoke into one's mouth so as to "killeth the worms, and assuageth the pain." It was not until 1757 that a dental treatise appeared that convincingly disputed the existence of worms in decayed teeth.[1]

The demise of the worms did not end the widespread usage of many quaint folk remedies for the cure of the toothache. Among the more popular were a celery root hung around the neck, roasted parings of turnips behind the ear, and opium tempered with the yolk of a hald-boiled egg.[2] Perhaps just as likely to work was the following instruction, presumably tongue-in-cheek, from the 1857 *Farmer's Almanac*: "Get a kettle of water. Let it come to a boil. Put your head into it and let simmer for precisely half an hour. Take out your head and shake all your teeth into a heap. Pick out the decayed ones and throw them away. The sound ones you can put back in again."[3]

In the early Christian era, Catholic clerics performed most dental surgery. In the Middle Ages, it was barbers. Dentistry did not become an occupation until the early nineteenth century and was not recognized as a medical

The Fluoride Wars: How a Modest Public Health Measure Became America's Longest-Running Political Melodrama   By R. Allan Freeze and Jay H. Lehr
Copyright © 2009 John Wiley & Sons, Inc.

profession until long after that. As late as 1897, those with medical aspirations could heed this advertisement in an agricultural journal: "Be Your Own Dentist: Family dental care, with filling for twenty teeth, instruments, and full instructions. Sent by mail on receipt of $2." Or, for a slightly higher fee of $5, one could purchase Dr. Hale's Home Dental Outfit, whereby "teeth are easily and painlessly filled at home without previous experience."[4]

All this concern about cavities and toothaches, from antiquity through the dawn of the modern era, reflected more on the painfulness of the affliction and the lack of a remedy (oil of cloves and cinnamon, notwithstanding) than it did on the frequency of its occurrence. Prior to the industrial revolution, dental caries was a relatively uncommon complaint. Some people never experienced it; others, perhaps once or twice in a lifetime. Then, in the late nineteenth century, what had in days past been a rarity became an epidemic. By the early years of the twentieth century, most people experienced tens of cavities. Over 20% of the population ultimately lost all their permanent teeth.[5] The selling and fitting of false teeth became big business. By midcentury, at the time when fluoridation appeared on the scene, dental caries was one of the most prevalent diseases in the United States, especially among children and teenagers, and anything that offered relief was bound to be considered a godsend. These were the days before painless anesthetics and modern drills, and a visit to the dentist still conjured up images of giant needles and scary-looking hooked metal tools that would soon be probing the deepest crevices of our teeth searching out the most sensitive and painful nerves. It is no surprise that one of the most effective scenes of horror ever filmed by Hollywood features Laurence Olivier as a Nazi on the run in *The Boys of Brazil*, opening up his leather packet of gleaming dental probes, ready to "experiment" on Dustin Hoffman, who is bound helplessly in Olivier's reclining dental chair.

Perhaps Ogden Nash* put it best in this immortal couplet:[6]

> One thing I like less than most things is sitting in a dentist chair
>   with my mouth wide open,
> And that I will never have to do it again is a hope that I am
>   against hope hopen.

The lure of fluoridation, then, is clear. It is not surprising that the early trials in Grand Rapids, Newburgh, and Brantford had strong public support, and that interest ran high across the country awaiting a favorable outcome. We have already learned of the success of these early trials in proving the value

---

*Ogden Nash, This Is Going to Hurt Just a Little Bit, *The Face Is Familiar: Selected Verse of Ogden Nash*, Garden City Publishing, 1941. Copyright © 1935 by Ogden Nash. Reprinted by permission of Curtis Brown, Ltd.

of fluoride in the reduction of dental caries in the test communities. But we also learned some of the shortcomings of those experiments. It is natural to wonder whether these early successes have been sustained in ongoing studies over the years. In this chapter we look at the later studies of the effectiveness of fluoridation and assess the value of these studies and their conclusions. Before doing so, however, we ought to learn a little more about tooth decay. What causes it? And what led to the twentieth-century epidemic in the United States? Then, if we are to credit fluorine for the eradication of this plague, we ought to learn more about this peculiar element. How does it occur in nature? What happens to it when we ingest it into the human body? And what are the mechanisms by which it might prove effective in the reduction of dental caries?

TEETH

In case you haven't counted them recently, and assuming that you haven't lost any, you have 32 teeth in your mouth. For ease of reference, dentists have both names and numbers for every one of them.[7] The numbering system used in the United States differs from that used internationally, but one is as good as another. The U.S. system begins with the upper-right-hand backmost tooth, and goes from one to 16, right to left, across your upper jaw. Then it runs from 17 to 32, from left to right, along your lower jaw. There are four quadrants in your mouth (upper left, upper right, lower left, and lower right), and each quadrant has eight teeth. Starting from the middle of your two front teeth, the dental profession identifies them as *central, lateral, cuspid, first bicuspid, second bicuspid, first molar, second molar,* and *third molar.* The third molars are widely known as the wisdom teeth, and if you had all four of them extracted in early adulthood, as many people do, you are now missing teeth numbers 1, 16, 17, and 32 and are destined to go through life with 28 teeth (not to mention less wisdom).

As the tooth fairy well knows, we go through two sets of teeth in our lifetime. The baby teeth, or *primary dentition* (sometimes called the *deciduous dentition*), actually begin to develop in the prenatal fetus and stay with us through infancy and early childhood. Adult teeth, or *permanent dentition,* also begin to develop shortly after birth and stay with us through adulthood. In late childhood, there is a period of *mixed dentition,* as the baby teeth are lost and the permanent teeth emerge. The primary teeth are generally replaced by permanent teeth by age 12.

Each tooth is a relatively complex physical, chemical, and biological system. Figure 7.1 identifies the many features that make up a tooth. The *crown* is that part of the tooth above the gum line; the *root* is that part of

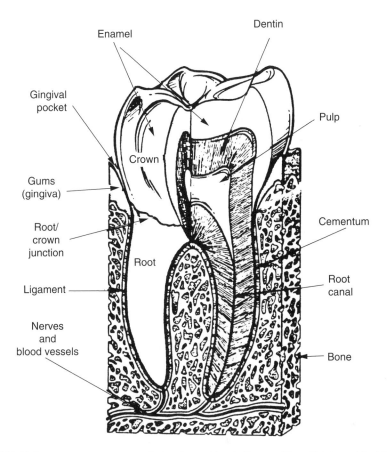

FIGURE 7.1 The tooth. (*Source*: T. McGuire, *Tooth Fitness: Your Guide to Healthy Teeth*, St. Michael's Press, 1994.)

the tooth below the gum line. The outer layer of the crown is made of hard *enamel*, the inner layers of softer *dentin* and softer-yet *pulp*. Electron microscope images of tooth enamel reveal that it consists of bundles of parallel rodlike structures, with each rod filled with crystals of the mineral apatite. The pulp contains cells, blood vessels, and nerves. Some teeth have one root, some have two, and others have three or more. Each root has a *root canal* at its center, a layer of *cementum* that covers the root, and *ligaments* that completely surround the cementum and attach the tooth to the bone. The gums, also known as *gingiva*, are a type of skin that covers and protects the bone between and around the teeth. The space between the crown and the gums is known as the *gingival crevice*.

The grinding surfaces on the tops of the molars and bicuspids are known as *occlusal surfaces*. (You may also hear your dentist refer to *proximal, distal, mesial, buccal, and lingual surfaces.*) The occlusal surfaces have more topography than the smooth vertical surfaces that we show off when we smile. The occlusal surfaces feature cusps and grooves, and the enamel on the cusps is thicker than that in the grooves. The bicuspids get their name from their twin cusps, with a single groove between. The molars feature more complex relief, with several cusps creating a branchlike network of grooves.

Teeth are constantly bathed in oral fluids. There is *saliva*, which is generated and circulated through the mouth, and there are *gingival fluids* that occupy the crevices between gums and teeth. Of even greater relevance to the occurrence of dental caries is the buildup of *plaque* that forms on tooth surfaces. This thin, sticky, colorless deposit is a mixture of bacteria (both dead and alive), saliva, food particles, and dead skin cells. It can be *subgingival* or *supragingival*, depending on whether it occurs above or below the gum line. If plaque is allowed to remain on the tooth surfaces, it may become calcified into *calculus* or *tartar*, which bonds to the teeth even more strongly than plaque.

The tooth surfaces that are most susceptible to dental caries are those where the enamel is thin or absent, and where plaque is most likely to build up. These include the occlusal grooves, the contact points where two teeth touch, roots that become exposed due to gum recession, tooth surfaces just above the gums, surfaces that exhibit pits or other defects, and areas underneath fillings or where fillings meet teeth.

There seems to be a wide variance among the population in susceptibility to dental caries. During the period when caries was more common than it is today, some people had tens of cavities whereas others had few or none. In trying to get a handle on what controlled this variance, dental researchers have carried out many surveys of dental health over the years in many parts of the country and in many parts of the world. In doing so, they needed a simple measure of caries occurrence that could be used to compare the prevalence of tooth decay from place to place and time to time. Early on, they began using the number of decayed, missing, and filled teeth as this measure, referring to it as the *DMF index*. In 1945, when the fluoridation trials first got under way, it was the DMF index that was used to keep account of caries incidence, and it is the mean scores of this index that appear on Tables 5.1 and 5.2, charting the progress of the trials in the various cities.

With time, some researchers felt the need for a more detailed index that would reflect the caries status for each tooth surface rather than for the tooth as a whole. Other researchers saw the value in differentiating between DMF scores for primary teeth and those for permanent teeth. As outlined in Table 7.1, there are now four different DMF scores in common use.[8] Those in capital letters (DMFT and DMFS) refer to *permanent* dentition; those in lowercase letters (dmft and dmfs) refer to *primary* dentition. Those with a T on

TABLE 7.1   Measures of Dental Caries

Measure	Definition
DMFT	Number of decayed, missing, or filled teeth, permanent dentition
dmft	Number of decayed, missing, or filled teeth, primary dentition
DMFS	Number of decayed, missing, or filled tooth surfaces, permanent dentition
dmfs	Number of decayed, missing, or filled tooth surfaces, primary dentition
% Caries-free	Percentage of persons in the population (or in a statistical sample of the population) who have no decayed, missing, or filled teeth

the end (DMFT and dmft) are based on the number of *teeth* affected, as in the original index. Those indices with an S on the end (DMFS or dmfs) are based on the number of affected *tooth surfaces*. Molars, cuspids, and bicuspids are considered as having five surfaces each, front teeth four surfaces. For people with 28 teeth, the maximum DMFT score is 28, the maximum DMFS score, 128. It is obvious that the two indices are quite different, yet there are occasions when one would like to compare the results of a survey that has used the DMFT index with one that has used the DMFS index. A method for doing so is available,[9] and we will see an example of its use later, in Table 7.2.

THE PEOPLE'S DISEASE

The tremendous numbers of cavities in school-aged children in the United States in the early twentieth century led the dental establishment to embark on a concerted campaign to clarify the causes of dental caries and to establish preventive protocols. So ubiquitous was dental caries, and so democratic in its attack on the children of all social classes, that the Public Health Service referred to it as the "people's disease."[10]

Early dental researchers tended to go in one of two directions when searching for the cause of dental caries. One group, having dispensed with worms as the cunning external agents, now wanted to pin the blame on a more modern and more likely set of culprits: the bacterial microorganisms that were by then known to inhabit the human mouth. At any given time, your mouth contains hundreds of different types of bacteria, and millions of individual microorganisms. In a mouth with prevalent tooth decay, there are even more of them. One dental text claims that there are "more germs in the diseased mouth than there are stars in the Milky Way galaxy."[11] In the early years of the twentieth century, dental scientists set out to determine which of these many bacteria might be most active in the attack on tooth enamel. In 1924, a British scientist,

J. Kilian Clarke, identified the microorganism *Streptococcus mutans* as the most likely candidate.[12] Subsequent work over the years has shown the importance of several other bacterial strains, but the position of *S. mutans* has never been challenged as the dominant microbial actor on the caries stage.

The other group of researchers zeroed in on diet, and in particular on the increasing popularity of sugar in the diet. White sugar, or sucrose, is a fermentable carbohydrate whose fermentation produces acids that are known to dissolve tooth enamel. Other sugars, such as lactose (which is found in milk), may also have a detrimental effect. Early observers of the caries epidemic recognized that it is a disease that is associated with increasing prosperity and acculturation.[13] Dental caries is not common in primitive societies, nor was it common in European society before the thirteenth century, when the arrival of refined sugar on the market first bred a love of sweet confections. We know this because, believe it or not, there are a group of dental archeologists, whose research involves the exhuming of the bodies of long-ago-buried children and the examination of caries prevalence in those whose teeth have been suitably preserved. Their findings confirm the absence of caries in prehistoric times, and a slow growth in the disease beginning in the Middle Ages and carrying on through the seventeenth and eighteenth centuries to modern times.[14]

Initially, only the rich imbibed the sweet white crystals. Queen Elizabeth I was said to be overfond of sugar and suffered greatly from dental caries as a result.[15] But eventually, all the classes, both high and low, got to share the pleasure (and the pain). With an improved lot in life came increased accessibility to sugar in the diet. In 1820, annual sugar consumption in England was less than 10 kilograms (kg) per person and dental caries was still fairly rare. In the early twentieth century, it was more than 40 kilograms per person and caries was rampant. Today, annual sugar consumption varies widely around the world. In the less developed world (e.g., Ethiopia, China, Thailand), annual sugar use is less than 10 kg per person. In the developed countries (e.g., Australia, Great Britain, United States), it is greater than 40 kg per person. There is a strong inverse correlation with the prevalence of tooth decay. By age 12, at the height of the caries epidemic, children in the less developed world averaged only one cavity per child; those in the developed countries, eight.[16]

Observers have also noted greater increases in the number of cavities in urban children than in rural children, and ascribed this fact to the more liberal access of urban children to highly sweetened junk food. Cases have also been documented where isolated population groups with no experience of caries developed the disease when exposed to sugar-rich Western diets. Australian Aborigines, New Zealand Maoris, and North American

Eskimos experienced little tooth decay before the arrival of European colo-
nists. More recently, further confirmation of the role of sugar was provided
by the sharp decline in dental caries that was observed in England and
Japan during World War II under the sugar rationing programs in place at
that time.

As it turns out, we now know that both groups involved in the search for
the cause of tooth decay were right. Modern science has clarified the conditions under which dental caries develops, and both microbiology and diet
play a role.[17] There are three requirements: a sucrose-rich diet, the presence
of microorganisms that like to metabolize sucrose, and susceptible teeth.
Bacteria of the *Streptococcus mutans* strain do the job. They colonize on teeth
surfaces, forming plaque. Protected from removal by the adhesive properties
of the plaque, they metabolize the sugar, fermenting it and releasing acid in
the process. Saliva is the body's natural protective mechanism. It protects
the teeth to some degree by neutralizing the acid, but if more acid is generated than the saliva can neutralize, the acid begins to dissolve the apatite
mineral crystals that comprise the tooth enamel, and cavities are initiated.
Carbonate impurities in the apatite crystal lattice, being more soluble than
the host mineral, are particularly susceptible to initial attack. If the lesions
occur where the enamel is thin, as in occlusal grooves, the caries process may
make its way through the enamel, and begin to attack the softer and less
resistant dentin in the interior of the crown.

These ideas emerged from the dental research world in the first half of
the twentieth century like pieces of a jigsaw puzzle randomly falling into
place. It was not really until 1955 that incontrovertible proof of the validity of
the sucrose–bacteria model was presented. In that year, a research team led
by Frank Orland, the director of the Zoller Memorial Dental Clinic at the University of Chicago, reported their results from a set of laboratory experiments
carried out on specially bred bacteria-free hamsters.[18] They observed that no
caries developed in the bacteria-free animals, even when they were fed a
sugary diet that always produces caries in normally bred members of this
species. In 1960, two scientists at the National Institute of Dental Research,
Robert J. Fitzgerald and Paul Keyes, carried out further experiments on the
growth of caries in these specially bred hamsters. They confirmed that one
needs *both* a sucrose diet *and* the presence of bacteria such as *S. mutans* to
produce tooth decay. With the sugar diet and no bacteria, caries did not
develop. With bacterial colonization and no sucrose, caries did not develop.
Only when both were present together did cavities arise on the hamster's
tiny teeth.[19]

There are other contributing factors, of course. It is now recognized that
chewing can be important in reducing caries. In prehistoric times (and in less

developed countries) the available cuisine required more chewing, whereas modern diets tend to reduce chewing. Lack of vigorous chewing may play a minor role in the growth of caries over the ages. It has even been suggested that regular chewing of (sugarless) gum may be beneficial in caries prevention.

In our current milieu of abundant sugar access, social conditions often control the amount and frequency of sugar intake and the level of oral care given to children's teeth. Caries rates are a fairly reliable indicator of socioeconomic status. Children from disadvantaged backgrounds suffer disproportionately from caries affliction. Changes in social conditions usually change the caries rate.

REVERSAL OF MISFORTUNE

With the mechanisms of dental caries understood, the preventive options clarified themselves. Three main approaches to combating the caries epidemic came to the fore. First, one can try to reduce or modify the intake of caries-promoting ingredients in the diet. In this class, fought at every turn by the sugar lobby, and never all that successful, were the many public campaigns to reduce the sugar intake of children. More successful in the long run was the search for a sugar substitute that could sweeten food without providing fodder for bacterial metabolization, a search that ultimately culminated in the development and wide use of the artificial sweetner dipeptide aspartame. Second, one can try to combat the buildup of caries-inducing microorganisms. This approach emphasizes improved oral hygiene through regular brushing and flossing and the use of mouthwashes and oral rinses containing antimicrobial agents designed to prevent the formation of plaque. Third, and most pertinent to our discussions, one can try to increase the resistance of the teeth to attack. Much research has been carried out on various types of sealants that can be applied to teeth to smooth and seal pits and fissures. But of course the greater effort has gone toward attempts to strengthen teeth through the optimization of fluoride intake.

From the beginning, there had always been two lines of thought on how best to get fluoride to the teeth. Up to this point, we have emphasized the *systemic* approach, whereby fluoride reaches the teeth only after it is metabolized into our bodily system following the ingestion of fluoridated water. However, there was also considerable support in the dental research community for *topical* applications of fluoride directly onto the teeth. This approach was pioneered by J. F. Volker of the University of Rochester (together with the ever-present Harold Hodge) and Basil Bibby of Tufts University, who experimented in the early 1940s with fluoride therapies that involved painting the teeth with a solution of sodium fluoride.[20] In 1945, John Knutson of the Minnesota State Department of Health and Wallace Armstrong of the University of Minnesota presented the results of a trial of topical fluoride therapy that was similar in design to the trials of community water fluoridation then being carried out in Grand Rapids and Newburgh. They reported a 40% reduction in caries in the Minnesota test communities within a year or two of the application of fluoride coatings on selected tooth surfaces.[21]

Topical fluoride therapy continued to grow in popularity during the same period that community water fluoridation was sweeping the nation. Congress allocated $1 million for the promotion of topical fluoride programs as early as 1949, and there was continued congressional support through the years. In the National Caries Program, which was a concerted attack on tooth decay carried out by the National Institute of Dental Research during the early 1970s, emphasis was placed on topical programs. The flagship study involved the participation of 75,000 students in 17 communities over a three-year period, during which time subjects were given a weekly oral rinse with a 0.2% solution of sodium fluoride. This program was judged a great success, and wider-ranging ventures followed. By 1981, over 13 million children in 44 states were participating in self-applied, school-based fluoride mouth-rinsing programs.[22]

Adding to the topical dosage was the widespread use of fluoridated toothpastes. Procter & Gamble were the first off the mark, introducing Crest toothpaste onto the market in 1955. Initially, it made little impact, but buoyed upward by the clever "Look, Ma. No Cavities!" advertising campaign, its market share climbed, and then with the controversial endorsement of Crest in 1960 by the American Dental Association, it exploded. By 1985, almost every toothpaste manufacturer had a fluoride brand on drugstore shelves, and the total market share of all fluoridated toothpastes in the United states had risen to over 90%.[23]

With all this fluoride targeted on the nation's teeth, the dental community felt that the prevalence of dental caries was sure to decline. They eagerly awaited the outcome of every study, anxious to see whether the promise of the early fluoridation trials would be fulfilled. When the results began to trickle in the 1960s and 1970s, and then became a torrent in the 1980s, they learned that their dreams had come true. Not only had the prevalence of dental caries declined, it had done so precipitously! Wondrously! And not only at home, but around the world (or at least in the developed countries around the world). One review article, written in 1988, listed 33 studies from 12 different developed countries (United States, United Kingdom, Ireland, Australia, New Zealand, Sweden, Denmark, Finland, Norway, Netherlands, Hungary, and Iceland) that were carried out during the 10-year period between 1979 and 1989, each of which documented a decline in caries. The reported rates of decline were as great as 60% and averaged more than 35%.[24] Another author, writing in 1982, went so far as to say that dental caries "may have been eliminated as a public health problem in the United States."[25]

One can get an idea of the universality of the decline by examining the data contained in the Global Oral Data Bank maintained by the World Health Organization at the WHO Collaborating Center at Malmo University in Malmo, Sweden (easily accessible on the Internet).[26] The data are listed as year-by-year mean DMFT values for 12-year-old children on a countrywide basis for hundreds of countries in the world. Some of these data are summarized in Table 7.2, which provides representative evidence of the caries decline in the industrialized countries in the second half of the twentieth century. The nationwide DMFT scores for 15 European countries fell from a median value of 5.9 when the first reckonings were made (during the period 1950–1975) to a value of 1.5 when the most recent calculations were carried out (during the period 1990–2000). The data for Sweden, also shown in Table 7.2, are representative. The median nationwide DMFT fell smoothly from 7.8 to 0.9 between 1937 and 1999.

TABLE 7.2   Decline in Dental Caries in the Developed Countries of the World as Indicated by DMFT Scores for 12-Year-Old Children During the Period 1937–2000

Country	Date	Estimate of Representative Nationwide DMFT		Source[a]
		Range	Median	
15 European countries	First nationwide calculation, 1950–1975	3.2–8.7	5.9	(1)
	Most recent nationwide calculation, 1990–2000	0.9–2.1	1.5	(1)
Sweden	1937		7.8	(1)
	1977		6.3	(1)
	1990		2.0	(1)
	1999		0.9	(1)
United States	1945	6.99–11.66	8.8	(2)
	1965–1967		4.0	(1)
	1979–1980		2.4	(3)
	1986–1987		1.7	(3)
	1991		1.4	(1)

[a](1) World Health Organization, Global Oral Data Bank.[26] (2) Four trial cities prior to fluoridation, from Table 5.1. (3) Second NIDR national survey of U.S. schoolchildren.[28] DMFS scores converted to DMFT scores.[27]

The United States has undergone a similar transformation, also noted in Table 7.2. If we take the pre-fluoridation DMFT values from the four fluoridation-trial cities as representative of the nation, the median nation-wide DMFT has declined from 8.8 in 1945 to 1.4 in 1991. The intermediate values listed in Table 7.2 for 1979–1980 and 1986–1987 come from detailed national surveys of caries prevalence in U.S. schoolchildren carried out by the National Institute of Dental Research. Their results, reported as DMFS scores, have been converted to DMFT scores to make the numbers consistent with the WHO data. There are lots of assumptions and difficulties involved in this con-version,[27] but the resulting figures are sufficiently robust for our purposes.

The NIDR surveys were massive undertakings that required consider-able organization, personnel, and money. The Second National Survey of Caries in U.S. Schoolchildren, carried out in 1986–1987, for example, involved the examination of over 39,000 children, aged 5 through 17, in hundreds of schools across the country. The protocols and interpretive methodology were much improved over those used in the original fluoridation trials, so that criticism on this front from the anti-fluoridation movement was largely deflected. The 14 dental teams that carried out the examinations were fully calibrated by the NIDR. They used standardized diagnostic criteria, and they performed replicate examinations by different examiners on a subset of the subjects at each location. The country was divided into seven geographic regions, and stratified further by median family income and urban versus rural lifestyle, so that possible confounding factors could be investigated. Information was obtained from parents for every child in the study docu-menting residence history, dental health history, and history of fluoride use from all sources. It was possible to identify those children who had lived continuously at a single residence in either a fluoridated or nonfluoridated community, and to separate out those children in either circumstance who had access to topical fluorides.

The results of the 1986–1987 NIDR survey were presented in a special issue of the *Journal of Dental Research* in February 1990.[28] Figure 7.2 is taken from that article. The solid line in the figure graphs the mean measured DMFS scores for all 39,000 children as a function of their age. Unsurprisingly, the total number of caries sites in a child's mouth increases with age, in this case from 0.07 at age 5 to 8.04 at age 17. The DMFS value for 12-year-old children (which was converted to a DMFT value of 1.7 in Table 7.2) is 2.66. The overall average DMFS value for all subjects of all ages in the 1986–1987 survey was 3.07.

The dashed and dotted lines on Figure 7.2 indicate the results from two earlier nationwide surveys: the first NIDR National Survey of Caries in U.S. Schoolchildren in 1979–1980, and an earlier study carried out during

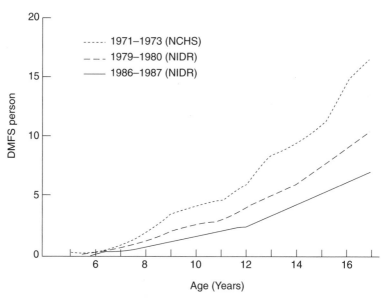

FIGURE 7.2 Age-specific incidence of dental caries in U.S. schoolchildren in three national epidemiological surveys, showing reduction in caries over period 1971–1987. (*Source*: J. A. Brunelle and J. P. Carlos, Recent trends in dental caries in U.S. children and the effect of water fluoridation, *J. Dent. Res.*, 69, 723–727, 1990.)

the National Caries Program by the National Center for Health Statistics. The overall average DMFS values for the earliest study was 7.01, and for the middle study, 4.77, indicating a decline in caries prevalence of 32% between 1973 and 1980, and a further decline of 36% between 1980 and 1987.

The full sweep of caries prevalence in the industrialized nations over recorded history is illustrated in Figure 7.3. This graph shows the near-absence of caries in prehistoric times, the slow growth of the disease through the Middle Ages as acculturation and sugar use increased, the epidemic levels reached by the turn of the twentieth century, and the precipitous decline since 1950. The rising side of the curve is based on the findings of the dental archeologists mentioned earlier, and in particular on a summary figure from an article by Elizabeth O'Sullivan and co-workers of the Department of Child Dental Health at the University of Leeds in England.[29] The falling side of the curve is a schematic plot of the data from Table 7.2. The rightmost point on the curve, for the year 2000, is based on WHO's Global Trends and Projections for Oral Health, which indicates a global weighted mean DMFT value for 12-year-olds of 1.74. This value is remarkably similar to estimated caries rates in prehistoric human beings. WHO further notes that 70% of the reporting countries, representing 85% of the world population, now have nationwide median DMFT indices below 3.0.[30]

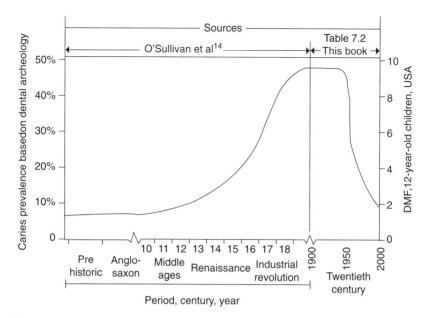

FIGURE 7.3   The rise and fall of dental caries in the industrialized nations from prehistoric times to the present day. (Note the nonlinear time scale.)

The dental community is unanimous in its view that the credit for this reversal of misfortune must be given to fluoride. Certainly, the synchronicity of the initiation of fluoridation and the decline in caries seems to provide an argument that is too powerful to question. However, there are two problems with this simple interpretation. Both have led to intense debate within the dental fraternity and in the hot-blooded world of pro- and anti-fluoridation politics.

The first issue is one that might initially appear to be of interest only to dental specialists, but in fact it has broader implications. The truth of the matter is that when the good news about caries decline first came to light and fluoride seemed the obvious choice as the catalyst of this pleasant turnaround, dental researchers still did not have a good handle on how fluoride might actually be doing the job. It was a source of some embarrassment in the dental community that the mechanisms by which the caries miracle had come to pass were so poorly understood. On the one hand, the effectiveness of drinking fluoridated water seemed to argue for the systemic effect. On the other hand, the johnny-come-lately topical applications, including the ever-more-popular fluoridated toothpastes, seemed to work just as well. Although the leaders of dental research organizations were quick to clarify that topical fluoride programs were intended to supplement, not compete with, community water fluoridation, this show of solidarity hid an intense debate about how fluoride actually works to reduce dental decay. Some researchers argued for the primacy of the systemic route, others for the topical route. Writing in 1993, the respected dental research scientist Louis W. Ripa stated that "despite nearly 50 years of fluoride use, the relative importance of these two modes of contact in the prevention of dental caries are still uncertain."[31] Ten years later, the debate continues, although some degree of consensus may be appearing on the horizon.

The second issue is very simple and will come as a shock to those who can't imagine how the evidence presented thus far could possibly lead to any doubts about the role of fluoride in the decline of caries. Well, there is a kicker. It turns out that the declines in dental caries observed, which are usually ascribed to community water fluoridation, have occurred not only in fluoridated communities but also in unfluoridated communities. Not only that, but many of the countries that have experienced significant declines in dental caries, including most of the 15 European countries noted in Table 7.2, do not have widespread community water fluoridation. Some of them have scarcely any. The caries decline in these unfluoridated countries of the developed world has been similar in timing and magnitude to that in fluoridated countries such as the United States.

Not surprisingly, anti-fluoridationists have been quick to leap on this fact and use it to proclaim that fluoridation is a huge hoax that is not in any way responsible for improved dental health. It is a staple argument in their rhetoric and in their written creed. Although the credibility of the more florid antis might be open to some question, that is not the case for some of the other doubters. There are several reputable researchers, both inside and outside the dental community, who have also raised the issue. Mark Diesendorf, a mathematics professor at the Australian National University, calls it "the mystery of declining tooth decay." His article under this title, which appeared in a 1986 issue of the prestigious scientific journal *Nature*, was one of the first to raise the flag.[32] By then, evidence of declining caries was becoming pretty solid, and Diesendorf does not dispute it. What he does dispute is the role of fluoridation as the sole contributor to the phenomenon. He relies heavily on the observation that caries rates are falling in unfluoridated areas just as they are in fluoridated areas. He claims, for example, that by 1983 the rate of caries prevalence in the Australian state of Queensland, which is only 5% fluoridated, was approximately equal to that in Western Australia, which is 83% fluoridated.

So we are left to ponder two questions. If fluoride is responsible for the decline in caries, just how does it work? And if it works, why are unfluoridated communities apparently getting just as much benefit as fluoridated ones? In the remainder of the chapter we address these questions in turn. However, if we are to understand the debates over these two issues and ponder the policy implications of any emerging consensus, we must first digress for a moment and learn a bit more about the chemical entity at the center of all the controversy, the fluoride ion itself.

THE FLUORIDE CYCLE: FROM APATITE TO APATITE

Fluorine is the seventeenth most abundant element in the Earth's crust. It is a member of the halogen family, sharing many properties with its sister elements on the periodic table: chlorine, bromine, and iodine. Fluorine is the most reactive of all the elements. It is so reactive that pure fluorine never occurs in nature. It always combines with other elements into compounds, many of which take the form of simple fluorides. It is *possible* to isolate pure fluorine in a laboratory, a feat that was first accomplished in 1886 and led to a 1905 Nobel prize for the chemist Henri Moisson, but it is not easy. At room temperature, fluorine is a pale yellow gas with a pungent odor. It is so corrosive that it cannot be held in most metal vessels. Many common materials such as wood or rubber held in a stream of fluorine gas at room temperature will burst into flames. Fluorine combines with hydrogen to form hydrogen fluoride gas, which we encountered in earlier chapters as a common air pollutant from certain industrial operations. Hydrogen fluoride and water produce hydrofluoric acid, which dissolves every metal except platinum and gold.[33]

Over the years fluorine has evolved from a laboratory curiosity to the point where it now holds an extremely valued place in modern industry. We have already learned the important role of uranium hexafluoride in the nuclear industry. Hydrofluouric acid is used widely in the etching and frosting of glass. Other fluorine compounds include the refrigerant Freon, the space-age plastic lubricant Teflon, and the fluorocarbons, which were widely used in aerosol spray dispensers until it was discovered that they may play a role in the depletion of the ozone layer, which shields the Earth from harmful shortwave solar radiation.

Fluorine occurs in nature primarily in the form of three minerals: fluorspar, cryolite, and apatite. *Fluorspar* is a calcium–fluoride salt that occurs as a transparent, cube-shaped, glasslike crystal that looks much like common salt. It has been used since the Middle Ages as a flux in metal-smelting operations. *Cryolite* is a relatively rare sodium–aluminum–fluoride mineral that was used in the early years of the aluminum-smelting industry in the process that separates aluminum from bauxite ore. *Apatite* is a calcium–phosphate mineral that occurs as a common rock-forming mineral in many granitic rocks. In addition to the calcium and the phosphate, the apatite crystal can accommodate chlorine, fluorine, or hydroxyl atoms in its lattice. The variety that hosts the fluorine atom is sometimes called *fluorapatite*. Apatite and fluorapatite are mined in many locations as a source of phosphate fertilizer. As we have already learned, apatite is also the mineral that makes up human tooth enamel. The fact that much of the fluoride used in community water fluoridation is derived from the waste streams produced during phosphate mining operations, together with the fact that much of the fluoride taken into the body as fluoridated water ends up in the tooth enamel, means that the fluoride that began as apatite also ends up as apatite.

The fluorine-bearing minerals in the Earth's crust are all sparingly soluble, so when groundwater flows through rocks containing these minerals, fluoride ions are released into the water. However, naturally occurring fluoride concentrations in groundwater are generally quite low, less than 0.5 ppm in most cases, rising to a few parts per million here and there (as we learned earlier was the case for well waters in Colorado Springs, Colorado; Bauxite, Arkansas; and Oakley, Idaho), and even as high as 30 to 40 ppm in isolated instances (primarily in Central Africa and the Indian subcontinent). Most freshwater streams in North America average less than 0.2 ppm, and the fluoride content of the ocean runs about 1 ppm or a little higher.[34] Fluoridated water supplies are adjusted to a concentration around 1.0 ppm. Most nonfluoridated water supplies have considerably lower concentrations.

Human beings take fluoride into their bodies through the air they breathe, the water they drink, and the food they eat. The metabolism of fluoride in the human body is relatively well understood and relatively simple.[35] In the first step, fluoride that is ingested as food or liquid is absorbed from the gastrointestinal tract into the bloodstream. Absorption is rapid and relatively complete; 80% of the food-based fluoride is absorbed and up to 97% of the liquid-based fluoride. Once in the bloodstream, fluoride ions are distributed rapidly to one of two destinations. Roughly 50% make it to the kidneys, from where they are excreted, almost entirely as urine. The other 50% are taken up by the mineral crystals of the body's hard tissues: the bones and the teeth. Fluorine is the most exclusive bone-seeking element known to medical science. It is the "bone-seeker par excellence."[36] Ninety-nine percent of all the fluorine in the human body occurs as fluoride in the calcified tissues of bones and teeth. The fluoride content of one's bones and teeth increases through life, although the *rate* of fluoride uptake slows with age.

So it is not really a surprise that ingested fluoride heads for the teeth, or perhaps even that the fluoride so incorporated into the teeth might make them more resistant to decay. What is needed from a scientific perspective, however, is not just the observation that this appears to be so, but a concrete and consistent explanation of how and why this resistance to decay comes to pass. To address this issue, we return once again to the first of the two contentious issues raised earlier: the debate over systemic versus topical fluoride therapy.

HOW FLUORIDE WORKS

When Frederick McKay and Trendley Dean first recognized the role played by the fluoride ion in reducing rates of dental caries in the United States in the 1930s, they thought that they were breaking entirely new ground. They were apparently unaware that there had already been considerable recognition of the value of fluoride in tooth health in earlier years in Europe, albeit in a grassroots rather than an academic vein. As early as 1874, articles had appeared in the European popular press promoting a role for fluoride to combat dental disease.[37] It was felt that a lack of sufficient fluorine in the diet might be responsible for the prevalence of tooth decay (and also apparently, appendicitis). To remedy the situation, it was recommended that 100 grams of finely powdered fluorspar be consumed daily. Historians of dental science have also drawn attention to the availability of calcium fluoride tablets that were marketed in Denmark in the early twentieth century under the brand name *Fluoridens*, claiming that they would "remedy the decay of the teeth." The distributors argued that tooth decay is "due mainly to the refined food-stuffs which do not contain a sufficient quantity of fluorine." A pamphlet from this era recommends that mothers sprinkle powdered Fluoridens onto their children's sandwiches in order to maintain the recommended daily dose.[38]

Whatever their knowledge may have been of these previous ideas, the early water fluoridation proponents had a conceptual rapport with their earlier kin. Taking Fluoridens tablets can clearly be classified as a systemic rather than a topical therapy, and when the idea of fluoride as a dental prophylactic first emerged in the United States in the 1930s, it was a systemic approach that was envisaged. The early proponents of community water fluoridation based their espousal of this approach on their belief that fluoride would reach the teeth under a systemic mechanism of delivery. The value of fluoride was assumed to lie in its incorporation into the apatite crystals of developing teeth. It was widely known in mineralogical circles at that time that the mineral *fluorapatite* is less soluble to acid attack than normal *apatite*. Normal apatite features a considerable proportion of hydroxyl groups in its crystal lattice. It was felt that the systemic uptake of fluoride by the teeth involved the replacement of the hydroxyl groups by fluoride ions, thus converting the normal apatite to fluorapatite, with a concomitant reduction in solubility. The lower solubility would provide greater resistance to acid dissolution and hence stronger, more resistant teeth.[39]

This conceptual model went hand in hand with a belief that water fluoridation would be of greatest value in the *pre-eruptive phase* of tooth development (i.e., for teeth that had not yet erupted into the mouth) rather than in the *post-eruptive phase*, after teeth have fully emerged into the mouth. On the basis of this reasoning, early fluoridation proponents felt that it was important that children receive fluoridated water from birth, so that developing teeth could experience the maximum possible fluoride uptake. They expected benefits to both the primary and permanent dentition, but they did not expect the benefits to manifest themselves until several years after the initiation of fluoridation in a community.

Even in the early years of the fluoridation trials, evidence came to light that should have called the pre-eruptive hypothesis into question. First, the dental researchers in charge of the trials themselves were surprised to find evidence of reduced caries after only two or three years of water fluoridation, and often in older children that had not had fluoride exposure during the pre-eruptive developmental period. Although results were equivocal in the early studies, it also appeared that beneficial effects were more pronounced in permanent teeth than in primary teeth. Clearer yet in their implications for the systemic theory were the findings coming out of Minnesota showing the benefits of topical fluoride applications. These benefits, similar in degree to those of water fluoridation, manifested themselves after only one or two years of therapy and without systemic ingestion of fluoride.

Despite this evidence, the systemic hypothesis remained in fashion in the dental community for several decades, and it was routinely heralded by fluoridation proponents in many a referendum battle. However, beginning in the 1980s, and gaining steam ever since, there has been a movement by dental researchers to look more carefully at the mechanisms of fluoride action. This movement was aided by the development of new analytical methods that allowed for more accurate determination of the fluoride content of teeth. Initial results were as expected. The average fluoride content of teeth in fluoridated communities was demonstrably higher than that in nonfluoridated communities. And as we have seen, the occurrence of dental caries was much reduced in the former communities relative to the latter. However, when studies were carried out on *individuals* within each community, results were *not* as expected. Investigator after investigator reported that there was no clear correlation between the fluoride levels in the tooth enamel of individual subjects and the dental caries experience of that person.

Moreover, the tooth–fluoride data provided additional evidence that did not sit well with the systemic hypothesis. It soon became clear that measured fluoride concentrations in tooth enamel were not large enough to have a significant effect on apatite solubility. The theoretical concentration of fluoride in pure fluorapatite is 38,000 ppm, and concentrations approaching this value would be needed to effect significant solubility reduction. However, the average whole-tooth concentrations of fluoride in tooth enamel in fluoridated communities seldom exceeded a few hundred parts per million. The idea of reduced apatite solubility as the primary mechanism of fluoride action was called into question.[40]

Furthermore, the pattern of fluoride concentrations in teeth did not square with a systemic uptake. If the mechanism of uptake were systemic, one would expect to find the fluoride distributed evenly throughout the tooth enamel, but detailed measurements have shown that this is not the case. Enamel thicknesses are on the order of 1000 micrometers (μm) or so, but high fluoride concentrations are found only in the outer 30 to 50 μm. Concentrations of fluoride in this outer layer of the enamel in fluoridated communities may approach 3000 ppm, but the remaining 95% of the tooth enamel is almost free of fluoride.[41] This finding offers strong support to those who believe in a topical mechanism that occurs at the tooth surface.

There are actually two quite independent topical mechanisms that have now been demonstrated by clinical and laboratory studies and which are now widely accepted in the dental community.[42] First, it is held that increased fluoride concentrations in the plaque reduce the ability of the plaque microorganisms to produce acid, thus reducing the severity of the attack on tooth enamel. Second, it is thought that increased fluoride concentrations in the oral fluids at the tooth surface promote the repair of the enamel at those points where lesions have been initiated by acid attack.

On the first front, fluoride is well known in microbiological circles as an inhibitor of enzyme activity in living cells. The fluoride that is topically absorbed into the plaque on tooth surfaces is taken up by the microorganisms in the plaque, where it interferes with their enzyme activity and inhibits the bacterial conversion of sugar to acid. The reduced levels of acid production are more easily neutralized by saliva, and less acid gets free to attack the tooth enamel.

The second mechanism relies on the concept of nature's striving for a chemical equilibrium at any solid–liquid interface. If the liquid at such an interface is undersaturated with respect to the chemical components that make up the solid, dissolution of the solid begins to take place. If the liquid becomes oversaturated with respect to these components, precipitation of the solid takes place. In our case, the solid is the mineral apatite in the tooth enamel, and the liquid is the oral fluid associated with saliva, plaque, and gingival fluids. Dissolution initiates the formation of lesions on the tooth surface; precipitation serves to repair the incipient lesions. As the acidity in the mouth rises and falls, there is a continuous cycle of *demineralization* through dissolution and *remineralization* through precipitation. The result is an ongoing process of crystals dissolving and re-forming on tooth surfaces. Large numbers of laboratory studies now confirm that the presence of fluoride ions in the oral fluids inhibits demineralization and facilitates remineralization, thus providing a double dose of protection against tooth decay. Furthermore, it has been clearly shown in these experiments that even very low fluoride concentrations in the plaque provide considerable protection.

Despite the emerging consensus, the systemic hypothesis is not entirely dead. It is pointed out by some observers that systemic and topical effects can easily be blurred; some systemic products have topical effects, and vice versa. And in one of the most careful studies carried out to date, a team of scientists from the Netherlands, using data for 15-year-olds exposed to fluoride since birth in the Tiel–Culemborg fluoridation trial, concluded that the caries reduction observed was 50% due to pre-eruptive systemic effects and 50% to topical post-eruptive effects.[43] The American Dental Association, in their *Fluoridation Facts* pamphlet, still credits systemic mechanisms equally with topical mechanisms.[44] However, the tide is turning. One widely used textbook states baldly that the dramatic decline in caries in the 1970s is "largely due to the post-eruptive exposure to fluoride," and that the pre-eruptive contribution is "likely to be small in comparison with the post-eruptive effect."[45] Yet another major review concludes that "the major cariostatic effect is post-eruptive and topical."[46] In the ultimate capitulation, even the U.S. Public Health Service is now on board, affirming that the "theory of pre-eruptive fluoride incorporation as the sole or principal mechanism of caries prevention has been largely discounted."[47]

So, if the mechanism of fluoride action on tooth enamel is topical and post-eruptive rather than systemic and pre-eruptive, the question arises as to whether the ingestion of fluoridated drinking water is doing us any good at all. There are some respected dental researchers who think not. Two Danish researchers who have published widely in this area, A. Thylstrup of the Royal Dental College in Copenhagen and Ole Fejerskov of the Department of Dental Pathology at Aarhus University, have both stated publicly that they believe the ingestion of fluoride is unnecessary and undesirable.[48] A Canadian researcher, Hardy Limeback, who is head of the Department of Preventive Dentistry at the University of Toronto and a former spokesman for the Canadian Dental Association, recently published an article with its subtitle in the form of a question. "Is There Any Anti-caries Benefit from

Swallowing Fluoride?" he asks.[49] Limeback is so convinced that the answer to this question is negative that he has become an active participant in the anti-fluoridation movement, one of the most prestigious scientists to take this career-threatening step.

This anti-fluoridation viewpoint is seen as extreme by the great majority of researchers and practitioners in the dental community. The explanation of the apparent conundrum, and it is now widely accepted throughout the dental profession, is that the ingestion of fluoridated water has topical as well as systemic impact. Even though it may remain in your mouth for only a few seconds before being swallowed, the swirling action involved in drinking and swallowing brings the fluoride into sufficient contact with the teeth to allow uptake by dental plaque. It is argued that the effect, while perhaps operative over a shorter time frame, is similar to that of oral rinsing with a fluoride solution. In fact, the very authors who promote the remineralization mechanism as the primary fluoride action are onboard with this view. Several of them are on record as stating that the remineralization mechanism is best promoted by the frequent introduction of low-concentration fluoride into the mouth.[50] They feel that the requisite fluoride levels can be obtained just as easily from fluoridated water as from any of the other available sources. A recent review goes so far as to say that "community water fluoridation is still the delivery vehicle of choice because it does more to enhance and maintain fluoride levels in oral fluids and is thus more compatible with the inhibition of demineralization and the promotion of remineralization than other vehicles."[51]

MORE STUDIES AND DIMINISHING RETURNS

Research projects that compare dental caries experience in fluoridated and nonfluoridated communities have been a cottage industry in the dental research world for over 50 years now. Beginning in 1945, right from the time of the first trials, the *Bulletin of the American Association of Public Health Dentists* (a precursor of the *Journal of Public Health Dentistry*) provided a special section in every issue devoted to the presentation of results of fluoridation studies. Thousands of articles and short reports appeared in this forum in the first 30 years of the fluoridation age.[52] And that is just the beginning. Michael Easley of the National Center for Fluoridation Policy and Research claims that there have been more than 3700 studies of the effectiveness of fluoridation since 1970.[53]

It would be a daunting task to monitor each of these thousands of articles presenting comparative results from individual studies. Luckily for us, there have been many reviews over the years that have attempted to digest and

TABLE 7.3   Major Institutional Reviews of the Effectiveness of Community Water Fluoridation, 1950–2000

Date	Sponsor[a]	Title
1951	NAS/NRC	*Risks and Benefits of Fluoride*[54]
1954	AAAS	*Fluoridation as a Public Health Measure*[55]
1958	WHO	*Report of Expert Committee on Water Fluoridation*[56]
1970	WHO	*Fluorides and Human Health*[57]
1976	British RCPL	*Fluoride, Teeth and Health*[58]
1977	NAS/NRC	*Drinking Water and Health*[59]
1979	AAAS	*Continuing Evaluation of the Use of Fluorides*[60]
1986	WHO	*Appropriate Use of Fluorides for Human Health*[61]
1991	USPHS	*Review of Fluorides: Benefits and Risks*[62]
1993	NAS/NRC	*Health Effects of Ingested Fluoride*[63]
1994	WHO	*Fluorides and Oral Health*[64]
1999	Ontario MOH	*Benefits and Risks of Water Fluoridation*[65]
2000	British SSH	*A Systematic Review of Public Water Fluoridation*[66]

[a]NAS/NRC, U.S. National Academy of Sciences, National Research Council; AAAS, American Association for the Advancement of Science; WHO, World Health Organization; British RCPL, Royal College of Physicians of London; USPHS, U.S. Public Health Service; Ontario MOH, Ontario Ministry of Health; British SSH, British Secretary of State for Health.

interpret all these data in order to pass some kind of judgment on the overall effectiveness of community water fluoridation. Table 7.3 lists 13 such reviews that have been carried out in the past half-century by major institutional bodies such as the U.S. National Academy of Sciences, the American Association for the Advancement of Science, and the World Health Organization.[54–64] Two very recent reviews, one carried out in 1999 for the Ontario Ministry of Health by David Locker, a dental researcher at the University of Toronto, and one carried out in 2000 for the British National Health Service by a team of scientists at York University in Britain, are especially valuable as independent, objective summaries of current thought.[65,66] The dental literature is also replete with many review articles prepared by prestigious research scientists who have participated in the fluoridation revolution. Table 7.4 lists seven such articles that have appeared since 1989.[67–74]

Most of the articles and reports in Tables 7.3 and 7.4 provide tables and graphs that summarize the results from some subset of the thousands of comparative studies that have been carried out in U.S. cities and towns and in the remainder of the developed world. Some of the reviews limit themselves to a particular period, others to a particular country or continent, still others to studies that meet the reviewers' concept of an acceptable standard of experimental design. Table 7.5 provides a representative listing of

TABLE 7.4 Review Articles on the Effectiveness of Community Water Fluoridation, 1989–2000

Date	Author (1)	Title
1989	Newbrun	Effectiveness of Water Fluoridation[67]
1990	Brunelle and Carlos	Recent Trends in Dental Caries in U.S. Children and the Effect of Water Fluoridation[68]
1990	Kalsbeek and Verrips	Dental Caries Prevalence and the Use of Fluorides in Different European Countries[69]
1990	Kaminsky et al.	Fluoride: Benefits and Risks of Exposure[70]
1993	Murray	Efficacy of Preventive Agents for Dental Caries[71]
1993	Ripa	A Half-Century of Community Water Fluoridation in the United States: Review and Commentary[72]
1994	Lewis and Banting	Water Fluoridation: Current Effectiveness and Dental Fluorosis[73]
1996	Petersson and Bratthall	The Caries Decline: A Review of Reviews[74]

TABLE 7.5 Summary of Studies Comparing Prevalence of Dental Caries in Fluoridated and Nonfluoridated Communities

Source	Number of Comparative Studies	Date of Comparative Study	Percent Difference in Caries Experience Between Fluoridated and Unfluoridated Communities[a] Range[b]	Median[c]
Early fluoridation trials (Table 5.2)	4	1951–1959	20 to 57	50
Review 1[71]	113	1956–1979	10 to 90	50
Review 2[67]	33	1979–1989	8 to 60	35
Review 3[73]	14	1989–1992	8 to 56	25
Ontario MOH Review[65]	29	1994–1999	0 to 64[d]	35
York University Review[66]	26	1951–1999	−5 to 64	15
1986–1987 NIDR Study of U.S. Schoolchildren	1	1987	—	18

[a]A positive difference implies less caries in fluoridated communities relative to nonfluoridated communities. A negative difference implies the opposite. In general, statistical analyses of the percent differences include all values reported from individual studies, regardless of whether they reflect DMFT, DMFS, dmft, or dmfs scores. The York University analysis differs from the others in that it is based on percent caries-free children rather than DMF scores.
[b]Range: the highest and lowest values reported in the studies covered by the review.
[c]Median: Half the studies covered by the review recorded a higher value, and half the studies, a lower value.
[d]One unlikely outlier of −69% is not included.

the results of several of these reviews. The original fluoridation trials are listed at the top as a baseline. In the middle are a set of five review papers that chart the results of comparative studies carried out during different time periods. The first review covers the earliest and longest time period (1956–1979); the second and third, the decade that followed (1979–1989 and 1989–1992); and the Ontario study, the more recent years (1994–1999). The York University study spans the period from 1951 until 1999. The first three reviews used all the studies they could find, whereas the Ontario and York assessments sifted through the available studies and selected only those that met a predetermined level of scientific sophistication. The final article listed in Table 7.5 reports the results of the huge nationwide survey of U.S. schoolchildren in 1986–1987. It is only one study, but the total number of subjects in this one study probably exceeds that of any 10 of the individual studies listed above it.

The question of experimental design deserves further mention. You may recall the many methodological flaws identified by critics of the original fluoridation trials. Those who designed these early studies were taken to task for failing to keep track of the oral health history of their subjects, failing to control for confounding factors such as socioeconomic status or dental hygiene practices, and failing to use examiners who were blind to the exposure status of each subject. Many of the same problems crop up in many of the studies that were put under review by the various review teams listed in Table 7.5. The Ontario and York University reviewers were the only ones who tried to establish a minimum acceptable set of standards for the inclusion of a study in their assessments. Both sets of acceptance criteria were based on establishing a hierarchy of studies, giving greater weight to those with the most careful controls. Those that took care to eliminate examiner bias received greater weight than those that didn't. Those that tracked individual subjects longitudinally through time received greater weight than those that sampled the population statistically without tagging individual subjects. Those that recorded careful histories for their subjects and used them to control for confounding factors received greater weight than those that did not. It is instructive to note that the York University review found only 214 studies out of the thousands that have appeared in print during the period 1951–1999 that met their acceptance criteria, and of these, only 26 provided a defensible analysis of the direct impact of fluoridation on dental caries.

The data in the second rightmost column in Table 7.5 reveal that every one of these exercises uncovered a large range in the percent difference in caries experience between fluoridated and nonfluoridated communities in the studies that were evaluated in that review. The right-hand column lists the median value of the percent difference for each set of studies (i.e., half the studies covered by that review recorded a higher value and half the studies a lower value).

Table 7.5 is set up with the reviews that cover the earliest comparative studies at the top and those that cover more recent studies at the bottom. In earlier years, the median difference was on the order of 50%. That is, on average, the children in fluoridated communities experienced 50% less tooth decay than their cousins in nonfluoridated communities. This is the value that has been used ever since in the pro-fluoridation camp to try to convince the public of the clear-cut advantages of community water fluoridation. The American Dental Association still highlights it in their pamphlet *Fluoridation Facts.*

However, as is clear from a perusal of the right-hand column of Table 7.5, and as is now widely accepted within the dental research community, the percent difference in caries experience between fluoridated and nonfluoridated communities has been declining over the years. The most recent review, that of the Ontario Ministry of Health, quotes a value of 35%. The lowest value in Table 7.5 suggests that the percent difference could be as low as 15%. This low value is associated with the York University review, which utilized only the best designed studies in its assessment (a commendable approach, but one that is also likely to bias the data set toward the recent era). Perhaps the most defensible measure of all is that from the nationwide 1986–1987 NIDR study of U.S. schoolchildren. The average DMFS value for children with a history of lifelong exposure to fluoride was 2.79, while that for children with no fluoride exposure at all was 3.39, a difference of 18%. This is still a statistically significant value, but it is a far cry from the 50% benefit claimed in earlier years.

In the same year that NIDR scientists published the results of the 1986–1987 study, John Yiamouyiannis, that perennial burr in the side of the pro-fluoridation movement, published his own analysis of the NIDR data, claiming that even the 18% difference could not be justified.[75] Yiamouyiannis states that he was unable to get any cooperation from NIDR in his attempt to assess their results, so he obtained the raw data through the U.S. Freedom of Information Act. He then carried out his own independent statistical analysis, coming to the conclusion that "there is no statistically significant difference" between the average DMFT rates for those with lifelong exposure to community water fluoridation and those with no history of exposure at all. He found this to be true in all regions of the country and for all ages. His work is widely quoted in anti-fluoridation circles as proof of how the medical establishment plays careless with the numbers.

Without taking on an independent analysis as detailed as the original studies themselves, it is difficult to determine why the Yiamouyiannis figures came out so differently from those of the NIDR. There are some methodological contrasts that might account for some of the discrepancy. For example, the NIDR study analyzed the raw data in terms of DMFS scores, whereas Dr. Y chose to interpret them in terms of DMFT scores. Furthermore, Dr. Y used an "age-standardized" caries rate, which appears to involve an averaging procedure that is different from that used by the NIDR scientists. There may well be other games afoot in these treacherous statistical waters, but if so, they are not evident to the casual reader. If one tries to judge credibility, I suppose the edge must be given to the NIDR scientists. They published their study in a widely circulated, peer-reviewed medical journal, whereas Yiamouyiannis's paper appeared in the closed-shop anti-fluoridation journal *Fluoride*. Both sides perhaps had motivation for bias, but I believe that by 1990, when these studies were published, the dental research establishment had largely bitten the bullet of declining impact and was prepared to let the chips fall where they may. Dr. Y, on the other hand, as we learned back in Chapter 2 with his *Lifesaver's Guide to Fluoridation*, and as we will see again in Chapter 8, has a documented propensity for single-minded argumentation.

Up until the appearance of the Ontario Ministry of Health report and the York University study, reviews of fluoridation effectiveness carried out by the medical establishment had always presented a rosy picture that fully supported pro-fluoridation claims of a large social benefit associated with community water fluoridation programs. These two new reports were much more muted in their findings. The Ontario study concluded somewhat hesitantly that "the balance of evidence suggests that rates of dental decay are lower in fluoridated than non-fluoridated communities," but it went on to say that "the magnitude of the effect is not large in absolute terms, is often not statistically significant, and may not be of clinical significance."[76] The York study concurred that "the best available evidence suggests that fluoridation of drinking water supplies does reduce caries prevalence," but it then hedged the point by declaring that "the degree to which caries is reduced is not clear from the data available." The York authors further warned that "the estimates of effect could be biased due to poor adjustment for the effects of potential confounding factors." In a final direct slap at the research community, they expressed consternation at the methodological shortcomings that continue to plague fluoridation studies. "Given the level of interest surrounding the issue of public water fluoridation," they lament, "it is surprising to find that so little high-quality research has been undertaken."[77]

When the York study was released in Britain, the British Medical Association and the British Dental Association both put out widely quoted press releases that implied business as usual on the fluoridation front. They crowed that yet another study had confirmed that "water fluoridation is safe and effective" and that fluoridation was once again endorsed as "the most effective way to reduce dental health inequalities." This brought Trevor Sheldon, professor of dentistry at York University and chairman of the advisory group for the York study, out of his chair. He sent letters to the British media accusing the BMA and the BDA of misleading the public about the findings of the review. Health campaigner Edward Baldwin (Earl Baldwin of Bewdley) put it even more plainly. "Anyone who considers this report a ringing endorsement," he declared, "is either dishonest, a fanatic, or scientifically illiterate." One journalist, writing in the *London Financial Times*, found this political wrangling among supposed scientific experts disquieting. "It is tempting to giggle at the sight of a trouserless hell-fire preacher explaining how he was wrestling with sin," he wrote, "but there are serious issues here of trust. The public is already skeptical of reassurances on health matters from official bodies. In the long term, such spinning on the contents of an inconvenient review will do nothing to improve that."[78]

There were also myriad letters to the editor of the *British Medical Journal*, where a summary of the York study was first published. Most of them came from well-known anti-fluoridation leaders, some of whom had apparently only seen the BMA and BDA press releases and were trying to belittle the York report, while others, better informed, crowed over the study's equivocal findings with respect to the benefits of fluoridation. Our personal favorite was submitted by Don Caron, who readers may or may not remember as one of the anti-fluoridation leaders from Spokane, Washington. "I guess the York study wasn't actually a study as studies go," he wrote, "because this study didn't study animals or people, it simply studied studies. Although this was touted to be the study to end all studies, almost immediately both the Green Party and the Fluoride Action Network published their studies of the York study. These were then studies of the study that studied studies. The studies of the study that studied the studies pointed out that this study that studied the studies had left some 3000 studies unstudied, and they called for a study of studies that would study all studies and therefore not necessitate a further study of the study of the studies as this study had done."[79] Suspicions run deep. The York group had hoped to garner kudos for their careful selection process, but instead, all they got were brickbats for their "unstudied studies."

THE HALO EFFECT

Regardless of where one comes down on the Yiamouyannis counteranalysis or the fuss over the York report, it is clear that even the results coming from the dental establishment itself seem to suggest that the level of effectiveness of community water fluoridation in fighting tooth decay is declining. This is certainly the interpretation that is put on this data by antifluoridation activists. However, this interpretation fails to take into account a truly gigantic confounding factor. As we have noted before, the DMF scores are declining across the nation in both fluoridated and unfluoridated communities, and any fair interpretation of the declining difference between them must take into account the fact that there is simply no longer as large a gap to be closed. Surely, an equally likely (or even more likely) interpretation of the available data is that the increase in fluoride exposure throughout society is causing the caries decline in *both* communities. Those in the dental research community believe that this is the case, and they call it the *halo effect*. It is their answer to the question that we posed some pages ago: *Why is it* that dental caries rates are declining in nonfluoridated communities just as they are in fluoridated communities?

First, they argue, one must accept that it is indeed fluoride that is responsible for the observed societal reduction in dental caries. It may be systemic fluoride, or it may be topical fluoride, but it is fluoride nevertheless. When the worldwide decline in tooth decay first became evident, dental research leaders from around the world gathered in Boston in 1982 to attend the First International Conference on the Declining Prevalence of Caries.[80] At that conference, speaker after speaker assessed all the possible explanations, then one after another, irregardless of their predilections, they came down on the side of fluoride as the most justifiable determinant. As one of the participants later stated: "No convincing evidence has been offered to refute the conclusion that the dramatic decrease in dental caries ... is primarily the result of exposure to fluoride."[81] In 1994, at the Second International Conference, they did it again. Some of the participants wanted to give all the credit to fluoride; some felt that fluoride was just one of many contributing factors; but none were willing to ignore it.[82] Let's face it. It is difficult for anyone, Nobel prizewinner or man on the street, to deny a role for fluoride when the precipitous decline in tooth decay occurs in perfect tandem with the introduction and spread of fluoride in society.

Second, they argue, one must accept that community water fluoridation works. It may work systemically, or it may work topically, but it works. To support this credo, they point to the undeniable reductions in caries that were achieved during the early trials, noting further that these successes occurred long before the widespread use of topical fluoride treatments. The conclusion that is drawn from all this by those with a pro-fluoridation viewpoint is that ingested fluoridated water clearly did the job in the early going, so surely it must be doing so still.

Third, they point to the introduction and growing popularity of topical fluoride, especially the now-almost-universal use of fluoridated toothpastes in the developed countries of the world. The topical delivery systems work, too, they argue, and coming online a decade or two after the beginning of community water fluoridation, they have had a delayed but almost equally effective impact. John Featherstone of the NIDR-funded Rochester Cariology Center in Rochester, New York believes that the two impacts were sequential and additive, with initial caries reductions on the order of 40 to 60% in the 1960s due to the initiation of community water fluoridation, and an additional 40 to 60% in the 1970s and 1980s due to the spread of fluoridated toothpastes.[83]

The halo effect is seen as a combination of two societal phenomena, dubbed *diffusion* and *dilution*.[84] *Diffusion* of the effects of fluoridation into nonfluoridated communities comes about through the widespread distribution of foods and beverages that are prepared using fluoridated water. As we have seen in the fluoridation statistics of Chapter 2, the implementation of community water fluoridation has been concentrated in the larger cities and towns of the nation. It is these cities and towns that are likely to host soft drink bottling plants and food processing plants. The food and beverages they prepare are then marketed throughout the region they serve, both in the fluoridated communities themselves and in the smaller unfluoridated communities and rural areas. The rise in fluoride concentrations of processed foods and beverages over the past 50 years is well documented, as is the increased intake of fluoride in the diets of those in both fluoridated and unfluoridated communities.

The *dilution* of the observed effectiveness of community water fluoridation is ascribed to the widespread availability and utilization of fluoride toothpastes, oral rinses, and supplements, and the greater numbers of children who now routinely receive topical applications of fluoride on a regular basis from their dentist. This increase in topical exposure has been documented in both fluoridated and unfluoridated communities. The impact of topical exposure dilutes the apparent impact of fluoridated water intake.

Proponents of the halo effect can point to several pieces of evidence that support their position. For example, you may recall the 1986–1987 NIDR study of U.S schoolchildren, which found 18% less caries in children who were lifelong residents of fluoridated communities relative to those with no fluoride exposure. It turns out that if children who had exposure to dietary fluoride supplements or topical fluoride applications are excluded from consideration, the percent difference between lifelong fluoride recipients and abstainers rises to 25%. These figures document the pro-fluoridation claim that measured differences between fluoridated and nonfluoridated communities are diluted by topical usage. The same study also found that the smallest differences in caries experience between the two populations occurred in the Midwest, where the percentage of children on community water fluoridation was greatest (72%), while the largest differences occurred in the Pacific region, where participation was least (18%). In other words, the more ubiquitous the fluoride, the greater the influence of the halo effect. The less widespread the fluoridation, the greater the gap still existing between the fluoridated and nonfluoridated groups.

There is another set of data that can be interpreted similarly. During the long course of political turmoil over the fluoridation issue, there have been many communities that started fluoridation but were later forced to stop. Dental researchers were quick to leap into the breach to see what happened to dental caries rates under these circumstances. It is instructive to review their analyses for cities and towns that discontinued their community water fluoridation programs at different points in time. Those that did so in the early years, such as Antigo, Wisconsin,[85] and Wicks, Scotland,[86] immediately experienced a rebound in dental caries incidence. The pro-fluoridation community has used this fact ever since as further proof of the value of fluoridation and the harm that comes to our children's oral health on its cessation. However, more recent experience does not support these earlier findings. In Tiel, the Netherlands, for example, surveys carried out as part of the long-running Tiel–Culumberg fluoridation trial, indicated the expected rebound of 18% in dental caries in 1980, seven years after the stoppage of fluoridation, but by 1988 there had actually been a decline in caries of 11% during the intervening eight years despite the absence of fluoridation.[87] Recent studies in Kuopio, Finland[88] and Cheminitz, Germany[89] indicate that caries rates in those cities continued to decline after the stoppage of fluoridation at much the same rates as they had during fluoridation.

Once again, these data must be viewed in the context of the overall declining trend of dental caries through the past half-century. In the early years, the few communities that were fluoridated experienced large declines in dental caries incidence, and huge differences existed between fluoridated communities and the nation at large. In that era, the cessation of fluoridation led to a measurable rebound in caries rates in previously fluoridated communities, as the caries rates moved back up toward the national average. In recent years, with caries rates falling precipitously across the board, communities that stop their fluoridation programs continue to benefit from the declining national trend even after they turn off their fluoridation equipment. Anti-fluoridationists exult in these recent data and declaim it as further proof of the worthlessness of community water fluoridation. Pro-fluoridationists see it as entirely consistent with their concept of the halo effect.

While the persuasive explanatory power of the halo effect is a boon to those who espouse fluoridation, it also has a downside. As has been pointed out by several frustrated dental statisticians,[90] if one accepts the ubiquitous diffusion of fluoride through society as the reason for reduced caries, it follows that one may no longer be able to measure differences in response from fluoridated and nonfluoridated communities. We may soon reach the position that John Yamouyiannis claimed that we had already reached in 1987, where there are no significant statistical differences between caries experience in cities with community water fluoridation and those without. The clash of absolutes will then be able to function in a pure vacuum of reason, with anti-fluoridationists claiming that fluoride does nothing, pro-fluoridationists claiming that fluoride does everything, and no way to prove either side right or wrong.

FLOSSERS AND CHEESEHEADS

Most credible anti-fluoridationists who have tried to argue that fluoride is not responsible for the declines observed in dental caries in the past half-century have based a large portion of their argument on the fact that caries has declined in nonfluoridated communities as well as in fluoridated commodities. This was the basis of Mark Diesendorf's classification of the caries decline as a "mystery," and it was also the basis of another influential article that appeared in the journal *Perspectives in Biology and Medicine* in 1997 entitled "Why I changed my mind about water fluoridation" by a former fluoridation advocate from New Zealand named John Colquhoun (pronounced "Co-houn").[91] Diesendorf and Colquhoun rejected the halo effect as an explanation of the phenomenon. They discount the diffusion argument on the basis of the European experience, where declines in dental caries have occurred despite the almost complete absence of community water fluoridation in many European countries. They discount the dilution argument on the basis of anecdotal evidence from their home countries. Diesendorf argues that much of the reported improvement in Australian dental health occurred before community water fluoridation began and before the widespread use of fluoridated toothpastes. He quotes a study in Sydney that showed that children with "naturally sound teeth" increased from 4% to 20% between 1961 and 1967, even though Sydney did not fluoridate its water supply until 1968. Colquhoun states that caries declined dramatically in nonfluoridated areas of New Zealand despite the fact that "very few children used fluoride toothpaste, many had not received fluoride applications to their teeth, and hardly any had been given fluoride tablets."

These arguments from Down Under have not gone uncontested by the dental establishment. Brian Burt, the respected leader of the University of Michigan's dental research program, was the lead author on a paper published in the *Journal of Public Health Dentistry* entitled "Water Fluoridation: A Response to Critics in Australia and New Zealand." In it, he strongly questions the validity of the Sydney data. He also chides Diesendorf for his "outdated view of how fluoride exerts its anticariogenic action," and he questions Colquhoun's interpretation of his anecdotal data. He concludes that "neither author has produced evidence to challenge the established safety and effectiveness of water fluoridation."[92]

One can take all this carping back and forth among experts for what it is worth, but the fact remains that anti-fluoridationists who deny the impact of fluoride on dental health are whistling in the dark unless they can produce an alternative explanation for the decline in dental caries that is at least as persuasive as the fluoride argument. This they have tried to do, relying on one or other of two general arguments. It is their contention that much of the decline in caries is due either to an improvement in dietary patterns, or to an improvement in dental hygiene, or both.

Arguments that credit improved diet for the decline in tooth decay usually begin with an examination of sugar consumption. At first glance, this argument would appear to fail, because the total per capita consumption of sugar in the United States and other developed countries of the world has remained relatively constant for several decades. If anything, it is rising slightly rather than falling. However, there *has* been a change in the *mix* of the types of sugar consumed. In 1970, sucrose accounted for 75% of the sugar consumed in the United States; by 1990, this figure was less than 50%.[93] The slack has been taken up by an increased use of high-fructose corn syrup (HFCS) in the production of processed foods and soft drinks. Although the relative cariogenicity of the various sugars has still not been fully deciphered, there is considerable evidence that HFCS is less cariogenic than sucrose.

Much of this argument relies on developments in the soft drink industry. The American thirst for soft drinks is apparently insatiable, with current usage approaching 200 liters per person per year (that's over 500 cans per person per year, or about one-and-a-half cans per person per day). In recent years, the industry has switched almost fully from sucrose to HCFS sugars in their nondiet drinks. In addition, the market for diet drinks sweetened with the sugar substitute aspartame rather than sugar has increased to the point where it now accounts for over 30% of soft drink consumption.[94]

The question is whether these changes in sugar use could possibly account for the precipitous decline in tooth decay that has been observed. Medical and dental nutritionists do not think so. One of the arguments against this explanation lies in the timing. The catalyst that led food and drink producers to switch from sucrose to HFCS was an instability in world sugar markets in the late 1970s. Evidence of reduced caries appeared much earlier than this.

Other changes in dietary patterns have also been mooted in the scramble to avoid the fluoride explanation. Diesendorf credits the general improvement in nutritional values and the widespread increase in consumption of whole-grain cereals and nuts. Colquhoun admits that he does "not know the answer for sure," but he draws attention to the tremendous increase in the consumption of fresh fruits and vegetables since the 1930s, due to the widespread introduction of household refrigerators. One dietary explanation, which appears fanciful on first encounter, but which apparently has some basis in fact, is the consumption of cheese. One review article identified 17 separate studies confirming the benefits of cheese.[95] It now seems well established that several types of cheese inhibit caries progression, apparently acting as an effective buffering agent that neutralizes plaque acids.

Another quasidietary explanation, suggested anecdotally by several observers, but apparently never tested in a controlled experiment, involves the increased medical use of antibiotics in coping with childhood diseases. It is suggested that irregular but frequent antibiotic use might have a deleterious impact on *Streptococcus mutans* and the other oral bacteria that produce the acid implicated in tooth decay.[96]

If improvements in diet do not quite convince as the sole causative agent of the caries miracle, the antifluoride forces then turn to improvements in dental hygiene as an additional explanatory factor. Included in this category are improvements in professional care in the dentist's chair, improved oral hygiene habits at home in the form of more effective toothbrushing routines and regular flossing, better dental education in the schools, and more accessible preventive programs for children by government dental health agencies. There seems little doubt that such improvements have taken place and that such improvements must count for something, but it is difficult to assess the absolute importance of their role. This is especially true if one discounts, as anti-fluoridationists do, the two improvements in oral hygiene that everybody else thinks are the most important: the availability of topical fluoride treatments in the dentist's office, and the use of fluoridated toothpaste at home.

In all fairness, it should be pointed out that there are some in the antifluoridation movement who do not discount the value of fluoride in reducing tooth decay. This minority group accepts the strong evidence supporting a role for fluoride in the caries miracle but continues to oppose community water fluoridation on other grounds. Some members of this group oppose community water fluoridation, not because it doesn't work, but because they feel that the health risks (which we examine in Chapter 8) outweigh the benefits. Others are offended by what they see as governmental coercion in community water fluoridation programs and would prefer that citizens be allowed to determine their own fluoride dose through topical use at home. Still others feel that current medical thinking, which downplays the systemic impact of fluoride in favor of topical impact, argues against the need for community water fluoridation.

There is one issue that both pro- and anti-fluoridation camps seem to agree on: that oral hygiene is poorer, and rates of dental caries higher, in those members of society who live in conditions of socioeconomic deprivation. However, the two camps put a different spin on this issue. Anti-fluoridationists claim that things are improving on this front, and that it may well be the transformation of hygienic practices in this sector of society, rather than fluoride, that is responsible for the improvement in national dental caries statistics. Pro-fluoridationists, on the other hand, use the deprivation data to argue for the continuation of community water fluoridation programs in order to meet the needs of this sector of society, which they feel is not likely to take on the cost and responsibility of proper home care.

This question of whether community water fluoridation brings equity in caries experience across socioeconomic groups has not gone unstudied in the dental research literature. Perusal of just two review articles identified 19 different studies that addressed this issue.[97] Despite all this attention, the issue remains unresolved. Some studies report significant steps toward equity; others report no effect at all. David Locker, the author of the respected Ontario Ministry of Health review, reports that the relationships that have been observed are equivocal and interpretations difficult. Overall, however, he was able to reach two generalizations. First, it appears that the difference in caries rates between children in fluoridated and nonfluoridated communities is consistently larger when the communities are at the lower end of the socioeconomic scale than when they are at the higher. Second, caries rates are highest of all in children from low-socioeconomic groups who live in nonfluoridated communities. These two points would seem to provide ammunition to pro-fluoridation arguments on this issue.

THE BACK OF THE COIN: THE INCREASE IN DENTAL FLUOROSIS

It has been known since early in the fluoridation movement that high concentrations of fluoride in drinking water can disfigure teeth. You will recall that the very discovery of fluoride's cavity-fighting power grew out of the studies that first identified fluoride as the cause of mottled teeth. Dental fluorosis is

caused by disruptions in enamel formation that occur during tooth development in early childhood. It is apparently a systemic effect caused by excessive
fluoride ingestion during the years when teeth are forming under the gums.
The tooth enamel becomes *hypomineralized*, a process by which the width of
the spaces between the apatite crystals in the enamel are enlarged, creating
an increase in porosity of the tooth surface. Once erupted, the affected teeth
exhibit opaque, paper-white spots that are in contrast to the glossy translu-
cence of normal enamel. In severe cases, staining appears and pitting can
occur in hypomineralized areas.[98] H. Trendley Dean, in his early studies of
mottled teeth, created a fluorosis index that is still in use today (although
there are other more recent classifications that are also widely used). He
distinguished between very mild, mild, moderate, and severe fluorosis, with
the mild varieties exhibiting only white spots, the moderate featuring some
staining, and the severe evincing serious tooth breakdown due to pitting.[99]
Of course, not all teeth are affected to an equal degree, and Dean's classification system is relatively conservative in this regard. The index for a
given subject is based on the condition of the two worst teeth in the subject's
mouth.

Right from the beginning, the dental research community knew that
community water fluoridation would lead to a trade-off between reductions
in tooth decay and increases in dental fluorosis. The reader may wish to flip
back to Figure 5.3, which is a plot of the data that led Harold Hodge in 1950 to
suggest that the optimal concentration of fluoridated water should be about
1.0 ppm. This diagram clearly illustrates the caries–fluorosis trade-off and
defines the "optimal" concentration explicitly in terms of this trade-off. Certainly, Trendley Dean recognized the trade-off in his early studies. It was his
stated opinion that widespread fluoridation at 1.0 ppm would lead to dental
fluorosis in 10 to 20% of the population.[100]

Dean was bothered by this prediction, and it may have contributed to his
tardy entry into the pro-fluoridation fold (see Chapter 5), but he ultimately
became a firm supporter of fluoridation, probably because he felt that the
increase in fluorosis would all be of the very mild to mild variety. It was
his view, and the strong view of the pro-fluoridation movement ever since,
that these low levels of fluorosis are unimportant, a mere cosmetic effect and
of no health concern. The American Dental Association's *Fluoridation Facts*
describe mild fluorosis as a condition that has no effect on tooth function, is
not readily apparent to the casual observer, and requires a trained specialist to detect.[101] In their decision on a health safety standard for fluoride in
water (see Chapter 9), the Environmental Protection Agency described the
mild varieties of dental fluorosis as a "cosmetic effect with no known health
effects." The U.S. Public Health Service states that dental fluorosis is "not

much of a dental public health concern," admitting only that it might be "an indication that the total fluoride exposure may be more than necessary to prevent tooth decay."[102]

The anti-fluoridation movement is outraged by this cavalier attitude. They see the occurrence of dental fluorosis as a "pandemic," a clear sign of "fluoride overdose in children," and an "indicator that the destructive effects of fluoride are occurring in bone, in connective tissue, and in immune and enzyme function."[103] John Colquhoun, one of the most widely known of the high-profile dental scientists who changed their mind about the value of fluoridation, stated that "the claim that only tooth forming cells are damaged by fluoride is extremely implausible, contrary to common sense, and can be disputed on scientific grounds."[104] Paul Conett, another well-known anti-fluoridation activist, has declared that "dental fluorosis is a warning that something else is going on."[105]

Even if it were certain that dental fluorosis did not constitute a health threat, the anti-fluoridationists would object on purely aesthetic grounds. It is their view that dental fluorosis can lead to embarrassment and self-consciousness on the part of young children and that even a few such cases are a few too many. They point to the findings of an ad hoc panel convened by the Environmental Protection Agency during their search for a meaningful health safety standard for fluoride, which concluded that people who have suffered impaired dental appearance as the result of moderate or severe dental fluorosis are at increased risk for psychological and behavioral problems and difficulties.[106] David Locker, in his objective assessment of fluoridation for the Ontario Ministry of Health, is not convinced that even mild or very mild fluorosis would necessarily be insignificant to the persons affected. He notes that under Dean's classification, those who suffer from *very mild* fluorosis may have opaque white areas scattered irregularly over as much as 25% of the affected tooth surfaces, and those with *mild* fluorosis, up to 50%. He doubts that such impacts would be considered as merely *cosmetic* by those for whom a simple smile becomes an embarrassment. He notes that Dean's definitions were coined in the 1930s, when concerns and awareness of appearance were less marked than they are today.[107]

The reasons for this fierce clash over the importance of dental fluorosis become clearer when one looks at the fluorosis statistics for the past few decades. These statistics show that dental fluorosis has been increasing significantly over time. The trend is clear and accepted by both camps, gleefully on the one hand, grudgingly on the other. To the anti-fluoridation camp, the fact of increasing fluorosis provides the most compelling available support for their view that community water fluoridation is doing something bad to the nation. For the pro-fluoridation camp, with their unshakable faith in the value of fluoridation, it requires a defensive posture that downplays this increase in dental fluorosis as unimportant.

Table 7.6 is based on the findings of the 1986–1987 study of U.S. schoolchildren carried out by the National Institute of Dental Research.[108] This survey of over 39,000 children looked not only at the prevalence of dental caries as reported earlier in the chapter, but also at the prevalence of dental fluorosis. As shown in the table, 22.3% of all U.S. schoolchildren suffered from dental fluorosis at the time of the survey. Almost all of it was of the very mild to mild variety, with only a 1.3% prevalence of moderate or severe fluorosis. The table indicates a clear relationship between the concentration of fluoride in drinking-water supplies and the prevalence of dental fluorosis. In optimally fluoridated communities, 29.9% of the children surveyed exhibited some indication of dental fluorosis.

Table 7.7 provides a comparison of the prevalence of dental fluorosis in fluoridated and nonfluoridated communities. It is based on David

TABLE 7.6   Prevalence of Dental Fluorosis in Communities with Different Fluoride Concentrations in Their Water Supply, 1986–1987 NIDR Study of U.S. Schoolchildren[108]

Concentration of Fluoride in Water Supply (ppm)	Prevalence of All Dental Fluorosis (%)	Prevalence of Moderate and Severe Dental Fluorosis (%)
<0.3	13.5	0.5
0.3–0.7	21.7	1.2
0.7–1.2[a]	29.9	1.3
>1.2	41.4	7.3
Overall	22.3	1.3

[a]Optimally fluoridated range.

TABLE 7.7   Comparison of the Prevalence of Dental Fluorosis in Fluoridated and Nonfluoridated Communities[a]

	Prevalence of All Dental Fluorosis (%)		Prevalence of Moderate and Severe Dental Fluorosis (%)	
	Fluoridated Communities	Nonfluoridated Communities	Fluoridated Communities	Nonfluoridated Communities
Range	9–79	0–53	0–27	0–25
Median	51.3	21.4	3.0	0.5

[a]Summary statistics of results from 1999 Ontario Ministry of Health review of 16 studies in nine countries.[109]

TABLE 7.8   Prevalence of All Dental Fluorosis in Optimally Fluoridated Communities (0.7–1.2 ppm) Over Time

Period	Reference	Prevalence (%)
1939–1940	H. Trendley Dean[110]	13.6
1978–1982	U.S. Public Health Service[111]	22.2
1986–1987	NIDR[108]	29.9[a]
1995–1999	Ontario Ministry of Health[109]	51.3[b]

[a]From Table 7.6.
[b]From Table 7.7.

Locker's review of 16 studies in nine countries carried out during the period 1994–1999. While the values reported by the various studies cover a wide range, the trend in the median values is very clear. A total of 51.3% of those surveyed from fluoridated communities exhibited some evidence of dental fluorosis. The figure for those from nonfluoridated communities was much less, 21.4%.[109] There is little question that people living in fluoridated communities live under greater risk of dental fluorosis than those in nonfluoridated communities.

Table 7.8 documents the growth in dental fluorosis in optimally fluoridated communities over the past several decades. The value for 1939–1940 is taken from Dean's 1942 study.[110] The value for 1978–1982 comes from an ad hoc committee on fluoride convened by the U.S. Public Health Service in 1991.[111] The two most recent values come from the 1986–1987 NIDR study presented in Table 7.6, and from Locker's study for the Ontario Ministry of Health summarized in Table 7.7. Table 7.8 indicates a clear growth in dental fluorosis in optimally fluoridated communities from 13.6% in 1940 to 51.3% in 1999. Most of this growth is in the very mild to mild categories of dental fluorosis. The prevalence of moderate to severe dental fluorosis is still fairly low but not insignificant. Similar results are reported in the York University review carried out for the British National Health Service, and in an independent review carried out by a Canadian dental researcher.[112]

Whereas the anti-fluoridation camp would like to place all of the blame for this increase in dental fluorosis on the shoulders of community water fluoridation programs, dental researchers in the pro-fluoridation camp argue for a shared responsibility with the other sources of increased fluoride intake in current vogue. A large number of studies have been carried out that show a strong and consistent association between dental fluorosis and early childhood use of fluoride toothpastes, early childhood use of fluoride supplements, and prolonged use of infant formula with a high fluoride content. These studies show that the odds of developing dental fluorosis are at least as great from any of these other activities as they are from drinking fluoridated water. In all four cases, taken singly, the probability of developing dental fluorosis increases two- to fourfold over that of an unfluoridated regimen. The real problem arises when children who live in a fluoridated community are also subjected to fluoride supplements and fluoride toothpastes. In these cases, the chances of developing dental fluorosis increase 10- to 20-fold. Another way of looking at the issue is to try to ascertain the risk attributable to the various factors. The bottom line here seems to be that the increase in dental fluorosis observed can be attributed about 50% to community water fluoridation and about 50% to the additional discretionary intake of fluoride by infants from other sources.[113]

Ultimately, one's final position on the importance of dental fluorosis is a value judgment. One either feels that the increase in fluorosis is an acceptable price to pay for ending the scourge of tooth decay, or one doesn't. One either feels that dental fluorosis is a public health problem or one doesn't. On the latter point, Burt and Eklund in their widely used textbook on dental health practice note that dental fluorosis is a serious public health problem in East Africa and India, where crippling skeletal fluorosis is also endemic. They conclude that "dental fluorosis cannot be classified as a public health problem in the United States" at this time, but "it would be a mistake ... to assume that it could not become so."[114] They argue that the problem is best avoided by prudent use of fluoride now. Not surprisingly, the two fluoride camps cannot agree on what constitutes "prudent use." Pro-fluoridationists argue that much of the increase in dental fluorosis could be avoided by ensuring that children in fluoridated communities do not receive additional fluoride supplementation, and they have been trying to get this message across to parents, community dentists, and dental hygienists.[115] Anti-fluoridationists take the opposite tack. If the double dose is too much, they argue, why not let people choose their own level of fluoride intake, and stop the community fluoridation?

THE BOTTOM LINE ON FLUORIDE AND TEETH

When all is said and done, it seems that the public's main interest centers more on the eradication of tooth decay than on concern over dental fluorosis. To this end, there seems little doubt that increased fluoride intake is the primary causative factor in the decline observed in dental caries since 1950. This precipitous decline in tooth decay has occurred in perfect tandem with the introduction and spread of fluoride in society, both through community water fluoridation and through topical applications, especially the use of fluoridated toothpastes. Although improvements in diet, dental hygiene, and professional dental care may have played a role, all evidence points to increased access to fluoride as the prime determinant in the caries turnaround.

The early fluoridation trials, which took place prior to the widespread introduction of fluoridated toothpaste and other topical applications, provide proof of the effectiveness of community water fluoridation in reducing dental caries. Recent research has clarified that the dental impact of fluoride is due primarily to topical effects on erupted teeth rather than systemic effects on pre-erupted teeth as thought originally. It is now recognized that teeth benefit most from the continuous presence of low-concentration fluoride in the oral fluids adjacent to the teeth, a condition that is enhanced by both fluoridated water and fluoridated toothpaste. Many dental experts, including David Locker in his Ontario Ministry of Health study, have gone on record with their opinion that community water fluoridation is still the delivery vehicle of choice because it does more than any other method to enhance and maintain fluoride levels in the oral fluids.[116]

The anti-fluoridation movement has tried to deny the impact of fluoride by observing that the decline in dental caries has occurred in all communities in North America, regardless of whether or not community water fluoridation has been present, and in all developed countries regardless of whether or not fluoridated water supplies have been prevalent. However, this argument is effectively trumped by the persuasive explanatory weight of the halo effect. The increased fluoride content of food and beverages in the United States, and the increased worldwide use of fluoridated toothpastes, have both been documented extensively and provide a convincing explanation of the widespread decline in dental caries.

Anti-fluoridationists are on firmer ground in raising the flag on dental fluorosis. It is clear from the evidence available that dental fluorosis is more prevalent in fluoridated than in nonfluoridated communities, and that it has increased over time across the United States in incidence and severity. Arguments still rage as to the dental, medical, and psychological importance of this trend, but there are few knowledgeable observers who are not worried about it to some degree.

If worries about dental fluorosis prove prescient, and if good diet, good hygiene, and carefully controlled use of fluoridated toothpaste were to become more or less universal, perhaps an argument could be made for the cessation of public water fluoridation. The experience in developed European countries that have little community water fluoridation might support such a step. It is apparent from the caries statistics coming from those countries that it is possible to achieve similar reductions in dental caries through self-administered topical use as it is through community water fluoridation.

Anti-fluoridationists might be better off to bite the bullet, accept a role for fluoride in the reduction of tooth decay, and zero in on the delivery mechanism. Indeed, some of the more responsible members of the anti-fluoridation camp have already done so. Edward Groth III, writing in an appendix to Brian Martin's softly anti-fluoride book *Scientific Knowledge in Controversy: The Social Dynamics of the Fluoridation Debate*, states his belief in the "almost indisputable evidence that fluoride is an effective anti-caries agent." Geoffrey Smith, who in his earlier years wrote in strident opposition to fluoridation, has mellowed with age, and by 1987 was willing to concede that "the success of fluoridation in combating tooth decay is well-documented and would appear beyond dispute." These authors go on to make their case against community water fluoridation, but they do so without tilting at the windmills of cause and effect.[117]

The continued growth of caries in unfluoridated third-world countries and the continued socioeconomic disparities at home make it clear that reductions in dental caries can only be achieved through access to low-level fluoride intake in one form or another. While anti-fluoridationists argue for freedom of choice through self-administered plans, the pro-fluoridation lobby keeps up the pressure to continue and expand community water fluoridation programs. Herschel Horowitz of the National Institute for Dental Research has been the most zealous advocate for the compelling advantages of a public health approach to disease prevention. He commends the safety, efficacy, and cost-effectiveness of such an approach, but his real passion is for the social equity that it provides. He points out that the entire community benefits, regardless of age, educational attainment, or socioeconomic status. The benefits are derived without any direct action on the part of each citizen and without dependence on professional dental services or the ability to afford them.[118] Perhaps a pro-fluoridation advocate, Brian Burt of the University of Michigan, has said it best: "The research challenge," he writes, "is to determine just how much fluoride is enough, what the best delivery combinations are, and how to get the fluoride to those who need it most."[119]

If the only question on the table were whether fluoride reduces tooth decay, this book would end here. We all know that life is not so simple. Like most social decisions related to health and environment, there are risks associated with fluoridation that must be assessed and weighed against the benefits. At the very least we are aware that increased fluoride intakes can lead to unsightly dental fluorosis. But what about the worst-case scenarios, exemplified by anti-fluoridation worries about cancer and heart disease and mental incapacitation. In Chapter 8 we set out to determine whether any of these health risks represent something to be concerned about and which ones we can discount out of hand. Once we have the toxicological issues in hand, we can move on in the following chapters to the issue of dosage. We have learned in this chapter that in the context of tooth decay, a little fluoride is good for you, but we will learn in Chapter 8 that in other contexts, too much fluoride is not good for you. Reputable scientists on both sides of the fence have raised the issue of the possible overfluoridation of society and have begun calling for a reassessment of the optimal concentration for community water fluoridation. We are beset by both good and bad things at every turn, benefits and risks that must be balanced, uncertainties to put us off our game, and many unreliable narrators who will try to deflect us down their own favored path through the maze.

REFERENCES

1. R. R. Harris, *Dental Science in a New Age: A History of the National Institute of Dental Research*, Montrose Press, Rockville, MD, 1989.

2. G. P. H. Foley, *Foley's Footnotes: A Treasury of Dentistry*, Washington Square East Publishing, Wallingford, PA, 1972. This book is a collection of pieces based on the author's columns in the *Journal of Dental Education* during the period 1961 to 1969 and the *Journal of the American Dental Association* during the period 1965 to 1972. For more quaint folk remedies, see C. Gysel, Toothache in the XVII century: classical therapy and new medicines, *Bull. Hist. Dent.*, 38, 3–7, 1990.

3. Foley, 1972, op. cit.

4. Ibid.

5. U.S. Public Health Service, Centers for Disease Control and Prevention, Achievements in public health, 1900–1999: fluoridation of drinking water to prevent dental caries, *MMWR*, 48(41), 933–940, 1999.

6. Ogden Nash, This is going to hurt just a little bit, *The Face is Familiar: Selected Verse of Ogden Nash*, Garden City Publishing, New York, 1941.

7. Much of the material in this section, including Figure 7.1, has been adapted from T. McGuire, *Tooth Fitness: Your Guide to Healthy Teeth*, St. Michael's Press, Grass Valley, CA, 1994.

8. B. A. Burt and S. A. Eklund, *Dentistry, Dental Practice, and the Community*, W. B. Saunders, Philadelphia, 1999; World Health Organization, http://www.whocollab.odont.lu.se.

9. S. Jarvinen, Epidemiologic characteristics of dental caries: relation of DMFS to DMFT, *Comm. Dent. Oral Epidemiol.*, 11, 363–366, 1986. The original idea, and the source of one of the correlative equations tested by Jarvinen, is a paper by J. W. Knutson, Epidemiological trend patterns of dental caries prevalence data, *J. Am. Dent. Assoc.*, 57, 821–829, 1958.

10. Harris, 1989, op. cit.

11. McGuire, 1994, op. cit.

12. J. K. Clarke, On the bacterial factor in the aeiology of dental caries, *Br. J. Exp. Pathol.*, 5, 141–147, 1924.

13. D. H. Leverett, Fluorides and the changing prevelance of dental caries, *Science*, 217, 26–30, 1982.

14. W. J. Moore and M. E. Corbett, The distribution of dental caries in ancient British populations, *Caries Res.*, 5, 151–168, 1971 (see also the same journal, 7, 139–153, 1973, and 9, 163–175, 1975); E. A. O'Sullivan, S. A. Williams, R. C. Wakefield, J. E. Cape, and M. E. J. Curzon, Prevalence and site characteristics of dental caries in primary molar teeth from prehistoric times to the 18th century in England, *Caries Res.*, 27, 147–153, 1993.

15. E. Newbrun, *Cariology*, 3rd ed., Quintessence Publishing, Hanover Park, IL, 1989.

16. Ibid.; L. M. Sreebny, Sugar availability, sugar consumption, and dental caries, *Comm. Dent. Oral Epidemiol.*, 10, 1–7, 1982.

17. J. D. Featherstone, The mechanism of dental decay, *Nutr. Today*, pp. 10–16, May–June 1987; Newbrun, 1989, op. cit.; G. Nikiforuk, *Understanding Dental Caries*, 2 vols., Karger, Basel, Switzerland, 1985; J. J. Murray, ed., *The Prevention of Dental Diseases*, Oxford University Press, New York, 1989; L. M. Silverstone, N. W. Johnson, J. M. Hardie, and R. A. D. Williams, *Dental Caries: Aetiology, Pathology, and Prevention*, Macmillan, New York, 1981.

18. F. J. Orland, J. R. Blaney, R. W. Harrison, J. A. Reyniers, P. C. Trexler, R. E. Ervin, H. A. Gordon, and M. Wagner, Experimental caries in germ-free rats innoculated with enterococci, *J. Am. Dent. Assoc.*, 50, 260–261, 1955.

19. R. J. Fitzgerald and P. H. Keyes, Demonstration of the etiologic role of streptococci in experimental caries in the hamster, *J. Am. Dent. Assoc.*, 61, 9–19, 1960.

20. J. F. Volker, H. C. Hodge, H. J. Wilson, and S. N. von Voorhis, The absorption of fluoride by the enamel, dentin, bone, and hydroxyapatite as shown by the radioactive isotope, *J. Biol. Chem.*, 184, 543, 1940; B. G. Bibby, Fluorine and dental caries, *NY J. Dent.*, 15, 99–103, 1945.

21. J. W. Knutson and W. D. Armstrong, The effect of topically applied sodium fluoride on dental caries experience, *Publ. Health Rep.*, 60, 1085–1090, 1945.

22. Harris, 1989, op. cit.

23. H. S. Horowitz, The effectiveness of community water fluoridation in the United States, *J. Publ. Health Dent.*, 56(5)(Special Issue), 253–258, 1996.

24. E. Newbrun, Effectiveness of water fluoridation, *J. Publ. Health Dent.*, 49, 279–289, 1989.

25. Leverett, 1982, op. cit.

26. World Health Organization, Global Oral Data Bank, http://www.whocollab.od.mah.se.

27. Jarvinen, 1986, op. cit.

28. J. A. Brunelle and J. P. Carlos, Recent trends in dental caries in U.S. children and the effect of water fluoridation, *J. Dent. Res.*, 69(Special Issue), 723–727, 1990.

29. O'Sullivan et al., 1993, op. cit.

30. M. H. Leclercq, D. E. Barmes, and J. Sardo-Infirri, Oral health: global trends and projections, *World Health Stat. Q.*, 40, 116–128, 1987.

31. L. Ripa, A half-century of community water fluoridation in the United States: review and commentary, *J. Publ. Health Dent.*, 53, 17–44, 1993.

32. M. Diesendorf, The mystery of declining tooth decay, *Nature*, 322, 125–129, 1986.

33. R. C. Weast, ed., *Handbook of Chemistry and Physics*, 53rd ed. CRC Press, Boca Raton, FL, 1972.

34. R. A. Freeze and J. A. Cherry, *Groundwater*, Prentice Hall, Englewood Cliffs, NJ, 1979; American Dental Association, *Fluoridation Facts*, http://www.ada.org; G. L. Waldbott, A. W. Burgstahler, and H. L. McKinney, *Fluoridation: The Great Dilemma*, Coronado Press, Lawrence, KS, 1978.

35. H. C. Hodge, Metabolism of fluorides, *J. Am Med. Assoc.*, 177, 313–316, 1971; M. G. Buonocore and L. W. Ripa, Pharmacologic and therapeutic aspects of fluoride, *J. Prev. Dent.*, 1, 12–23, 1974; B. A. Burt and S. A. Eklund, *Dentistry, Dental Practice, and the Community*, W. B. Saunders, Philadelphia, 1999.

36. Hodge, 1971, op. cit.

37. J. J. Murray, A. J. Rugg-Gunn, and G. N. Jenkins, *Fluorides in Caries Prevention*, 3rd ed., Butterworth-Heinemann Publishers, Boston, MA, 1991.

38. K. Hunsfadbraten, Fluoride in caries prophylaxis at the turn of the century, *Bull. Hist. Dent.*, 30, 117–120, 1982.

39. Ripa, 1993, op. cit.

40. E. D. Beltran and B. A. Burt, The pre- and post-eruptive effects of fluoride in caries decline, *J. Publ. Health Dent.*, 48, 233–240, 1988.

41. Ibid.; Nikiforuk, 1985, op. cit.; J. R. Mellburg and L. W. Ripa, *Fluoride in Preventive Dentistry: Theory and Clinical Applications*, Quintessence Publishing, Hanover Park, IL, 1983.

42. J. D. Featherstone, Prevention and reversal of dental caries: role of low-level fluoride, *Comm. Dent. Oral Epidemiol.*, 27, 31–40, 1999; R. P. Shellis and R. M. Duckworth, Studies on the cariostatic mechanisms of fluoride, *Int. Dent. J.*, 44(3)(Suppl 1), 263–273, 1994; Ripa, 1993, op. cit.; Murray et al., 1991, op. cit.; Burt and Eklund, 1995, op. cit.; O. Fejerskov, J. Ekstrand, and B. A. Burt, eds., *Fluoride in Dentistry*, 2nd ed., Munksgaard Publishing, Copenhagen, Denmark, 1996.

43. A. Groeneveld, A. Van Eck, and O. Backer-Dirks, Fluoride in caries prevention: Is the effect pre-or post-eruptive? *J. Dent. Res.*, 69(Special Issue), 751–755, 1990.

44. American Dental Association, *Fluoridation Facts*, http://www.ada.org.

45. Murray et al., 1991, op. cit.

46. D. Locker, *Benefits and Risks of Water Fluoridation*, Ontario Ministry of Health, Toronto, Ontario, Canada, 1999; available at http://www.gov.on.ca/health.

47. U.S. Public Health Service, *Review of Fluoride: Benefits and Risks*, U.S. PHS, Washington, DC, 1991. The results of this report are summarized in *J. Am. Med. Assoc.*, 266, 1061–1067, 1991.

48. As qoted in Murray et al., 1991, op. cit.

49. H. Limeback, A re-examination of the pre-eruptive and post-eruptive mechanism of the anti-caries effects of fluoride: Is there any anti-caries benefit from swallowing fluoride? *Comm. Dent. Oral Epidemiol.*, 27, 62–71, 1999.

50. Beltran and Burt, 1988, op. cit.; Murray et al., 1991, op. cit.

51. Locker, 1999, op. cit.

52. V. L. Richmond, Thirty years of fluoridation: a review, *Am. J. Clin. Nutr.*, 41, 129–138, 1985; R. G. Rozier, A new era for community water fluoridation? Achievements after one-half century and challenges ahead, *J. Publ. Health Dent.*, 55, 3–5, 1995.

53. M. W. Easley, Fluoridation: a triumph of science over propaganda, *Priorities*, 8(4), 1996.

54. U.S. National Academy of Sciences, National Research Council, Committee on Toxicology, *Risks and Benefits of Fluoride*, National Academies Press, Washington, DC, 1951.

55. J. H. Shaw, ed., *Fluoridation as a Public Health Measure*, American Association for the Advancement of Science, Washington, DC, 1954.

56. World Health Organization, *Report of Expert Committee on Water Fluoridation*, WHO Technical Report Series 146, WHO, Geneva, Switzerland, 1958.

57. P. Adler et al., *Fluorides and Human Health*, World Health Organization, Geneva, Switzerland, 1970.

58. Royal College of Physicians of London, *Fluoride, Teeth and Health*, Pitman Medical Publishing, London, 1976.

59. U.S. National Academy of Sciences, National Research Council, Safe Drinking Water Committee, *Drinking Water and Health*, National Academies Press, Washington, DC, 1977.

60. E. Johansen, D. R. Taves, and T. O. Olsen, eds., *Continuing Evaluation of the Use of Fluorides*, American Association for the Advancement of Science, Westview Press, Boulder, CO, 1979.

61. J. J. Murray, ed., *Appropriate Use of Fluorides for Human Health*, World Health Organization, Geneva, Switzerland, 1986.

62. U.S. Public Health Service, 1991, op. cit.

63. U.S. National Academy of Sciences, National Research Council, Board on Environmental Studies and Technology, *Health Effects of Ingested Fluoride*, National Academies Press, Washington, DC, 1993.

64. World Health Organization, *Fluorides and Oral Health*, WHO Technical Report Series 840, WHO, Geneva, Switzerland, 1994.

65. Locker, 1999, op. cit.

66. M. McDonagh et al., *A Systematic Review of Public Water Fluoridation*, NHS Centre for Reviews and Dissemination, University of York, prepared for the British National Health Service, 2000. See also *Br. Med. J.*, 321, 855–859, 2000.

67. Newbrun, 1989, op. cit.

68. Brunelle and Carlos, 1990, op. cit.

69. H. Kalsbeek and G. H. W. Verrips, Dental caries prevalence and the use of fluorides in different European countries, *J. Dent. Res.*, 69(Special Issue), 728–732, 1990.

70. L. S. Kaminsky, M. C. Mahoney, J. Leach, J. Melins, and M. J. Miller, Fluoride: benefits and risks of exposure, *Crit. Rev. Oral Biol. Med.*, 1, 261–281, 1990.

71. J. J. Murray, Efficacy of preventive agents for dental caries, *Caries Res.*, 27(Suppl. 1), 2–8, 1993.

72. Ripa, 1993, op. cit.

73. D. W. Lewis and D. W. Banting, Water fluoridation: current effectiveness and dental fluorosis, *Comm. Dent. Oral Epidemiol.*, 22, 253–158, 1994.

74. G. H. Petersson and D. Bratthall, The caries decline: a review of reviews, *Eur. J. Oral Sci.*, 104, 436–443, 1996.

75. J. A. Yiamouyannis, Water fluoridation and tooth decay: results from the 1986–1987 National Survey of U.S. Schoolchildren, *Fluoride*, 23, 55–67, 1990.

76. Locker, 1999, op. cit.

77. McDonagh et al., 2000, op. cit.

78. J. Burne, Fluoridation findings set teeth gnashing, *London Financial Times*, January 27, 2001.

79. D. Caron, Letter to the editor, *Br. Med. J.*, October 12, 2000.

80. R. L. Glass, ed., Proceedings of the First International Conference on the Declining Prevalence of Dental Caries, *J. Dent. Res.*, 61(Special Issue), 1304–1383, 1982.

81. Brunelle and Carlos, 1990, op. cit.

82. Proceedings of the Second International Conference on the Declining Prevalence of Dental Caries, *Int. Dent. J.*, 44, 365–458, 1994.

83. Featherstone, 1987, op. cit.

84. Ripa, 1993, op. cit.; Horowitz, 1996, op. cit.

85. C. W. Lemke, J. M. Doherty, and M. C. Arra, Controlled fluoridation: the dental effects of discontinuation at Antigo, Wisconsin, *J. Am. Dent. Assoc.*, 80, 782–786, 1970.

86. K. W. Stephen, D. R. McCall, and J. I. Tullis, Caries prevalence in northern Scotland before and 5 years after water defluoridation, *Br. Dent. J.*, 163, 324–326, 1987.

87. H. Kalsbeek, G. W. Kwant, A. Groeneveld, O. Backer-Dirks, A. Van Eck, and H. M. Theuns, Caries experience of 15-year-old children in the Netherlands after discontinuation of water fluoridation, *Caries Res.*, 27, 201–205, 1993.

88. L. Seppa, S. Karkainen, and H. Hausen, Caries frequency in permanent teeth before and after discontinuation of water fluoridation in Kuopio, Finland, *Comm. Dent. Oral Epidemiol.*, 26, 256–262, 1998.

89. W. Kunzel and T. Fischer, Rise and fall of caries prevalence in German towns with different fluoride concentrations in drinking water, *Caries Res.*, 31, 166–173, 1997.

90. Lewis and Banting, 1994, op. cit.; Rozier, 1995, op. cit.

91. Diesendorf, 1986, op. cit.; J. Colquhoun, Why I changed my mind about water fluoridation, *Perspect. Biol. Med.*, 41, 29–44, 1997.

92. B. A. Burt and E. D. Beltran, Water fluoridation: a response to critics in Australia and New Zealand, *J. Publ. Health Dent.*, 48, 214–219, 1988.

93. B. A. Burt, Relative consumption of sucrose and other sugars: Has it been a factor in reduced caries experience? *Caries Res.*, 27(Suppl. 1), 56–63, 1993.

94. Ibid.

95. Featherstone, 1987, op. cit.; E. L. Herod, The effect of cheese on dental caries: a review of the literature, *Aust. Dent. J.*, 36, 120–125, 1991.

96. Diesendorf, 1986, op. cit.; Petersson and Bratthall, 1996, op. cit.

97. References to the 19 articles can be found in Locker, 1999, op. cit., and Burt and Beltran, 1988, op. cit.

98. ADA *Fluoridation Facts*, op. cit.; Ripa, 1993, op. cit.

99. H. T. Dean, The investigation of physiological effects by the epidemiological method, in *Fluorine and Dental Health*, edited by F. R. Moulton, American Association for the Advancement of Science, Washington, DC, 1942; Ripa, 1993, op. cit.; R. G. Rozier, Epidemiological indices for measuring the clinical manifestations of dental fluorosis; overview and critique, *Adv. Dent. Res.*, 8, 39–55, 1994.

100. Leverett, 1982, op. cit.

101. ADA, *Fluoridation Facts*, op. cit.

102. U.S. Public Health Service, 1991, op. cit.

103. E. Babiuk, *Submission to City Council, Calgary, Alberta, 1997*, as posted by the Health Action Network, http://www.fluoridation.com.

104. Ibid.

105. F. Henry, The invisible fear, *Cleveland Plain Dealer*, Sunday supplement, March 26, 2000.

106. National Federation of Federal Employees Chapter 280 *Amicus Curiae* brief filed in support of *Natural Resources Defense Council, Inc., petitioner* v. *Environmental Protection Agency, respondent*, Civ. No. 85-1839, in the U.S. Court of Appeals for the District of Columbia Circuit, September 3, 1986.

107. Locker, 1999, op. cit.

108. Brunelle and Carlos, 1990, op. cit.

109. Locker, 1999, op. cit.

110. Dean, 1942, op. cit.

111. As reported in Ripa, 1993, op. cit.

112. McDonagh, 2000, op. cit.; D. C. Clark, Trends in prevalence of dental fluorosis in North America, *Comm. Dent. Oral Epidemiol.*, 22, 148–152, 1994.

113. Lewis and Banting, 1994, op. cit.; A. I. Ismail and R. R. Bandekar, Fluoride supplements and fluorosis: a meta-analysis, *Comm. Dent. Oral Epidemiol.*, 27, 48–56, 1999; J. J. Warren and S. M. Levy, A review of fluoride dentifrice related to dental fluorosis, *Pediatr. Dent.*, 21, 248–254, 1999.

114. Burt and Eklund, 1999, op. cit.

115. D. G. Pendrys, Risk of fluorosis in a fluoridated population: implications for the dentist and hygienist, *J. Am. Dent. Assoc.*, 126, 1617–1624, 1995.

116. Locker, 1999, op. cit.

117. E. Groth III, The fluoridation controversy: Which side is science on? in *Scientific Knowledge in Controversy: The Social Dynamics of the Fluoridation Debate*, State University of New York Press, Albany, NY, 1991; G. E. Smith, Fluoridation: forty years on, *Endeavour*, 11, 16–20, 1987.

118. Horowitz, 1996, op. cit.

119. B. A. Burt, The future of the caries decline, *J. Publ. Health Dent.*, 45, 261–269, 1985.

CHAPTER 8

FLUORIDE AND HEALTH

When it comes to assessing the impact of chemicals on human health, one has to peel the layers away carefully. We are at the intersection of science, medicine, and politics, with a strong flourish of human emotion thrown in to tangle the knot. Doubt and uncertainty rule, and clear-cut answers do not come easily. The ground is ripe for contention.

If there is a feeling that we do not know as much as we should about the toxicology of fluoride, it is not for lack of the written word. Over the years, there have been several book-length treatises on the subject,[1] many detailed review papers,[2] and literally hundreds of articles, pro and con, on every deleterious health impact that could possibly be laid at the door of fluoride. The anti-fluoridation camp combs this literature looking for ammunition. The pro-fluoridation camp takes up defensive positions awaiting the next firefight.

In this chapter we explore the minefield. The first few sections lay the groundwork, providing an introduction to the toxicologist's terms and tools, and emphasizing some of the issues that allow the medical conflicts to fester. In later sections we summarize the evidence and assess the current state of understanding with respect to a wide host of possible health impacts of fluoride. The coverage begins with the known toxicities, primarily those relating to skeletal fluorosis and bone health, and then moves through the various health claims of the anti-fluoridation movement, from those where equivocal information still leaves room for doubt to those based on zeal rather than fact.

EXPOSURE, INTAKE, AND DOSE

To a large degree, the conflict revolves around questions of exposure, intake, and dose. *Exposure* to fluoride may result from either *inhalation* of gaseous

The Fluoride Wars: How a Modest Public Health Measure Became America's Longest-Running Political Melodrama   By R. Allan Freeze and Jay H. Lehr
Copyright © 2009 John Wiley & Sons, Inc.

219

fluoride compounds or *ingestion* of liquids or solids containing fluoride. Bodily response is controlled in part by the *level of intake* and in part by the *duration* of the exposure. Toxicologists consider the duration of exposure to be especially important in assessing the health impact. They differentiate carefully between an *acute* exposure that takes place over a short period of time, and a *chronic* exposure that takes place over a long period of time. As we shall see, there is little question that acute exposures to fluoride through inhalation or ingestion of a sufficiently high intake over a sufficiently short time period are harmful to human health. Similarly, it is agreed by all parties that chronic exposures at lesser intake rates, but above some definable level, and experienced over a sufficiently long period, are also unhealthy. The contention arises with respect to chronic exposure to very low intake rates, and in particular, the chronic exposure that comes from the lifetime ingestion of fluoridated water at a fluoride concentration of about 1.0 ppm.

Of course, it is not just *exposure* and *intake* that control the bodily response to an ingested chemical, but also the size of the body that does the ingesting. Toxicologists have long recognized that children may be more susceptible to harm than adults, and infants more susceptible than older children. To this end, they define the *dose* as the intake per kilogram of body weight. *Acute dose*, which arrives more-or-less instantaneously, has units of milligrams of fluoride per kilogram body weight (mg/kg). *Chronic dose*, which arrives over time, has units of milligrams of fluoride per kilogram body weight per day. Toxicologists also recognize the importance of a *dose–response* relationship. Not all chemicals will produce an undesirable effect at the same dose, and not all bodily organs will respond to a given dose of a given chemical in the same way. Health response is chemical-, dose-, and organ-specific.

Proponents of fluoridation see fluoride compounds as beneficial to human health in small amounts but harmful in large amounts. In this, they claim, fluorides are similar to many other chemical compounds. Most of us recognize the painkilling value of an acetaminophen tablet, for example, but few of us would down an entire bottle at one sitting. Everyone recognizes the value of low concentrations of chlorine in our drinking water, but none of us would agree to drink a cup of undiluted hydrochloric acid. Opponents of fluoridation, on the other hand, are fearful of deleterious health effects from even the smallest dose. They liken fluoride to some of the metals, or organic solvents such as vinyl chloride, which are thought to be harmful at any dose.

This disagreement as to whether harm shown at *any* dose is indicative of harm at *all* doses will reverberate through many of the following discussions. Health care professionals from the medical establishment usually recognize the existence of a threshold level, a *toxic dose*, below which no harm will come.

Those from an alternative or holistic medical background are suspicious of such thresholds and are more inclined to recommend complete abstinence. The anti-fluoride camp has no compunction in parading the results of *acute* fluoride poisoning events before the public as proof of its *chronic* dangers. The pro-fluoride camp sees this strategy as scientifically naive, misleading, and unfair.

THE ROOTS OF CONTENTION

It is not as easy as one might think to make an unequivocal determination of whether exposure to a given chemical is harmful to human health. Toxicologists generally turn to one of three approaches in attempting to make such determinations, and all of them are fraught with problems. Let us look briefly at each of the three in turn: epidemiological studies of human illness, laboratory animal studies, and physiology-based medical reasoning.

There are several different types of *epidemiological study*: (1) studies of the impact on humans of acute accidental exposure, (2) occupational health studies on groups of industrial workers who have experienced chronic exposures larger than the general population, (3) public health studies that compare health impacts on exposed populations with those of unexposed control groups, and (4) forensic studies of documented cases of public health degradation. The first two types of study have provided the basic information currently available on the toxic impacts of fluoride at high dosages. The final two types of study have been much used in trying to clarify the possible chronic health impacts of the lower dosages that arise from fluoridation. The third approach, for example, was the basis of the analyses carried out in the original Bartlett–Cameron health studies, and in the health studies carried out as part of the Newburgh–Kingston fluoridation trial. The fourth approach, which is designed to uncover correlations between the incidence of disease and possible contributing factors to that disease, has been used widely by anti-fluoridation analysts to try to implicate fluoridation as a causative factor in certain diseases.

All epidemiological studies have the advantage that they deal directly with human beings. However, many issues arise. Studies of acute exposure may not be representative of chronic exposure. Occupational exposure may not be representative of public exposure. In comparative public health studies of chronic exposure, the selection of appropriate populations can be very difficult. Even nearby communities may have different demographics, different levels of industrialization, and different environmental baselines. It may not be possible to separate out the effects of age, gender, race, and other possible confounding factors. In forensic studies, the determination of the fluoride status of a community may be complicated by the presence of complex water-transfer agreements with other communities, widespread use of bottled water, fluoridated toothpaste use, and the halo effect.

Moreover, most epidemiological studies are statistical in nature. There is much room for the misuse of statistics, whether intended or accidental. Bias and wishful thinking may intrude on objective calculations. Hypotheses may be poorly formulated. Statistical significance may be overstated. And when all is said and done, it must be remembered that any positive correlation uncovered by a forensic study is a statistical relationship and nothing more. It does not prove a cause–effect relationship. Proof of a cause–effect relationship requires individual case–control study, with careful tracking of individual subjects over time and full knowledge of their distinct environmental circumstances. Unfortunately, the most common type of epidemiological study is the *ecological* study, which uses statistical measures to compare health impacts between fluoridated and nonfluoridated communities. The results of such studies are often equivocal and always controversial.

Given all these problems, it is not surprising that the pressures to reach judgment have led many researchers away from the epidemiological approach toward *laboratory animal studies*. Animal studies attempt to extrapolate the impact of *large doses* of fluoride imparted over a *short time period* to *small animals* (usually, mice or rats) to the impacts that would be experienced from *small doses* imparted over much *longer time periods* to much *larger animals* (human beings). Although widely used in the scientific world, this extrapolation is a crude and flawed approach and there is little scientific consensus on the validity of either the procedures or the results.

Animal experimentation for fluoride toxicity is invariably limited to a single strain of laboratory animal, a single disease, and a single target organ (e.g., the kidney or the heart). There are invariably questions about the predisposition of the various available strains of laboratory animals to the disease under investigation, about the possible impurities in the diets of the animals, or about the possible influence of other uncontrolled confounding factors on the results. Almost every experimental animal study that has reported clear-cut results in the fluoridation debate has come under attack from other experimentalists, who pillory the experimental design.

Given the problems associated with both epidemiological studies and animal experimentation, some toxicologists have turned to *physiology-based medical reasoning* to try to reach defensible conclusions about cause–effect mechanisms. Medical science has clarified much about the workings of the human body, and it seems logical to try to bring this knowledge to bear on toxicological issues. For example, as we learned in Chapter 7, fluoride is an effective bone-seeking element in the human body. Over 99% of the fluoride intake that is not excreted through the kidneys ends up in the body's hard tissues: the bones and teeth. It is not surprising, then, that the primary documented deleterious health impacts of fluoride relate to the bones and teeth. With respect to the body's soft tissues, there is much ongoing medical research into the causal mechanisms that lead to kidney damage, or attacks on the central nervous system, or the initiation and promotion of cancer. In some of these cases, there are mechanistic reasons that might lead one to suspect a role for fluoride in these pathologies; in others, there are not. The idea of using the results of basic science to solve forensic toxicological problems is appealing, but as yet immature. Someday it may be possible to develop dose–response relationships based on a mechanistic understanding of the impact of every possible chemical intake on every organ, but such an approach is still far from reality.

ACUTE FLUORIDE POISONING

Much of what we know about the harmful effects of fluoride on the human body comes from incidences of acute exposure in industrial accidents. We learned in Chapter 6 that *inhalation* of hydrogen fluoride gas, as happened at the Deepwater, New Jersey plant, and may have happened at Donora, Pennsylvania and in the Meuse Valley in Belgium, can lead to respiratory damage, dermal burns, and ocular irritation. More pertinent to our interests, it is well documented that *ingestion* of fluoride compounds, even in small amounts, can lead to nausea and gastrointestinal distress. In larger amounts, ingestion of fluorides can lead to organ damage and even death. The *acute lethal dose*, which is defined as the dose that is likely to produce fatal fluoride poisoning, is estimated to be in the range 32 to 64 mg/kg. Thus, a one-time ingestion of 2.5 to 5.0 grams of fluoride (1 to 2 ounces) would be fatal to an 80-kg (180-pound) adult, as would 0.6 to 1.2 grams (less than half an ounce) for a 20-kg (45-pound) child.[3] The *acute toxic dose*, which is defined as the minimum dose that is likely to cause toxic symptoms requiring immediate therapeutic intervention, is thought to be about 5 mg/kg (a one-time ingestion of about 400 mg for an adult or 100 mg for a child).[4]

Poison control centers across the United States report several incidences of fluoride overdoses each year, primarily by children, and usually due to ingestion of too much fluoride toothpaste or some other home fluoride product, such as mouthwash or pills. A full bottle or full tube of any of these home-based supplemental fluoride products contains more fluoride than the acute toxic dose for a child. In Chapter 12 we look more carefully at the risks associated with such products. Suffice it here to say that most acute poisoning events of this type are relatively mild, and the overall societal risks are probably quite low. Nevertheless, rare deaths have occurred. Home fluoride products should be handled with care. The recommended first-aid treatment for someone who swallows a potentially toxic fluoride dose is to induce vomiting as quickly as possible, and to drink milk, which may bind some of the fluoride before it enters the bloodstream.

Acute fluoride overdoses can also arise from rare natural events. Volcanic eruptions in Iceland emit gaseous fluoride compounds that have led to documented health impacts. On the coastal plains of North Africa, violent winds known as "darmous" sweep across outcrops of rock rich in fluorophosphate minerals, creating toxic fluoride dust storms. Cultivated crops and garden vegetables become tainted, drinking-water supplies are muddied, and symptoms of fluorosis abound.[5]

Although the fluoride values quoted above that result in toxicity may at first glance appear alarmingly small, the American Dental Association is quick to point out that they have no relevance to the ingestion of fluoridated drinking water. The amount of fluoride that is ingested from a single 8-ounce glass of fluoridated tap water is 10,000 to 20,000 times less than the acute lethal dose.

KAJ ROHOLM'S LEGACY

Anti-fluoride activists like to make much of fluoride's *acute* dangers, but it is really the question of *chronic* exposures that should concern us most. The history of chronic fluoride toxicology can be dated to the clinical observations of a Danish physician, Kaj Roholm, who in 1937 was the deputy city health officer of the city of Copenhagen, Denmark. He was asked to look into the deteriorating health of a group of cryolite workers from a local aluminum plant who suffered chronic exposure to fluoride-laden industrial dust. He was the first to identify the most important ill effects of chronic fluoride poisoning as being associated with the bones and the teeth. He noted the high degree of dental fluorosis in most of the subjects. More ominously, he observed a diffuse hardening of the bones throughout the skeleton, a condition known as *osteosclerosis*. Ligaments tended to become calcified. There was often a reduction in spinal column motility, in some cases amounting to almost complete fixation.[6] To make matters worse, patients suffered from general ill-health, loss of weight, skin and eye irritations, and a never-satisfied, tormenting thirst.

Roholm was the first to try to estimate the *chronic toxic dose* for fluoride, the maximum dose that can be accepted by the body over a long period of time without ill effect. Later observations by others have led to some revision of his original values. The currently accepted value lies in the range 0.10 to

0.25 mg/kg per day. For an 80-kg adult, this translates into a maximum allowable intake of 8 to 20 mg/day.[7] The U.S. Food and Nutrition Board, which has the responsibility for setting a *tolerable upper intake level* for dietary nutrients have settled on a value of 10 mg/day for adult Americans. The implication is that adults who are exposed to dose rates greater than 10 mg/day over periods of 10 to 20 years are at risk for the development of osteosclerosis and the other symptoms of chronic fluoride poisoning. Those exposed to dose rates lower than 10 mg/day should be safe from any harm.

The World Health Organization (WHO) has decided that a lifetime exposure is more likely to last 40 to 80 years than just 10 to 20, so they recommend an even lower maximum allowable intake, 2 to 5 mg/day.[8] In this regard, it is worth noting that the average intake of fluoride for someone who regularly drinks fluoridated water is about 1.0 mg/day, which seems alarmingly close to the low end of the WHO limit. Fluoride foes point to these figures as proof of the menace of fluoridation. However, most knowledgeable observers find the WHO limits unduly conservative and point to the much larger margin of safety afforded by the FDA limits. All available evidence suggests that the fluoride intake of lifelong residents of fluoridated communities should lie well within the tolerable limits. People who spend many years in a community where the drinking water contains a high natural fluoride concentration, greater than 10 ppm, say, have more to worry about. They are candidates for chronic toxic impacts of the type Kaj Roholm first observed in the Copenhagen cryolite workers.

Kaj Roholm is probably the only establishment medical figure to be revered by both pro- and anti-fluoridation camps. Anti-fluoridationists are happy to quote his gruesome descriptions of fluorosis victims. Pro-fluoridation toxicologists recognize the careful foundation he laid for their specialty. Harold Hodge later dedicated one of his works to Roholm, describing him as "a talented and vigorous scientist, a devoted and dedicated clinician and public health officer, and a genuine and gracious human being."[9] Roholm died at a young age in 1948. The symptoms that he identified and documented in Copenhagen in the late 1930s are the precursors to a disease that is now known as *crippling skeletal fluorosis*.

THE TRAGEDY OF CRIPPLING SKELETAL FLUOROSIS

Crippling skeletal fluorosis (CSF) is a tragic disease that ages people before their time. It is the severest possible form of osteosclerosis. It is endemic in many third-world countries, most notably India, China, and some of the countries of North Africa. It is caused by excessive fluoride intake, usually from drinking water that is particularly high in natural fluoride (much higher than that of artificially fluoridated water). Phase 1 of the disease is described as involving sporadic pain and stiffness of joints; phase 2 leads to chronic joint pain, arthritic symptoms, and calcification of ligaments; and phase 3 displays limitation of joint movement, crippling deformities of the spine, and muscle wasting. In advanced cases, there are often neurological defects, usually ascribed to the compression of the spinal cord.[10] People who suffer from CSF have significantly reduced life expectancies.

The World Health Organization[11] estimates that over 100 million people in India and China drink water with naturally elevated fluoride levels, in many cases as high as 20 to 30 ppm fluoride. Over 1 million of them suffer from advanced stages of CSF. In the Guizhou province of China, some of the widespread skeletal fluorosis observed there may be caused by eating foods that are dried over coal-burning stoves that burn high-fluoride coal.[12] There are other contributing factors that tend to make CSF a third-world disease. For one thing, the disease is more prevalent in tropical climates that induce greater consumption of drinking water. For another, it is closely associated with nutritional deficiencies of calcium, magnesium, and vitamin C, which are common in the underdeveloped parts of the world.

Crippling skeletal fluorosis is extremely rare in the United States. There have only been five documented cases in the last 35 years. Two of these subjects are known to have been heavy water drinkers of high-fluoride water, with a total fluoride intake on the order of 15 to 20 mg/day.[13] Several health studies carried out in the United States over the years attest to the rarity of skeletal fluorosis in this country. The first health study to target fluoride, carried out in the 1940s in Bartlett and Cameron, Texas, found no significant difference between the high- and low-fluoride town with respect to arthritis, osteoporosis, or bone fractures. In the children's health study that accompanied the Newburgh–Kingston fluoridation trial, annual x-rays of the wrists and knees of each child found that all children were within the normal range of skeletal maturation. A study of the x-ray files of 170,000 people in Texas and Oklahoma who drink water with elevated fluoride levels (in the range 4 to 8 ppm) identified 23 cases of osteosclerosis, but none of crippling skeletal fluorosis.[14]

The pro-fluoridation camp, fully supported by all national health agencies and the entire medical establishment, feels that the evidence is very clear. In their view, 60 years of experience in the United States confirms the fact that chronic exposure to the low-fluoride dose delivered by fluoridated drinking water does not increase the risk of developing crippling skeletal fluorosis. The disease is essentially unknown in this country, and there is no evidence of a present or emerging problem. The anti-fluoride camp continues to warn that increasing levels of fluoride in the human environment, and increasing levels of dental fluorosis, are harbingers of an increase in CSF. Perhaps they believe this and perhaps they don't, but it is hard to put aside the suspicion that they harp on this horrible disease primarily for the shock value.

FLUORIDE AS MEDICINE: THE OSTEOPOROSIS EXPERIMENTS

Currently, over 25 million Americans suffer from the bone disease *osteoporosis*. It is particularly prevalent among postmenopausal women. Each year osteoporosis patients suffer 1.5 million bone fractures (primarily of the vertebrae, hip, and wrist). A woman at age 60 has an average residual lifetime risk of osteoporotic fracture of 56%. The annual costs associated with repairing osteoporotic fractures run to over $10 billion.[15]

Osteoporosis is the opposite of osteosclerosis. Where osteosclerosis features a hardening of the bones, an increase in bone density, and a decrease in porosity, osteoporosis features a softening of the bones, a decrease in bone density, and an increase in porosity. As we have seen, excessive fluoride intake is known to cause osteosclerosis, and although this is not a good thing when it is a precursor to skeletal fluorosis, it might be a good thing for someone who is suffering from osteoporosis. It is not surprising, therefore, that medical practitioners quite early in the game began to think about the possibility of using fluoride therapy for osteoporosis patients. If a lifetime of high-fluoride intake hardens the bones to excess, perhaps a controlled intake over a shorter period could be used to help strengthen bones weakened by osteoporosis and reduce the risk of bone fracture in later years.

Under the therapeutical regimen that was developed in the 1970s, osteoporosis patients were fed 50 to 60 mg/day fluoride, together with calcium and estrogen supplements. Note that this fluoride dose is more than five times the FDA's maximum acceptable daily dose, and considerably more than the dose that is known to cause dental and skeletal fluorosis. Nevertheless, in a number of controlled clinical trials, the subjects were tracked over the short term by assaying possible increases in their bone mass density, and over the long term, by comparing the incidence of bone fractures against a control group of untreated osteoporosis patients. Several review articles have summarized the results of these studies.[16]

The measurements of bone mass density (BMD) in most of the clinical trials were made by means of x-ray radiography. Initial results were encouraging and indicated an unequivocal increase in BMD for patients undergoing fluoride therapy. However, as time went on, and the fracture data began to come in, the initial enthusiasm was quickly dampened. In some of the clinical trials, fracture incidence seemed to be marginally lower in treated patients; in others it was marginally higher. Successive studies carried out by the same experimental team often reported favorable results in one paper, unfavorable results in the next. The only consistent finding was that fracture incidence appeared to be dependent on fracture site, with vertebral fractures perhaps more favorably influenced by fluoride therapy than fractures of the hip, neck, or wrist.

Kathy Phipps, Executive Director of the Oregon Pacific Area Health Education Center in Newport, Oregon, has provided a convincing explanation of the fracture-site findings in her review paper in the *Journal of Public Health Dentistry* in 1995.[17] She points out that 80% of skeletal bone is *cortical bone*, the solid mass of bone found in the shafts of long bones and the outer wall of most other bones. The other 20% is *trabecular bone*, which forms the latticework of rods, plates, and arches that complete the skeletal detail. Bone is being replaced and renewed continuously in a process known as *bone remodeling*. The turnover rate for trabecular bone remodeling is 26% per year, whereas that for cortical bone is only 3% per year. It follows that the fluoride that is taken into the apatite crystals in the bone structure is more likely to find a place in trabecular bone than in cortical bone. This is indeed what is observed, with increases in BMD being greater in trabecular than in cortical bone. The vertebral bones are largely trabecular, so it is not surprising that whatever small advantage might accrue from fluoride therapy would accrue there.

Overall, however, the judgment of the medical fraternity has been negative. Some studies seem to indicate that despite the increase in density, newly formed, fluoride-rich bone often exhibits reduced strength and increased fragility, leading to more rather than fewer bone fractures. In 1989, an advisory committee of the Food and Drug Administration was the first to conclude that fluoride therapy was not effective for the treatment of osteoporosis.[18] Almost every review since then has concurred. In his review of fluoride issues for the Ontario Ministry of Health, David Locker concluded that the results of fluoride treatment studies are inconsistent and that the therapy is of "uncertain value."[19] Not only is there no consistent proof of good, but the therapeutical dose rates are so high that they could possibly engender harm. At least for now, fluoride therapy is on the back shelf. Help for victims of osteoporosis will have to come from elsewhere.

BONE HEALTH AND HIP FRACTURES: LEGITIMATE QUESTIONS AND EQUIVOCAL ANSWERS

If fluoride intake cannot be shown to improve bone strength, it is only a small jump to question whether it might harm it. Anti-fluoridationists have been very vocal in their claim that increased intake of fluoride may be responsible for the large number of hip fractures that are experienced by elderly people in the United States. According to the Centers for Disease Control, there are over 340,000 hospital admissions per year for hip fractures, 75% of them elderly women. One in four of these women die within a year, and one in two never regain an independent existence. The annual Medicare costs for hip fractures is estimated at almost $3 billion.[20]

Given the undenied affinity of fluoride for bone, this charge falls within the nexus of legitimate medical concern. It has spawned a veritable flood of epidemiological studies since 1990 comparing the incidence of hip fractures in fluoridated and nonfluoridated communities. The results of these studies have been equivocal, to say the least. Locker's Ontario Ministry of Health review, for example, identified 15 separate studies. Of these, seven showed no discernible association between hip fracture incidence and community fluoridation status, five showed an increase in fracture incidence in fluoridated communities, and three showed a decrease.[21] The University of York review carried out for the British National Health Service identified 29 studies of bone problems, nine of which provided a comparative analysis of hip fracture data. Of these, four studies claimed to have identified an increased risk of fracture with fluoridation, five studies a decreased risk.[22]

Regular consumption of fluoridated water cannot even be shown to have a clearly established effect on bone mineral density. Locker identified five studies of this issue, with only two of them showing higher BMDs in fluoridated communities relative to nonfluoridated communities. Of these two, one was significantly higher, the other only slightly higher. The other three studies were unable to find any association at all.

It is possible that these generalizations hide some important details. The individual studies are far from identical, and across-the-board comparisons undoubtedly take something away from the uniqueness of each analysis. Different hip-fracture and BMD studies looked at different age groups, different bone sites, different geographical regions, and different durations of fluoride exposure. One association that is suggested by several of the studies is in keeping with the results from the osteoporosis trials. It appears that the most positive results (higher BMD, less fractures) tend to come from trabecular bone sites such as the spine rather than cortical bone sites such as the hip.

Overall, the reviewers of this body of work are unconvinced that any association between fluoridation status and the incidence of bone fractures has been identified. Locker feels that the anti-fluoride claims are "implausible." He concludes that "the studies conducted to date do not provide systematic and compelling evidence of an adverse effect on bone."[23] Joseph Raheb of the Health Department of Western Australia, in a particularly incisive review of this issue, notes that osteoporosis is widely regarded as the primary contributor to hip fractures in the elderly, and that it cannot be argued that fluoride plays any adverse role in the development of osteoporosis, as it has exactly the opposite influence on bone.[24] The University of York study concludes simply that there is "no clear association of hip fractures with fluoridation."[25]

THE SPECIAL CASE OF KIDNEY DIALYSIS

Half of the fluorine that makes it into the human bloodstream is excreted as urine through the kidneys. For this reason, fluoride toxicologists have always paid special attention to the possibility of kidney disease. Their concerns can be expressed in two separate questions. First, is there any evidence that fluoride intake could be responsible for a loss of renal function in otherwise healthy people? Second, can excess fluoride intake do harm to people who already suffer from kidney disease, especially those undergoing kidney dialysis treatment? The answer to the first question appears to be negative, that for the second question, positive.

The evidence seems clear-cut that even fairly significant levels of fluoride intake do not harm healthy kidneys. First, kidney damage has never been observed in aluminum plant workers who have suffered a fluoride overdose from exposure to hydrogen fluoride gas. Second, there has been no evidence of kidney damage in epidemiological studies carried out on lifetime residents of communities where drinking water has natural fluoride concentrations up to 8 mg/liter. Third, kidney damage has not been common in osteoporosis patients treated with fluoride doses up to 50 mg/day. And finally, experimental animal studies have never indicated renal toxicity at drinking water concentrations below 50 ppm.[26] Given these various lines of evidence, there seems little doubt that the ingestion of fluoride at the levels used in community water fluoridation programs is unlikely to produce kidney damage in humans. The National Kidney Foundation is on record to the effect that drinking fluoridated water does not harm the kidneys.[27]

However, for kidney patients who have already suffered a significant loss of renal function, the picture is quite different. The successful management of fluoride by the human body depends on its elimination by the kidneys. Impaired renal function leads to decreased fluoride clearance, a buildup of fluoride in the bones, and an increased risk of skeletal fluorosis and other bone diseases.[28] Defective bone development that is associated with impaired kidney function is known as *renal osteodystrophy*.

The primary candidates for renal osteodystrophy are kidney patients who are undergoing long-term hemodialysis. Under hemodialysis treatment, a patient's blood is exposed to as much as 150 gallons of water per week in an artificial kidney machine. If the water is not deionized, dissolved ions such as calcium, magnesium, aluminum, and fluoride can diffuse freely into the patient's blood. In the early years of development of the dialysis methodology, the dangers associated with fluoride diffusion were not realized, and there are several documented cases from the 1960s and 1970s of kidney patients on hemodialysis who developed symptoms of skeletal fluorosis.[29]

Some deaths have also been reported. The case of a 41-year-old nurse from Rochester, New York, was written up in 1965.[30] She died after her 14th hemodialysis treatment using fluoridated Rochester tap water. An autopsy showed her bone fluoride content to be 5500 ppm (more than twice normal). In Canada, in the late-1960s, a kidney specialist with several patients on identical hemodialysis regimens in Ottawa (where the water is fluoridated) and Montreal (where it is not), lost four of his Ottawa patients to complications brought on by osteosclerosis.[31]

News of these events diffused slowly through the kidney dialysis community, and by the mid-1970s the need for deionized water in hemodialysis treatment was widely recognized. Deionization removes not only fluoride, but also many other potentially harmful dissolved metals, notably aluminum, which have also been implicated in dialysis complications. In 1980, the U.S. Public Health Service issued a Surgeon General's advisory recommending the use of deionized water in all dialysis treatments.[32] It is now safe to say that all of the 175,000 Americans currently on dialysis are being treated without risk of developing symptoms of skeletal fluorosis, using deionized water in their kidney machines.

Sadly, this is not the end of the story. Deionization systems require regular replacement of their ion-exchange resins. In July 1993, a maintenance failure of a deionization system in a Chicago hospital led to the delivery of highly fluoridated water to 12 patients in a hemodialysis unit. Eleven of them became ill, and three of them subsequently died of cardiac arrest.[33] Hemodialysis treatment requires vigilant care. With proper protocols in place and barring serious human error, there is no longer any reason why hemodialysis patients should be at risk from fluoride poisoning.

ALLERGIC REACTIONS AND PSYCHOLOGICAL DISTRESS

Historically, the first claims of adverse health effects from drinking fluoridated water revolved around the issue of allergic reactions. They were brought to the fore by George Waldbott, a practicing physician who was chief of the allergy clinics in four Detroit hospitals during the period that the fluoridation movement was taking hold. Waldbott became convinced that the allergic reactions suffered by many of his patients were due to the increased dose of fluoride provided by newly fluoridated water supplies. He began keeping careful records and eventually published his case histories in a book that became the early bible of the anti-fluoridation movement.[34] He was also the founder of the International Society for Fluoride Research, and the first editor of its journal *Fluoride*. He was, without doubt, the titular leader of the scientific wing of the anti-fluoridation movement in the early years.

Critics are quick to note that Waldbott's case histories are anecdotal in nature. The symptoms that he claimed as evidence of fluoride poisoning (such as abdominal pain, headaches, skin rashes, numbness in the extremities, muscular weakness, and gastric distress) are common symptoms of many other minor diseases. Many of his histories involve patients whose complaints disappeared after they switched from fluoridated to nonfluoridated water. Such anecdotal recoveries are far from double-blind. Doubters claim that Waldbott's clinical services may have been more psychological than physiological.

The argument against allergic sensitivity to fluoride is in its own way also anecdotal. Pro-fluoridation activists ask why it is that all those who claim a hypersensitivity to fluoride seem to gravitate to the very small number of anti-fluoridation allergists who will take up their cause. Why is there no apparent impact on the millions of regular fluoride users? Or on the tens of thousands of Americans who move every year from nonfluoridated to fluoridated communities? Why aren't widespread allergic responses documented in the many fluoride trials that have been undertaken around the world? Why are allergic reactions not widely observed in the many carefully monitored school mouth-rinsing programs? Simply put, it is difficult to accept the isolated anecdotal claims of harm in light of the much larger numbers of people exposed to considerably more fluoride without effect.

The medical establishment is united in its view that allergic reactions to fluoride are unproven and unfounded. A careful review of past studies carried out in 1996 found no evidence of any negative immunological response following fluoridation, nor any confirmed, replicated diagnoses of allergic reactions.[35] The World Health Organization is on record that claims of allergic reactions to fluoride can be explained away as symptoms of "a variety of unrelated conditions."[36] The American Academy of Allergy, Asthma, and Immunology has concluded that "there is no evidence of allergy or intolerance to fluoride as used in the fluoridation of community water supplies."[37]

Pro-fluoridationists also gloat over what they see as clear proof of the psychological nature of allergy claims against fluoridation. In Cleveland, Ohio in 1956, newspapers reported that the recently approved fluoridation program for that city would began operation on June 1. However, for a variety of technical reasons the startup was delayed until July 15. During the intervening period, health officials received many complaints of physical ailments that were attributed to fluoridation before the fluoridation program had actually begun.[38] In another case, in Kuopio, Finland, after a "distressing dispute over the fluoridation issue," the city council announced that they would stop fluoridating the city water supply on December 31, 1992. In actuality, the fluoridation system was turned off on November 30 without public disclosure. A study carried out by the local medical research establishment monitored reports to local health authorities of symptoms ascribed by complainants to fluoridation. They found that a clear break in the number of such claims occurred after December 31, the announced date of cessation, not November 30, the actual date. They concluded that "fluoridation may have psychological effects which present themselves as perceived symptoms."[39]

The primary factor behind the strong stand by the medical establishment against fluoride allergies is the lack of a convincing immunological mechanism. They see an allergy as a reaction to a substance that the body recognizes as *foreign*. The fluoride ion, like other simple dissolved ions such as calcium and magnesium, is not foreign to the human body in an immunological sense. As a result, they contend that "no allergy to fluoride exists, or can exist."[40]

Anti-fluoridationists believe that they have found the necessary mechanism. They point to a paper published in the *Journal of the American Chemical Society* in 1981 by a team of biochemists led by J. Emsley of Kings College, London.[41] Emsley and his co-workers showed that a very strong molecular bond can develop *in vitro* (i.e., in laboratory experiments carried out on human cells) between fluoride ions and chemical entities known as *amides*. Amides are found at the junctions between the hundreds of amino acids that make up protein molecules. If fluorides can break the usual hydrogen bonding that occurs at such junctions, the body's immune system might treat the invading fluoride as foreign. If it does so, it will attempt to destroy the foreign intrusion, creating autoimmune allergic reactions in its wake. In fact, the Emsley team claims, the strong-bonding mechanism might also help explain many of the other purported adverse effects of fluoride on biological systems. They point out that hydrogen bonds are important in DNA cells, too, and hypothetically, interference with them could lead to genetic damage. Fluoride attack on collagen-producing cells could in principle help explain bone brittlization and arteriosclerosis. Needless to say, the scientific wing of the anti-fluoride movement is mightily intrigued.

The only problem is that the Emsley hypothesis has not proved convincing to other fluoride toxicologists. Immediately following publication of the Emsley paper, W. D. Armstrong, the dean of dental biochemists in the United States, attempted to replicate Emsley's findings without success. Despite careful study, he could find no evidence of the purported strong bonding between fluoride and amides.[42] Gary Whitford, author of the leading textbook on fluoride metabolism in the human body, performed similar studies with similar negative results. He concluded that it is extremely unlikely that strong fluoride–amide bonds develop in the human body.[43]

So we are left with another loose end. As usual, the anti-fluoride forces are forced to grasp at the only straw available, while the weight of medical thinking comes down on the other side.

AFFAIRS OF THE HEART

In 1972, an article appeared in George Waldbott's *National Fluoridation News* that claimed to have uncovered a link between the use of fluoridated water and increased heart disease.[44] The author of the article was a registered nurse from Antigo, Wisconsin, named Isobel Jansen. The town of Antigo (population 9000 at the time) fluoridated their water in 1949, discontinued the practice in 1960, and reinstituted it in 1965. Jansen was the president of the Citizen's Action Program, the group that led the local opposition to fluoridation over this period. Jansen's study, which she carried out on her own initiative, showed that during the period 1949–1970, while heart mortality rates across the nation rose slightly from 340 (per 100,000) to 366, the rates in Antigo rose dramatically, from 359 to 542. Jansen ascribed this rise in the cardiovascular death rate to the initiation of fluoridation in Antigo.

The National Institutes of Health were quick off the mark to repudiate Jansen's results. In a publication entitled "Misrepresentation of Statistics on Heart Deaths in Antigo, Wisconsin," they showed that a simple age correction accounted for the data.[45] Between 1949 and 1970, the percentage of the Antigo population greater than 75 years of age rose from 3.5% to 7.2% (from 1.5 times the state average to 3.4 times the state average). As Harold Hodge mused in his discussion of this finding: "Is there any wonder that the Antigo heart death rates were higher than average in 1950 and higher still in 1970?"[46] The NIH concluded that Jansen's purported association between fluoride and heart disease was illusory.

In the years that followed, perhaps prodded more by cancer mortality claims than by those associated with heart disease, several studies were carried out using national mortality statistics to determine whether there were any differences between fluoridated and nonfluoridated communities.[47] No such evidence was ever uncovered in these studies. The largest study was carried out by a group of experts at the National Heart, Lung and Blood Institute of the National Institutes of Health and was reported in the *American Journal of Epidemiology*.[48] It used data from the 20-year period 1950–1970 and involved examination of mortality rates in 227 fluoridated communities and 187 non-fluoridated communities. All crude differences in mortality experience were fully explained by corrections for age, gender, and racial composition. There was no difference between fluoridated and nonfluoridated communities in general mortality rates or in the specific mortality rates for heart disease. The American Heart Association has concluded that "there is no evidence that adjusting the fluoride content of public water supplies to a level of about 1.0 ppm has any harmful effect on the cardiovascular system."[49]

FLUORIDE AND GENETICS

Anti-fluoridationist claims that the ingestion of fluoridated water can cause genetic damage to unborn children rests on two studies, the first an epidemiological study carried out in the mid-1950s, and the second a laboratory animal study carried out in the mid-1970s. The pro-fluoridation medical establishment argues that both studies were flawed. The epidemiological study claimed an association between fluoridation and the occurrence of Down's syndrome, a genetic disease that indicates the presence of chromosomal aberrations in a patient's DNA. The study was carried out by Ionel Rapaport, a French-trained endocrinologist who worked at the Psychiatric Institute of the University of Wisconsin at Madison from 1954 to 1961. He studied the incidence of Down's syndrome in four midwestern states and concluded that mongoloid births occurred twice as often in fluoridated communities as in unfluoridated communities. He wrote up the results of his study and published them in a medical journal in France.[50] They might have remained buried were it not for the obsessive zeal of anti-fluoridation activists, some of whom discovered the work, had it translated from French into English, and began using its findings in anti-fluoridation battles across the nation.

Rapaport always claimed that he had no prior interest in fluoride and that he had been led to it by his search for the causes of Down's syndrome. He noticed that a disproportionate number of Down's syndrome patients at one of the Wisconsin state institutions had been born in Green Bay (much higher, for example, than for epileptics at the same institution). When he learned that Green Bay had a much higher natural fluoride content in its water supply than most other cities in the state, he began to read up on fluoride toxicity. It was his opinion that many of the clinical and biochemical features of Down's syndrome patients are similar to the chronic toxic effects of fluoride. Most notably, it appears that most Down's syndrome children have a low incidence of dental caries relative to the public at large and relative to their own healthy siblings. Many subsequent studies have confirmed the latter fact, although most of them have ascribed this odd finding to the impact of institutionalization.[51]

Rapaport, described as a quiet man who suffered "many internal scars,"[52] died in 1972, just before the mid-1970s publication of a spate of studies that contradicted his findings. A study carried out using birth records from Massachusetts for the period 1950–1966 showed no statistical significance between the incidence of Down's syndrome in fluoridated and nonfluoridated communities. In this study, the most highly correlated contributory factor was the age of the mother at the time of birth of the Down's child. The incidence of Down's syndrome was found to increase by about 0.2 case per 1000 births for each year of maternal age. All statistical differences that were observed between communities were fully explained by the influence of this correlation.[53] Later studies by J. D. Erickson of the U.S. Public Health Service, one of them a comprehensive study of Down's syndrome births in 44 U.S. cities, confirmed the influence of maternal age and found no difference in the prevalence of any type of congenital malformation between fluoridated and nonfluoridated cities.[54]

The laboratory animal study that underlies anti-fluoridationist claims of genetic damage from fluoride was carried out in the mid-1970s by a graduate student working under the direction of an experimental geneticist, Aly Mohamed, in the Department of Biology at the University of Missouri at Kansas City. Mohamed had published several earlier papers attesting to the mutagenicity of hydrogen fluoride gas on various vegetable crops and on the fruit fly, *Drosophila*. Other workers had reported chromosomal impacts from very high doses of sodium fluoride on mammalian cells in vitro. However, the work in question was the first to use rodents as experimental subjects. In the experiment, Mohamed and his co-worker claimed that they observed the development of dose-dependent chromosomal abnormalities in the bone marrow and sperm cells of laboratory mice who were fed fluoridated drinking water at concentrations between 1 and 100 ppm fluoride. Mohamed presented the results at a meeting of the American Chemical Society in San Francisco in 1976. However, the work did not appear in published form until six years later, and then only in the journal *Fluoride*, which is well known for its anti-fluoride bent.[55]

Nevertheless, claims of genetic damage like that presented by Mohamed represented a direct threat to the fluoridation movement. Shortly after the San Francisco meeting, the Public Health Service dispatched a two-person review panel to Kansas City, consisting of George Martin, the chief biochemist of the National Institute of Dental Research, and D. R. Taves, a well-known toxicologist from the University of Rochester. They pointed out that Mohamed's experiment was not double-blind, and they identified many instances in his protocols of what they held to be statistical distortions and inaccuracies. They concluded that the experimental team lacked objectivity and that the results indicated an undue degree of subjective judgment. Taves summarized these criticisms in the National Academy of Sciences' publication *Drinking Water and Health*, which was published in 1977.[56] Martin followed up with a paper in 1979 in which he and his co-workers stated that they were unable to replicate Mohamed's results.[57] These two studies, both of which appeared in print several years before Mohamed's work itself, concluded that there was no evidence that fluoride intake has any undesirable effect on rodent or human genetics.

In 1994, some 18 years after the original controversy, Aly Mohamed was part of a team of scientists that carried out an attempted replication of his long-ago work. It was a carefully controlled study of possible chromosomal aberrations in the bone marrow of mice under various regimens of fluoride intake. In a paper published in the highly regarded journal *Mutagenesis*, the team reported that fluoride intake could *not* be shown to induce genetic damage in the mice at any concentration. The authors state, with Mohamed presumably concurring, that "the results of the study do not confirm the positive responses reported earlier for similar treatment regimens in mice."[58] Although you will not find this news on any antifluoridation website, it appears that Mohamed has quietly but firmly repudiated the work that he and his graduate student reported back in 1976. It now appears that claims of genetic damage from fluoride intake have little experimental support.

Of course, as soon as one health fear wanes, another always seems to wax into its place. In the same year that Aly Mohamed was repudiating his claims of *mutagenic* impacts (damage to chromosomes, genes, and DNA), another scientist raised the specter of *teratogenic* impacts from fluoridation (involving birth rates). A risk analyst named Stan Freni, working at the National Center for Toxicological Research of the Food and Drug Administration, carried out an epidemiological study suggesting that birth rates in fluoridated communities may be reduced relative to those in nonfluoridated communities. He studied the total fertility rate for women between the ages of 10 and 49 over the period 1972–1988 in 30 regions of the country covering nine states. He found that in 20 of the regions, a county-by-county analysis of fertility rates showed decreasing fertility with increasing fluoride levels, while only 10 of the regions showed the reverse trend. The analysis takes into account many of the usual demographic confounding factors, including family income, unemployment rate, and education level, although apparently not such equally pertinent factors as attitudes toward contraception and abortion. Freni's results are statistically significant, but not strongly so. They are food for thought and will undoubtedly lead to more studies. Freni is not a maverick out to rattle the establishment cage. He recognizes the potential implications of his findings and the slippery statistical slope on which they are built. He recommends "caution" in interpreting his results.[59]

FLUORIDE, CANCER, AND CREDIBILITY

There is no more dreaded disease than cancer, and the anti-fluoridation movement has not been reticent in playing on the widespread public fear of this disquieting pandemic. As we shall see, the evidence that connects fluoride to cancer is very thin, but it has a history almost as long as the fluoridation movement itself. The first scientific study to claim a connection between fluoride and cancer was carried out in 1950 by Alfred Taylor of the Clayton Biochemical Institute at the University of Texas in Austin, Texas. Taylor claimed that when he fed fluoridated drinking water to a strain of cancer-prone mice, they developed tumors at an earlier age than mice that were fed distilled water. At the request of the Texas State Dental Health Officer, he initially agreed to keep these preliminary findings secret until confirmatory experiments could be performed. However, word leaked out. The story was picked up by local newspapers, and then by the Associated Press. Several Texas cities that were on the verge of instituting fluoridation, including Austin, Dallas, and Fort Worth, hastily postponed their programs.[60]

The National Cancer Institute immediately sent a team of investigators to Austin. They found fault with every aspect of Taylor's experiment. They claimed that the strain of mice was inappropriate and that the number of mice was insufficient to produce results of statistical significance. Most damning of all, they found that the animals' feed contained such a high concentration of fluoride that it would obliterate any possible effects that might have been discernable from the fluoridated water. They judged the experiments to be worthless and the purported relationship between fluoride intake and cancer initiation completely unproven. Despite these severe criticisms of his results, Taylor continued to speak publicly of them, most notably as an expert witness in the congressional hearings on fluoridation that were held in Washington in 1952. In his testimony, he did not mention the mouse chow issue.

Anti-fluoridation polemicists seldom mention Taylor's 1950 work. They prefer to highlight his second try, carried out 15 years later with his wife, Nell Carmichael Taylor, using a more appropriate strain of mice and fluoride-free feed. In this study the Taylors implanted carcinomas in mice and then measured the rate of tumor growth. They claimed an increased rate of tumor growth in the presence of sodium fluoride than in its absence.[61] However, this observation apparently held only at lower fluoride doses; at higher doses, tumor growth was actually inhibited. The loss of reputation from the earlier work, together with their proffering of this unlikely and never-replicated dose–response relationship, doomed the Taylors to further scolding from the medical establishment. Harold Hodge described their findings and conclusions "unthinkable."[62] Nowadays, their work carries no weight in the scientific community. It is kept alive solely through wish-fulfilling references to it in the anti-fluoridation literature.

Historically, the work of the Taylors is but a blip on the radar screen. The magnitude-10 earthquake came in 1975 with John Yiamouyiannis's claim that consumption of fluoridated water was responsible for 25,000 excess cancer deaths per year in the United States. This announcement came shortly after Yiamouyiannis had been removed from his editorial duties with the American Chemical Society because of his anti-fluoride activism. He announced these findings from his new pulpit as the science director for the National Health Federation, a group that made its name by opposing the medical establishment and espousing alternative health therapies. The entire affair was timed to hit the presses in the heat of the Los Angeles fluoridation referendum, and the resulting hubbub is widely credited with causing the defeat of that referendum. Yiamouyiannis based his claims on a study that he had carried out on the mortality data from 20 large American cities, 10 of which had been fluoridated since at least 1956 and 10 of which had never been fluoridated as of 1970. He claimed that the mean cancer mortality rate, summed over nine specific types of cancer, was 119.5 per 100,000 population in the fluoridated cities and only 95.5 per 100,000 in the nonfluoridated cities. He calculated that the difference of 25 per 100,000 would produce over 25,000 excess cancer deaths per year nationwide and that these deaths could be laid directly at the feet of the fluoridation movement.[63]

The medical establishment was flabbergasted by what they saw as a patent disregard for scientific objectivity. In their opinion, the report that Yiamouyiannis released during the Los Angeles referendum was little more than a "propaganda flyer," with its conclusions "emblazoned as slogans." It was not viewed as a "serious scientific effort." There were no "cautions or restrictions" noted. The bias was "pervasive and obvious," and the mistaken logic was "gross and naive."[64]

More tellingly, critics pilloried Yiamouyiannis for using crude mortality statistics in his study that were uncorrected for age. Cancer mortality is highly dependent on age. The annual incidence of breast cancer in women, for example, goes from near zero at age 20, to over 100 per 100,000 population at age 50, to almost 200 per 100,000 at age 70. Prostate cancer rates for men are almost zero at age 50, and rise to almost 300 per 100,000 by age 70.

Crude mortality statistics have little meaning if they are not corrected for the age distribution of the population studied. To a lesser degree, results are also sensitive to other demographic variables, such as gender and race. Men have higher cancer mortality rates than women, and blacks higher than whites.

Facing almost universal skepticism toward his findings, Yiamouyiannis turned to an unlikely source for help. Dean Burk was the recently retired chief chemist of the National Cancer Institute. He had been one of the founders of NCI and had spent almost 35 years with the agency. Burk was widely regarded as one of the world's leading cancer researchers. He had won innumerable national and international awards for his work on cancer metabolism, and was the co-author of papers with four different Nobel prize winners.[65] In the latter part of his career, however, he became interested in nonconventional cancer therapies, and often embarrassed his NCI colleagues by his support of questionable cancer drugs such as laetrile. On retirement, he founded the Dean Burk Foundation "devoted to research on health, nutrition, and chronic and degenerative diseases, including cancer." He was initially skeptical about Yiamouyiannis's study, but he was interested enough to join him in carrying out a reanalysis of the data that would address the issues raised by critics. Surprisingly, in Burk's opinion, Dr. Y's conclusions survived the reassessment, and Burk became a committed anti-fluoridationist.

Yiamouyiannis and Burk never published their study in a mainstream medical journal. Their results first appeared in the house organ of Yiamouyiannis's organization, the *Bulletin of the National Health Federation*, and later in the anti-establishment journal *Fluoride*.[66] It didn't matter. The impact of their work didn't come from these obscure articles, in any case. It came from their interactions with the U.S. Congress. In late 1975, they convinced an anti-fluoridation congressman James J. Delaney to read the results of their study into the *Congressional Record*. The press leaped on the story with glee. Anti-fluoridation activists boasted of "congressional approval" of their arguments against fluoride. In 1977, at another set of congressional hearings on fluoridation, they again made their case in friendly surroundings with much press coverage.

In the meantime, members of the medical establishment had taken up the cudgels. John Small, a spokesperson for the U.S. Public Health Service on fluoride matters, approached Marvin Schneiderman, the chief epidemiologist of the National Cancer Institute, and asked him to look into the Yiamouyiannis and Burk findings. Schneiderman assigned Robert Hoover to the task. Hoover and his NCI team looked carefully at the standard mortality ratios (SMRs) for the 20 cities used in the Burk and Yiamoutiannis study. The SMR is defined as the ratio of the number of deaths *observed* in a given city from a given disease, to the number of deaths *expected*, as determined from the national average. The SMR values for large cities are always greater than 1.0 because of the disproportionate number of older people and blacks who live in such cities and possibly also because of the higher levels of industrialization found there. In keeping with Yiamouyiannis and Burk, Hoover determined that the average SMR value for cancer in 1970 was indeed greater in the fluoridated cities (1.25) then in the non-fluoridated cities (1.15). However, Hoover's studies uncovered another fact of even greater importance: namely, that this difference in mortality ratios also existed in 1950 and there had been no change in their relative values over the period of study between 1950 and 1970. In other words, there had been no change in the patterns of cancer incidence in either fluoridated or nonfluoridated cities during the first 20 years of the fluoridation movement.[67]

Moreover, Hoover found that the nonfluoridated cities tended to be younger, whiter, and less industrialized than the fluoridated cities. The difference in cancer incidence between the two sets of cities was fully explained by these demographic differences in age, gender, and race. Another study based on the same data, carried out by a well-known British team of cancer epidemiologists, used 10-year age brackets, four categories of fluoride intake, and organ-by-organ cancer statistics (thyroid, kidney, stomach, esophagus, colon, rectum, bladder, bone, and breast). This study found no correlation with fluoridation status in any organ in any age bracket.[68] At least three other large-scale epidemiological studies carried out in the United States in the late 1970s failed to find any relationship between cancer and fluoride intake.[69]

Since that time, over 50 epidemiological studies have evaluated the possibility of an association between cancer mortality and water fluoridation. The overall conclusion from these studies is that there is no credible evidence that water fluoridation increases the risk of cancer. Independent studies by the U.S. Public Health Service, the U.S. National Academy of Sciences, the American Association for the Advancement of Science, the International Agency for Research on Cancer, and the World Health Organization all disclaim the existence of any relationship. The consensus of the scientific community is that the contrary results of Yiamouyiannis and Burk are attributable to "errors in data, errors in analytical technique, and errors in scientific logic."[70]

The American Cancer Society is on record that "scientific studies show no connection between cancer rates in humans and adding fluoride to drinking water."[71] The National Cancer Institute states that "studies to date have produced no credible evidence of an association between fluoridated drinking water and an increased risk of cancer."[72]

THE OSTEOSARCOMA CONTROVERSY

In making these statements that deny any relationship between fluoride and cancer, the medical establishment could be accused of glossing over some equivocal evidence relating to a rare type of bone cancer known as *osteosarcoma*. Given fluoride's propensity to lodge in the human skeleton, it is not unreasonable to search for a cancer impact in the form of malignant tumors of the bone. However, as we shall see, the evidence for such an impact is very controversial.

The story begins in 1977 at the congressional hearings on fluoridation carried out under the chairmanship of Congressman L. H. Fountain. These were the hearings where Yiamouyiannis and Burk presented their provocative cancer-link analysis and did battle with Robert Hoover and his team from the National Cancer Institute. As a result of the apparent discrepancies between these two studies, the congressional subcommittee that sponsored the hearings made a recommendation to the Public Health Service to carry out toxicological and epidemiological studies that would determine if there was any causal relationship between fluoride intake and cancer. It took over five years for the PHS to implement this recommendation, but in 1982 they began to do so under the auspices of the National Toxicology Program. They contracted the Battelle Memorial Institute of Columbus, Ohio to carry out animal-based toxicological studies on fluoride. Between 1982 and 1987, Battelle carried out two sets of studies, delivering their draft report to the NTP in 1988. The NTP didn't get around to releasing the final report to the public for another two years, but in 1990 they did so, some 13 years after the congressional mandate.

Buried within the mass of experimental data, most of which failed to indicate any relationship between fluoride and cancer intake, was one small nugget of concern. In one experiment where rats of a particular strain were fed fluoridated drinking water at the elevated concentrations of 11, 45, and 79 ppm, four rats (out of a total of 522) developed observable osteosarcomas. All of the affected rats were on the higher dosages, and all of them were male.[73] In 1990, an NTP Peer Review Committee termed this higher-than-expected incidence of osteosarcoma in male rats as "equivocal evidence of carcinogenic activity."[74] In the same year, just to muddy the waters, another experimental team attempting to replicate the NTP results did not observe the development of any osteosarcomas in any rats of either gender at any dose.[75]

In the meantime, on the epidemiological front, the National Cancer Institute was in the process of completing two studies using two different national registries of cancer mortality data. In the first study, they used their nationwide, county-by-county registry to analyze over 2.3 million cancer deaths that occurred in the United States during the period 1950–1985. This analysis allowed for the isolation of bone cancer statistics but not of specific types of bone cancer such as osteosarcoma. The study concluded that the risk of death from bone cancer 35 years after the widespread initiation of fluoridation was the same as in the years prior to fluoridation.[76]

The second study used the cancer registry of the NCI's Surveillance, Epidemiology and End Results (SEER) program. This registry, started in 1973, represents only about 10% of the U.S. population, but it provides more detailed data. In the case at hand, it allowed analysts to look more specifically at the incidence of osteosarcoma in two localized areas, the city of Seattle and the state of Iowa. What they found was a slight increase in the incidence of osteosarcoma in males under 20 years of age between the period 1973–1980 and the period 1981–1987 (from 3.6 cases per 100,000 population to 3.8). They also found a slightly higher incidence of osteosarcoma in fluoridated communities relative to unfluoridated communities. Notwithstanding the latter finding, the report concluded: "Although the reason for the increase in young males remains to be clarified, an extensive analysis reveals that it is unrelated to the introduction and duration of fluoridation."[77]

In 1991, the Public Health Service published its long-awaited *Review of Fluorides: Benefits and Risks*. It was based largely on the NTP experiments and the NCI epidemiological studies. The report concluded that the experimental studies "fail to establish an association between fluoride and cancer." Furthermore, the "extensive human epidemiological data available to date, including the new studies prepared for this report," provide strong evidence that "optimal fluoridation of drinking water does not pose a detectable cancer risk to humans."[78] The "equivocal" evidence concerning osteosarcoma was given little credibility.

The year after publication of the PHS *Review of Fluorides*, a health officer named P. D. Cohn, working with the New Jersey Environmental Health Service, published a brief report of his epidemiological findings from seven municipalities in New Jersey. He reached the same conclusion as that in the SEER study: that osteosarcoma rates in young males were significantly higher in fluoridated than in nonfluoridated communities.[79] However, similar studies carried out during the same period in New York and Alberta found no such relationship.[80]

The trouble with all the epidemiological studies, especially the very local ones, is the tiny size of the available statistical sample. In 1985, for example, there were over 450,000 cancer deaths in the United States, but only 1400 of these were bone cancers and only 750 were osteosarcomas. Osteosarcoma accounts for only 0.2% of all cancer deaths. One or two cases more or less in a local study, or even a national one, can skew the statistics significantly.

You will recall from discussions at the start of this chapter that case–control studies (studies that track individual patients) are far superior in reaching conclusions about cause–effect relationships than either laboratory animal experiments or human epidemiology studies. In 1995, three separate case–control studies on osteosarcoma patients appeared in the medical literature. The authors of all three reported that they could find no association between the development of osteosarcoma and exposure to fluoridated water.[81] The results of these studies deserve considerable weight when trying to reach a conclusion on osteosarcoma.

In his review for the Ontario Ministry of Health, David Locker states unequivocally that these case–control studies lay to rest the osteosarcoma concerns raised originally by the NTP rat experiments. He concludes that there is no reason to believe that exposure to fluoridated water increases rates of cancer, either of the bone or of any other body tissues.[82] The York University review, carried out for the British National Health Service, concludes that there is no clear association between water fluoridation and cancer incidence and mortality, including osteosarcoma and bone–joint cancers.[83]

Despite this seemingly unequivocal testimony, nagging worries remain. In an attempt to lay these worries to rest, the National Institute of Environmental Health Sciences (a branch of the National Institutes of Health) decided to fund a 15-year epidemiological study on the possible role of fluoride intake on the incidence of osteosarcoma. The grant was awarded to the Harvard School of Dental Medicine, with Chester W. Douglass as principal investigator. Much to the chagrin of the project's leaders, the first results, contained in the 2001 doctoral thesis of a graduate student, Elise Bassin, indicated a "robust" relationship between fluoride exposure and osteosarcoma in young males (5 to 10 years old). Douglass, for his part, considered this work preliminary. He did not encourage early publication of the results in a technical publication, nor did he report them to NIEHS in a 2004 overview report to the agency. It is his contention that Bassin's results have not been replicated in subsequent stages of the overall study.

In June 2005, the Environmental Working Group (EWG), an advocacy group whose primary goal is "to protect the most vulnerable segments of the human population from toxic contaminants," found out about Bassin's thesis and demanded that NIEHS carry out an investigation to determine whether Douglass's actions constituted a cover-up of facts that could pose a risk to society (and to the fluoridation movement).[84] Learning of the EWG charges, Paul Connett of the Fluoride Action Network called for Douglass's immediate removal. William Hirzy (a strong anti-fluoride leader whom we meet in Chapter 9) called for a nationwide moratorium on fluoridation until the issue is resolved.

At the behest of NIEHS, Harvard University set up an inquiry panel to review Douglass's actions. One year later, in August 2006, the panel reported the results of their deliberations. They exonerated Douglass, finding that he did not "intentionally omit, misrepresent, or suppress the findings" of his graduate student. Anti-fluoridation websites have honed in not on the exoneration, but on the word "intentionally." In the same year, Bassin's results were finally published in the journal *Cancer Causes and Control*.[85] Douglass was not a coauthor on the paper. In fact, he submitted a letter to the editor that was published in the same journal urging caution and warning against "overinterpretation or generalization" of these early results of the planned long-term study at Harvard.[86]

ALZHEIMER'S, INTELLIGENCE, CRIME, AND ADDICTION

In 1999, Roger Masters, an emeritus professor with the Foundation for Neuroscience and Society at Dartmouth College, together with a consulting chemical engineer, Myron Coplan, published the first of a series of papers that implicate the chemicals used in water fluoridation as a cause of diminished brain development and behavioral dysfunction. Masters and Coplan claim that the silicofluorides added to public water supplies (in the form of either fluosilicic acid or sodium silicofluoride) mediate the increased transfer of lead and other heavy metals from the gastrointestinal tract into the bloodstream, and from the bloodstream into the brain. It is widely recognized that heavy metals, especially lead, compromise normal brain development, leading to long-term learning deficits and problems of antisocial behavior in children. In attempting to tie silicofluorides into this web, Masters and Coplan are indicting the chemicals of choice in over 90% of America's fluoridation systems as a potential causitive factor in a high-profile public health issue that generates considerable parental dread. The underlying message seems obvious: If fear of lead was sufficient to bring about the demise of leaded housepaint and leaded gasoline, fluoridation should be the next to fall.

Masters and Coplan have not been shy in making their case. In 1999 alone, they presented their results at the annual meetings of the New York Academy of Medicine, the 17th International Neurotoxicology Conference in Little Rock, Arkansas, and the Association for Politics and the Life Sciences in Atlanta, Georgia. Their tone was shrill. "If further research confirms our findings," they stated, silicofluorides may be recognized as "the worst environmental poison since leaded gasoline." Surely, they argued, "innocent children should not be poisoned by public water supplies."[87]

Masters and Coplan have not carried out experimental studies to investigate the mechanisms by which silicofluorides might mediate lead uptake. Their work is statistical in nature, based on data provided to them by others. In one such study, they examined the results of 150,000 analyses of lead levels in the blood of children up to 6 years old from 105 midsized New York cities provided by the New York State Department of Children's Health for the period 1994–1998. After adjusting the data for age, race, and several other possible confounding factors, they found a statistically significant elevation in blood-lead concentrations for children from communities in which the water was fluoridated using silicofluorides, relative to those from nonfluoridated communities or communities that used sodium fluoride as the fluoridating chemical.[88]

The lead-uptake theories of Masters and Coplan are hotly contested by more traditional scientists. The pro-fluoridation camp whisks aside their work, pointing instead to more recent studies claiming that "no credible evidence exists to show that water fluoride has any quantifiable effects" on lead uptake.[89] However, Masters and Coplan claim more than just a theory of lead uptake by the brain; they claim to be able to document its societal impacts. In other studies carried out in Massachusetts and New York, they found that silicofluoride communities experience higher crime rates (1480 per 100,000 population compared to 1100 per 100,000 in nonfluoridated communities), a higher percent of criminals using cocaine at the time of their arrest (44% to 32%), and a higher rate of attention deficit disorder in children (with a risk ratio of 1.38).[90] Others have picked up on their lead, with one study purporting to show a strong correlation between water fluoridation and crime in the United States[91] (although the author is careful to note that his work represents a "data-based hypothesis about one possible cause of crime; it is not a definitive statement about crime causality"). All these authors argue the need for more cross-disciplinary research that integrates neurotoxicology, environmental chemistry, and the study of human behavior.

Masters and Coplan are not the only researchers to try to draw a connection between fluoridation and neurological matters. Two papers from China that appeared in the journal *Fluoride* attempted to develop a correlation between fluoride exposure and reduced intelligence in children.[92] These papers have been roundly criticized for working with crude statistical data that are uncorrected for any of the standard confounding factors. By the same token, a paper that appeared in the much more prestigious journal *Neurotoxicology*, which claimed that higher fluoride levels are actually *protec-*

tive against Alzheimer's disease, is open to the same criticism.[93] Yet another epidemiological study completed in 1986 in New Zealand concluded that there was no evidence to indicate that exposure to optimally fluoridated drinking water has any detectable adverse effect on children's health or behavior.[94]

These attempts to find neurotoxicological disorders associated with fluoride intake are not entirely off the wall. Plant workers exposed to acute fluoride poisoning from industrial accidents often become mentally disoriented as well as physically ill.[95] Furthermore, about 10% of all cases of crippling skeletal fluorosis are known to involve neurological complications. For these reasons, there have been several laboratory animal experiments designed to investigate possible impacts on the central nervous system from excessive fluoride intake. Two of these studies have suggested a positive relationship and so are much beloved by the anti-fluoridation movement.

Phyllis Mullenix, a neurotoxicologist working at the Forsythe Dental Center in Boston in the early 1990s, found that rats fed a high-fluoride diet exhibited behavior-specific changes related to cognitive deficits.[96] Neurotoxic effects were observed regardless of whether the rats were given the fluoride as adult animals, as young animals, or through the placenta before birth. However, the effects varied. Those rats given fluoride as young and adult animals exhibited depressed activity patterns. Those given fluoride before birth were unexpectedly hyperactive. Post-experimental autopsies indicated elevated fluoride levels in the brain tissues of the rats.

Critics of her work claim that Mullenix's fluoride dosages were too high to allow extrapolation of her results from rats to humans, but Mullenix argues that these dosages produce the same plasma fluoride levels in rats as a 5- to 10-ppm dosage would in humans. Other critics point to perceived inadequacies in experimental design: in particular, the lack of control groups. As one set of reviewers proclaimed: "We do not believe that the study by Mullenix can be interpreted in any way as indicating the potential for sodium fluoride to be a neurotoxicant."[97] In his 1996 book on fluoride toxicology, Gary Whitford states that "it seems more likely that the unusually high brain fluoride concentrations reported by Mullenix were the result of some analytical error."[98] For her part, Mullenix is firmly convinced that her rat study has flagged the potential for fluoride-induced motor dysfunction, IQ deficits, and learning disabilities in humans.

The other laboratory experiment that is widely quoted in anti-fluoride circles bears a resemblance to Masters and Coplan in its working hypothesis. J. A. Varner and co-workers report in the journal *Brain Research* that their rat experiments indicate that fluoride may mediate an increased transfer of aluminum to the brain, just as Masters and Coplan claim it does for lead.[99]

Elevated aluminum levels in the brain are widely suspected of playing a role in the development of Alzheimer's disease. The American Dental Association, through its Health Media Watch, has fiercely repudiated Varner's work.[100]

It must be emphasized that all of these studies attempting to implicate low-level chronic fluoride intake as a neurotoxicant are speculative. The epidemiological studies that suggest a relationship between fluoridation and social behavior are based on results that are at the lower levels of statistical significance, and they are open to the same issues of wishful thinking and interpretive manipulation as are all such studies. The results of the experimental studies have not been replicated by other scientists. There have been charges of inadequate experimental design. The protocols are open to the usual charge that experimental dosage was too high to allow reasonable translation of the results from rats to humans. Certainly, the experimental doses far exceed those received by people who ingest fluoridated water. None of the laboratory experiments can be fairly said to address the possible chronic effects of low-level fluoride intake by humans from fluoridated water. Nevertheless, the various studies provide food for thought. Anti-fluoridationists have for years warned of mind control, and now they have a few glimmers of scientific support for such neurotoxicologic suspicions. The issue is not going to go away soon. More experimental results can be expected, and more epidemiological studies are undoubtedly on the books.

As with most of these health issues, absolute proof of neurotoxicological harm is difficult to come by, but so is absolute proof of safety. Further detailed work will undoubtedly clarify the issues somewhat, but to our mind there are more general questions that still remain unanswered, and they come to the fore here perhaps more than in any of the other medical conundrums. Can we count on value-free research from scientists, who tend to sit on one side of the fence or the other? Can we expect a fair balance of research funding from agencies that have political positions to defend? Who out there is actually questing for the medical truth? In the next few chapters we investigate this clash of cultures as science comes up against sociopolitical reality.

REFERENCES

1. E. J. Largent, *Fluorosis: The Health Aspects of Fluorine Compounds*, Ohio State University Press, Columbus, OH, 1961; J. R. Marier and D. Rose, *Environmental Fluoride*, 2nd ed., Publ. 16081, National Research Council of Canada, Toronto, Ontario, Canada, 1977; R. Y. Eagers, *Toxic Properties of Inorganic Fluorine Compounds*, Elsevier, New York, 1986; U.S. National Academy of Sciences, National Research Council, Board on Environmental Studies and Technology, *Health Effects of*

Ingested Fluoride, National Academies Press, Washington, DC, 1993; G. M. Whitford, *The Metabolism and Toxicity of Fluoride*, Karger, Basel, Switzerland, 1996.

2. F. J. McClure, A review of fluorine and its physiological effects, *Physiol. Rev.*, 13, 277–300, 1933; H. C. Hodge and F. A. Smith, Some public health aspects of water fluoridation, in *Fluoridation as a Public Health Measure*, edited by J. H. Shaw, American Association for the Advancement of Science, Washington, DC, 1954; H. C. Hodge and F. A. Smith, Biological properties of inorganic fluorides, in *Fluorine Chemistry*, edited by J. H. Simons, Academic Press, New York, 1965, Vol. 4, pp. 1–42; G. M. Whitford, The physiological and toxicological characteristics of fluoride, *J. Dent. Res.*, 69, 539–549, 1990.

3. Hodge and Smith, 1954, op. cit.; B. A. Burt and S. A. Eklund, *Dentistry, Dental Practice, and the Community*, W.B. Saunders, Philadelphia, 1999; Public Health Service, Agency for Toxic Substances and Disease Registry, *Toxicological Profile for Fluorine, Hydrogen Fluoride, and Fluorides*, U.S. PHS, Washington, DC, 2003.

4. American Dental Association, *Fluoridation Facts*, http://www.ada.org.

5. F. J. McLure, *Water Fluoridation: The Search and the Victory*, National Institute of Dental Research, Bethesda, MD, 1970.

6. K. Roholm, *Fluorine Intoxication*, H. K. Lewis, London, 1937.

7. Hodge and Smith, 1954, op. cit.; Burt and Eklund, 1999, op. cit.

8. P. Adler et al., *Fluorides and Human Health*, World Health Organization, Geneva, Switzerland, 1970.

9. Hodge and Smith, 1954, op. cit.

10. S. S. Jolly, B. M. Singh, C. C. Mathur, and K. C. Malhotra, Epidemiological, clinical and biochemical study of endemic dental and skeletal fluorosis in Punjab, *Br. Med. J.*, 4, 427–429, 1968; S. P. S. Teotia and M. Teotia, Endemic fluorosis in India: a challenging national health problem, *J. Assoc. Phys. India*, 32, 347–352, 1984.

11. Adler et al., 1970, op. cit.

12. R. B. Finkleman, H. C. W. Skinner, G. S. Plumlee, and J. E. Bunnell, Medical geology, *Geotimes*, 46(11), 20–23, November 2001.

13. ADA, *Fluoridation Facts*, op. cit.

14. Ibid.

15. K. Phipps, Fluoride and bone health, *J. Publ. Health Dent.*, 55, 53–56, 1995; D. Locker, *Benefits and Risks of Water Fluoridation*, Ontario Ministry of Health, Ottawa, Ontario, Canada, 1999, available at http://www.gov.on.ca/health.

16. J. Raheb, Water fluoridation, bone density, and hip fractures: a review of recent literature, *Comm. Dent. Oral Epidemiol.*, 23, 309–316, 1995; Phipps, 1995, op. cit.; M. Kleerekoper, Fluoride and the skeleton, *Crit. Rev. Clin. Lab. Sci.*, 2, 139–161, 1996.

17. Phipps, 1995, op. cit.

18. L. Ripa, A half-century of community water fluoridation in the United States: review and commentary, *J. Publ. Health Dent.*, 53, 17–44, 1993.

19. Locker, 1999, op. cit.

20. See the Leading Edge International Research Group, http://www.trufax.org; P. Connett, Letter to the editor, *Br. Med. J.*, October 11, 2000.

21. Locker, 1999, op. cit.

22. M. McDonagh et al., *A Systematic Review of Public Water Fluoridation*, NHS Centre for Reviews and Dissemination, University of York, prepared for the British National Health Service, 2000. See also *Br. Med. J.*, 321, 855–859, 2000.

23. Locker, 1999, op.cit.

24. Raheb, 1995, op. cit.

25. McDonagh et al., 2000, op. cit.

26. V. L. Richmond, Thirty years of fluoridation: a review, *Am. J. Clini. Nutr.*, 41, 129–138, 1985; U.S. National Academy of Sciences, National Research Council, Board on Environmental Studies and Technology, *Health Effects of Ingested Fluoride*, National Academics Press, Washington, DC, 1993.

27. Ripa, 1993, op. cit.

28. L. I. Juncos and J. V. Donaldo, Renal failure and fluorosis, *J. Am. Med. Assoc.*, 222, 738–752, 1972.

29. A. Vilber, O. Bello, and H. J. Gitelman, High fluoride exposure in hemodialysis patients, *Am. J. Kidney Dis.*, 15, 320–324, 1990; P. E. Corday, R. Gagnon, D. R. Taves, and M. Kaye, Bone diseases in hemodialysis patients with particular reference to the effect of fluoride, *Trans. Am. Soc. Artif. Internal Organs*, 197–202, 1974.

30. D. R. Taves, R. Terry, F. A. Smith, and D. E. Gardner, Use of fluoridated water in long-term hemodialysis, *Arch. Internal Med.*, 115, 167–172, 1965.

31. G. A. Posen, J. R. Marier, and F. Jaworski, Renal osteodystrophy in patients on long-term hemodialysis with fluoridated water, *Fluoride*, 4, 114–128, 1971.

32. U.S. Public Health Service, Surgeon General's Advisory: *Treatment of Water for Use in Dialysis: Artificial Kidney Treatments*, U.S. Government Printing Office 872-021, U.S. PHS, Washington, DC, June 1980.

33. P. M. Arnow, L. A. Bland, S. Garcia-Houchins, S. Fridken, and S. K. Fellner, An outbreak of fatal fluoride intoxication in a long-term hemodialysis unit, *Ann. Intern. Med.*, 121, 339–344, 1994.

34. G. L. Waldbott, A. W. Burgstahler, and H. L. McKinney, *Fluoridation: The Great Dilemma*, Coronado Press, Lawrence KS, 1978.

35. S. J. Challacombe, Does fluoridation harm immune function? *Com. Dent. Health*, 13 (Suppl. 2), 69–71, 1996.

36. World Health Organization, *Fluorides and Oral Health*, WHO Technical Report Series 840, WHO, Genera, Switzerland, 1994.

37. American Academy of Allergy, Asthma and Immunology, A statement on the question of allergy to fluoride as used in the fluoridation of community water

supplies, *J. Allergy. Clin. Immunol.*, 47, 347–348, 1971. Reaffirmed February 1980; see also the AAAAI website, http://www.aaaai.org.

38. R. Sprague, M. Bernhardt, and S. Barrett, Fluoridation: Don't let the poisonmongers scare you!, as posted by Quackwatch, http://www.quackwatch.com.

39. M. Lamberg, H. Hansen, and T. Vartiansen, Symptoms experienced during periods of actual and supposed water fluoridation, *Comm. Dent. Oral Epidemiol.*, 25, 291–295, 1997.

40. H. C. Hodge, Evaluation of some objections to water fluoridation, in *Fluorides and Dental Caries: Contemporary Concepts for Practitioners and Students*, edited by E. Newbrun, Charles C Thomas, Springfield, IL, 1986.

41. J. Emsley, D. J. Jones, J. M. Miller, R. E. Overill, and R. A. Waddilove, An unexpectedly strong hydrogen bond: ab initio calculations and spectroscopic studies of amide-fluoride systems, *J. Am. Chem. Soc.*, 103, 24–28, 1981.

42. W. D. Armstrong, Is fluoride hydrogen-bonded to amides? *J. Dent. Res.*, 61, 292, 1982.

43. Whitford, 1996, op. cit.

44. I. Jansen, Heart ailments linked to fluoride in Wisconsin study, *National Fluoridation News*, 18, 1, 1972. See also I. Jansen, Heart deaths and fluoridation, *Fluoride*, 7, 52–57, 1974.

45. National Institutes of Health, Division of Dental Health, *Misrepresentation of Statistics on Heart Deaths in Antigo, Wisconsin*, Publication PPB-47, NIH, Bethesda, MD, 1972.

46. Hodge, 1986, op. cit.

47. J. D. Erickson, Mortality in selected cities with fluoridated and non-fluoridated water supplies, *N. Engl. J. Med.*, 298, 1112–1116, 1978.

48. E. Rogot, A. R. Sharrett, M. Feinleib, and R. R. Fabsitz, Trends in urban mortality in relation to fluoridation statistics, *Am. J. Epidemiol.*, 107, 104–111, 1978.

49. American Heart Association, *Minerals, Inorganic Substances: Fluoridation*, http://www.americanheart.org.

50. I. Rapaport, Contribution a l'étude du mongolisme: rôle pathogénique du fluor, *Bull. Acad. Nat. Med. (Paris)*, 140, 529–531, 1956; I. Rapaport, A propos du rôle pathogénique du fluor, *Bull. Acad. Nat. Med. (Paris)*, 143, 367–370, 1959.

51. G. Orner, Dental caries experience among children with Down's syndrome and their sibs, *Arch. Oral Biol.*, 20, 627–634, 1975.

52. A. L. Gotzsche, *The Fluoride Question: Panacea or Poison*, Davis-Poynter, London, 1975.

53. H. L. Needleman, S. M. Pueschel, and K. J. Rothman, Fluoridation and the occurrence of Down's syndrome, *N. Engl. J. Med.*, 291, 821–823, 1974.

54. J. D. Erickson, G. P. Oakley, Jr., J. W. Flynt, Jr., and S. Hay, Water fluoridation and congenital malformations: no association, *J. Am. Dent. Assoc.*, 93, 981–984, 1976; J. D. Erickson, Down's syndrome, water fluoridation, and maternal age, *Teratology*, 21, 177–180, 1980.

55. A. H. Mohamed and M. E. W. Chandler, Cytological effects of sodium fluoride on mice, *Fluoride*, 15, 110–118, 1982.

56. D. R. Taves, section on fluoride, in *Drinking Water and Health*, National Academy of Sciences, Washington, DC, 1977.

57. G. Martin, K. S. Brown, D. W. Matheson, H. Lebowitz, L. Singer, and R. Ophaug, Lack of cytogenic effects in mice or mutations in *Salmonella* receiving sodium fluoride, *Mutation Res.*, 66, 159–167, 1979.

58. E. Zeiger, D. K. Gulati, P. Kaur, A. H. Mohamed, J. Revazova, and T. G. Deaton, Cytogenic studies of sodium fluoride in mice, *Mutagenesis*, 9, 467–471, 1994.

59. S. C. Freni, Exposure to high fluoride concentrations in drinking water associated with decreased birth rates, *J. Toxicol. Environ. Health*, 42, 109–121, 1994.

60. D. R. McNeil, *The Fight for Fluoridation*, Oxford University Press, New York, 1957; Waldbott et al., 1978, op. cit.

61. A. Taylor and N. C. Taylor, Effect of sodium fluoride on tumor growth, *Proc. Soc. Exp. Biol. Med.*, 119, 252–255, 1965.

62. Hodge, 1986, op. cit.

63. U.S. National Academy of Sciences, National Research Council, Safe Drinking Water Committee, *Drinking Water and Health*, National Academics Press, Washington, DC, 1977.

64. Fluoridation: the cancer scare, *Consumer Reports*, pp. 392–396, July 1978, and pp. 480–483, August 1978.

65. H. L. McKinney, Obituary: Dean Burk (1904–1988), *Fluoride*, 22, July 1989.

66. J. Yiamouyiannis and D. Burk, A definite link between fluoridation and cancer death rate, *Bull. Nat. Health Fed.*, 21, 9, 1975; J. Yiamouyiannis and D. Burk, Fluoridation and cancer, *Congressional Record*, 191, H 7172–7176, July 21, 1975, and H 12731–12734, December 16, 1975; J. Yiamouyiannis and D. Burk, Fluoridation and cancer: age dependence of cancer mortality related to artificial fluoridation, *Fluoride*, 10, 102–123, 1977.

67. R. N. Hoover, F. W. McKay, and J. R. Fraumeni, Fluoridated drinking water and the occurrence of cancer, *J. Natl. Cancer Inst.*, 57, 757–768, 1976.

68. R. Doll and L. Kinlen, Fluoridation of water and cancer mortality in the U.S.A., *Lancet*, i, 1300–1303, 1977.

69. P. D. Oldham and D. J. Newell, Fluoridation of water supplies and cancer—a possible association? *Appl. Stat.*, 26, 125–135, 1977; Erickson, 1978, op. cit.; Rogot et al., 1978, op. cit.

70. Ripa, 1993, op. cit.; J. Clemmesen, The alleged association between artificial fluoridation of water supplies and cancer: a review, *Bull. World Health Org.*, 61, 871–883, 1983; K. P. Cantor, Drinking water and cancer, *Cancer Causes Control*, 8, 292–308, 1997. See also Table 7.3 and references therein.

71. American Cancer Society, *A Statement on Cancer and Drinking Water Fluoridation*, ACS, New York, 1998.

72. National Cancer Institute, *Fluoridated Water: Cancer Facts*, http://www.cancernet.nci.nih.gov.

73. J. R. Bucher, M. R. Hejtmancik, J. D. Toft II, R. L. Persing, S. L. Eustis, and J. K. Haseman, Results and conclusions of the National Toxicology Program's rodent carcinogenicity studies with sodium fluoride, *Int. J. Cancer*, 48, 733–737, 1991.

74. Ripa, 1993, op. cit.; Burt and Eklund, 1999, op. cit.

75. J. K. Mauer, M. C. Cheng, B. G. Boysen, and R. L. anderson, Two-year carcinogenicity study of sodium fluoride in rats, *J. Natl. Cancer Inst.*, 82, 1118–1126, 1990.

76. R. N. Hoover, S. Devesa, K. Cantor, and J. F. Franmeni, Time trends for bone and joint cancers and osteosarcomas in the SEER Program, in *Review of Fluorides: Benefits and Risks*, U.S. Public Health Service, Washington, DC, 1991, pp. F1–F7.

77. Ibid.

78. U.S Public Health Service, *Review of Fluorides: Benefits and Risks*, U.S. PHS, Washington, DC, 1991. See also *J. Am. Med. Assoc.*, 266, 1061–1067, 1991.

79. P. D. Cohn, A brief report on the association of drinking water fluoridation and the incidence of osteosarcoma in young males. New Jersey Department of Health, Environmental Health Services, Trenton NJ, 1992.

80. S. E. Hrudley, Drinking water fluoridation and osteosarcoma, *Can. J. Publ. Health*, 81, 415–416, 1990; M. C. Mahoney, Bone cancer incidence rates in New York, *Am. J. Publ Health*, 81, 475, 1991.

81. S. McGuire, C. Douglass, and J. DaSilva, A national case–control study of osteosarcoma and fluoridation. Phase I: Analysis of prevalent cases, *J. Dent. Res.*, 74, 98, 1995; M. E. Moss, M. S. Kanarek, and H. A. Anderson, Osteosarcoma, seasonality, and environmental factors in Wisconsin, 1979–1989, *Arch. Environ. Health*, 50, 235–241, 1995; K. H. Gelberg, E. F. Fitzgerald, S. Hwang, and R. Dubrow, Fluoride exposure and childhood osteosarcoma: a case-control study, *Am. J. Public Health*, 85, 1678–1683, 1995.

82. Locker, 1999, op. cit.

83. McDonagh et al., 2000, op. cit.

84. Professor at Harvard is being investigated: fluoride–cancer link may have been hidden, *Washington Post*, July 13, 2005.

85. E. B. Bassin, D. Wypij, R. B. Davis, and M. A. Mittleman, Age-specific fluoride exposure in drinking water and osteosarcoma (United States), *Cancer Causes Control*, 17, 421–428, 2006.

86. C. W. Douglass and K. Joshipura, Caution needed in fluoride and osteosarcoma study, *Cancer Causes Control*, 17, 481–482, 2006.

87. R. D. Masters, Poisoning the well: neurotoxic metals, water treatment, and human behavior, plenary address to Annual Conference of the Association for Politics and the Life Sciences, Atlanta, GA, September 2, 1999. Available at http://www.rvi.net.

88. R. D. Masters, M. J. Coplan, B. T. Hone, and J. E. Dykes, Association of silicofluoride treated water with elevated blood lead, *Neurotoxicology*, 21, 1091–1100, 2000; R. D. Masters and M. J. Coplan, Water treatment with silicofluorides and lead toxicity, *Int. J. Environ. Stud.*, 56, 435–449, 1999.

89. E. T. Urbansky and M. R. Schock, Can fluoridation affect water lead levels and lead neurotoxicity? *Proc. American Water Works Association Conference*, Denver, CO, June 11–15, 2000. Also in *Int. J. Environ. Stud.*, 57, 597–637, 2000.

90. Masters, 1999, op. cit.

91. J. Seavey, Water fluoridation and crime in America, *Fluoride*, 38(1), 11–22, 2005.

92. X. S. Li, J. L. Zhi, and R. O. Gao, Effect of fluoride exposure on intelligence in children, *Fluoride*, 28, 1995; L. B. Zhao, G. H. Liang, and X. R. Wu, Effect of high fluoride water supply on children's intelligence, *Fluoride*, 29, 190–192, 1996.

93. C. N. Still and P. Kelly, On the incidence of primary degenerative dementia vs. water fluoride content in South Carolina, *Neurotoxicology*, 1, 125–131, 1980.

94. F. T. Shannon, D. M. Fergusson, and L. J. Horwood, Exposure to fluoridated public water supplies and child health and behaviour, *N. Z. J. Med.*, 99, 416–418, 1986.

95. B. Spittle, Psychopharmacology of fluoride: a review, *Int. Clin. Psychpharm.*, 9, 79–82, 1994.

96. P. J. Mullenix, P. J. Denbesten, P. K. Schunior, and W. J. Kernan, Neurotoxicity of sodium fluoride in rats, *Neurotoxicol. Teratol.*, 17, 169–177, 1995.

97. J. F. Ross and G. P. Daston, Letter to the editor, *Neurotoxicol. Teratol.*, 17, 685–686, 1995.

98. Whitford, 1996, op. cit.

99. J. A. Varner, K. F. Jensen, W. Horvath, and R. L. Isaacson, Chronic administration of aluminum fluoride or sodium fluoride to rats in drinking water: alterations in neuronal and cerebrovascular integrity, *Brain Res.*, 784, 284–298, 1998.

100. Health Media Watch, Study linking fluoride and Alzheimer's under scrutiny, *J. Am. Dent. Assoc.*, 129, 1216–1218, 1998.

CHAPTER 9

EPA AND THE MCLs

On June 29, 2000, William Hirzy stood before a subcommittee of the U.S. Senate to explain why Chapter 280 of the National Treasury Employees Union, of which he was a vice-president, opposed the fluoridation of public drinking water supplies.[1] On the face of it, his appearance before the subcommittee would not seem all that noteworthy. Union presidents often speak before Senate subcommittees, arguing for or against various government proposals that they feel might affect their membership for better or for worse. This particular subcommittee was looking into the chemical quality of drinking water and the appropriateness of certain drinking water standards, including that for fluoride. What made Hirzy's appearance before the subcommittee noteworthy was the fact that the union that he represented is not a union of mechanics, truck drivers, or longshoreman. NTEU Chapter 280 is a union that represents the professional employees at the headquarters location of the U.S. Environmental Protection Agency in Washington, DC. Hirzy himself is a Ph.D. chemist, and a great number of the other members of his union boast Ph.D.'s or master's degrees in toxicology, biology, chemistry, and engineering. The members of NTEU Chapter 280 are the very people who carry out the scientific studies, toxicological analyses, and risk assessments that are used by EPA management to set drinking water standards. Given that the EPA had already set a drinking water standard for fluoride some years earlier, and that fluoride concentrations commonly delivered to consumers after water fluoridation are well below that standard, it must be seen as odd indeed that this group of EPA employees—this *particular* group of EPA employees—would see fit to speak against fluoridation in such a public forum. In doing so (and they have been doing so for many years), the EPA headquarters scientists have made

The Fluoride Wars: How a Modest Public Health Measure Became America's Longest-Running Political Melodrama By R. Allan Freeze and Jay H. Lehr Copyright © 2009 John Wiley & Sons, Inc.

themselves the most visible and the most reputable of all the groups that have publicly repudiated fluoridation.

FLUORIDE AS JEKYL AND HYDE

The federal government has always felt a responsibility to provide information to the public on dietary and nutritional practices that *enhance* public health. On the other hand, it has also felt a responsibility to protect the public against deleterious substances in the nation's water supplies that might *threaten* public health. Surprisingly, the two goals are not always easily meshed, and fluoride is a case in point.

On the nutritional front, the government has long sung the praises of such healthy practices as a hearty breakfast, a balanced diet that includes goodly portions of fruits and vegetables, and daily intake of vitamins A and D. The government publicizes this nutritional advice in the form of a table of *dietary reference intakes* (formerly known as *recommended dietary allowances*) which are prepared by an agency known as the Food and Nutrition Board (FNB). The FNB was established in 1940 as a unit of the Institute of Medicine, a part of the National Academy of Sciences. The FNB is made up of a multidisciplinary group of biomedical scientists with expertise in such areas as nutrition, food science, public health, epidemiology, food toxicology, and food safety. The major focus of the FNB over the years has been to evaluate the emerging knowledge of nutrient requirements, and to study the relationships between diet and the reduction of risk of common chronic diseases. They are the authoritative national voice on food intake, nutrition, and health.[2]

As part of the National Academy of Sciences, the FNB is not a line agency of any federal department. They receive funding from such agencies as the Food and Drug Administration, the National Institutes of Health, and the Centers for Disease Control, but their role is advisory rather than regulatory. It may seem odd that control over something as central to daily living as the dietary reference intakes is placed in the hands of an off-line board such as the FNB rather than coming directly from the Food and Drug Administration or the Public Health Service, but that is how it evolved historically, and given the funding setup, the board certainly goes out of its way to maintain close relationships with these line agencies.

The great fluoride breakthrough came early in the history of the Food and Nutrition Board. Given the wide publicity surrounding the early fluoridation trials, the strong evidence of reduced dental caries in children who drank fluoridated water, and the enthusiastic endorsement of the Public Health Service, it is not surprising that the FNB regarded fluoride intake as a good thing. In fact, they regarded it as such a good thing that fluoride was initially placed in the category of an *essential nutrient*. The dietary reference intake was set to reflect the intake that would be received by someone who drank 2 liters a day of fluoridated water at a concentration of 1 ppm fluoride, the concentration considered by the PHS to be optimal for protection against dental caries.

The Food and Nutrition Board continued to treat fluoride as an essential nutrient well into the 1970s, but by the late 1980s they had downgraded its status to that of a *beneficial element*. They backed away from their original position because an essential role for fluoride in human growth studies could not be confirmed, and because they felt that the role of fluoride in reducing tooth decay, valuable as that might be, did not justify classifying fluoride as an essential element. Nevertheless, the dietary reference intake continues to imply the need to supplement fluoride intake through the consumption of fluoridated water. And while the appellation *beneficial* doesn't quite bear the imprimatur of *essential*, it still represents strong support for the nutritional value of fluoride.[3]

The FNB is not the only group to support the beneficial value of fluoride intake. The American Dietetic Association also affirms that "appropriate fluoride supplementation, through its beneficial effects on dental health, has an important positive impact on health."[4]

During the same period that the Food and Nutrition Board was laboring over which chemical entities had demonstrable nutritional value to the human body, other agencies within the health and safety sphere of the federal government were looking at the other side of the coin, trying to establish which chemical entities could do demonstrable harm to the human body. In this regard, particular emphasis had always been placed on protecting the public against the presence of harmful substances in the nation's municipal water supplies. As early as 1914, the Public Health Service set the first drinking water standard. It was for bacteriological quality, reflecting the concerns of the day with respect to sanitation and its role in the development and spread of communicable diseases. In subsequent years the PHS added requirements with respect to the turbidity, color, taste, and odor of the water delivered to the nation's taps. The first *chemical* limit was placed not on an individual chemical constituent but on *total dissolved solids*, a measure of the overall salinity of water.

By 1962, in addition to these omnibus bacteriological, physical, and salinity measures, a total of 28 specific dissolved chemical constituents had been added to the regulated list.[5] However, the timing of this early list predated the widespread recognition of environmental degradation from industrial sources. The lessons of Donora were still sinking in; the Love Canal findings were yet to come. Almost all of the constituents on the 1962 list were inorganic chemical species that occur to some degree in all natural waters. Many of them were metals such as lead, arsenic, mercury and chromium, which can occur in natural waters in trace amounts and which were known even then to be harmful to health at higher concentrations. The rest were common anions such as sulfate and nitrate that were thought to have upper bounds on their healthy intake. Among the latter group, and most pertinent to our discussions, was fluoride.

There were actually two halogens on the list, chloride and fluoride, and they stood out from the other regulated chemicals as the only ones that are purposely added to water in order to enhance their natural concentrations for the purposes of health protection. Each is a two-edged sword. At low concentrations they do good; at high concentrations they have the potential to do harm. In the case of chloride, the use is of such long standing, and the good that is done is so great, that little public opposition has been encountered for many years. The public is well aware that chlorination saves lives through the prevention of diseases that are spread by bacteria. In the public eye, the chloride concentrations at which harm might occur are thought to be much larger than those that are generated through water chlorination (although recent concerns over trihalomethanes may be eroding that peace of mind). In the case of fluoride, on the other hand, the good is measured in terms of cavities prevented rather than lives saved, and concentrations at which harm might occur are not much greater than those generated in the fluoridation process. The setting of a drinking water standard for fluoride requires one to walk a challenging technical and political tightrope. Dr. Jekyl must meet Mr. Hyde halfway.

In the late 1960s, things came unstuck on the water quality front. National surveys showed that many municipal water systems were out of compliance with existing drinking water standards. More alarmingly, the torrent of new synthetic organic chemicals that had been coming onto the market since World War II, particularly organic solvents such as trichloroethylene and carbon tetrachloride, began to show up in water supplies at measurable concentrations. Toxicological evidence was mounting that implicated many of these new chemicals as possible carcinogens, yet there wasn't even a drinking water standard in place for most of them. The burgeoning environmental movement educated the public about these many threats in a shrill voice. The political fallout from all this was the establishment in 1970 of the Environmental Protection Agency, with an early charge to the new agency to bring drinking water standards up to date.

The establishment of drinking water standards may sound like a straightforward technical task, but it is not. Even the first step, the listing of a chemical for consideration, can send shockwaves through the constituencies affected. An EPA listing can potentially end the demand for a particular chemical, as customers scurry to the alternatives served up by competitors, some probably just as hazardous to health but not yet on the list. As the EPA geared up to the task, lobbying was intense. On the one hand, the environmental lobby urged the EPA to be tough and vindictive with corporate polluters; industry, on the other hand, urged them to go slowly and be cognizant of corporate economic realities. The two parties were seldom happy.

Even the reassessment of the original 28 substances was fraught with controversy, and none more so than fluoride. The pro-fluoridation community, with the vociferous support of the Public Health Service, pointed to fluoride's status as an *essential nutrient* for human health (as it was then considered to be). The anti-fluoridation community pointed to its apparent status as a *contaminant*, by virtue of its long-standing presence on the list of regulated chemicals. Proponents spoke of the salvation of dental caries. Opponents spoke of the scourge of dental fluorosis. Even when fluorosis was admitted, proponents of fluoridation spoke of the condition as a cosmetic issue, while opponents viewed it as a harbinger of serious disease.

BRINKSMANSHIP

The legislative instrument on which the EPA chose to hang its hat is known as the Safe Drinking Water Act. It was signed into law on December 16, 1974. Under the SDWA, the EPA was authorized to set national health-based standards for both naturally occurring and human-made chemical constituents that pose a threat to public health. EPA was given discretion with respect to which chemical constituents to list and the time frame for bringing the program to fruition. As a first step, in 1975 the EPA announced the National Interim Primary Drinking Water Standards, which included most, but not all, of the original 28 substances listed in the old Public Health Service standards, but did not yet include many of the new synthetic organic contaminants. It was understood that these *interim* standards would soon be made *final*, and that these *primary* standards, which were designed to protect public health, would soon be accompanied by *secondary* standards for the regulation of aesthetic properties of drinking water such as taste, odor, and appearance. Moreover, it was determined that the standard-setting process would occur in two steps. For each chemical that made it onto the list, the first step would involve the setting of an RMCL (recommended maximum contaminant level), which was defined as the concentration below which there is no known or expected adverse health impact.[6] The RMCL would be the health-based target, and it might be very low, perhaps even zero in a few cases, but it would not be an enforceable standard. The second step would see the establishment of an enforceable MCL (maximum contaminant level) that would be set as close to the RMCL as technologically feasible, taking cost into consideration. It was recognized that for many chemicals the MCL would be significantly higher than the RMCL because it was just not practical or economical to set the enforceable standard at the targeted value.

Regardless of where an MCL or an RMCL might be set, the presence of the c-word in these widely used regulatory acronyms identified the listed constituents, including fluoride, as *contaminants*. This choice of terminology greatly pleased the anti-fluoridation lobby, and they regularly used it to their advantage in the literature they distributed during referenda campaigns.

Between 1974 and 1985, the EPA set about their work, considering new chemicals for inclusion, reassessing old chemicals, setting RMCLs, making interim RMCLs final, and navigating the slippery slope toward enforceable MCLs. All this had to be done on a chemical-by-chemical basis. The work was slow. Lobbying was intense. Few new standards were put in place. Congress chafed. In 1978, a coalition of environmental groups, including the Natural Resources Defense Council, the Environmental Defense Fund, and the National Audubon Society, brought suit against the EPA demanding quicker action. The result was a consent decree between the EPA and the plaintiffs under which EPA was required to establish a priority pollutant list within a year's time and then begin to actively set enforceable MCLs for the contaminants on the list. The EPA came up with the priority pollutant list in 1979. It included 129 contaminants, 114 of them organic chemicals, and the other 15, metals. Fluoride was a notable absence. Despite the threat of court action under the consent decree, the setting of MCLs remained stalled.

In 1986, the Safe Drinking Water Act came up for reauthorization. Frustrated by EPA's lack of progress, Congress took away their discretion with respect to the time frame for standard setting. They decreed that EPA must set RMCLs and MCLs for 83 of the contaminants on the priority pollutant list within a fixed schedule. They also declared that the interim standards set in 1975 would be declared final. To confuse matters further they changed the terminology for the nonenforceable health-based targets from RMCLs to MCLGs, maximum contaminant level goals.

All during this period, EPA received intense lobbying from both sides of the fluoridation movement over the drinking water standard for fluoride. The interim standard for fluoride, set in 1975, was based on the old

Public Health Service standard. This standard, which dated from the early fluoridation years, was set at twice the optimum value for the prevention of dental decay. The PHS felt that such a standard struck an acceptable balance between the the prevention of dental caries and the occurrence of dental fluorosis. When the PHS had first set the optimum value at 1 ppm, there had been much ado about the fact that people in warmer southern climates were likely to drink more water than those in the cooler north, thus receiving greater fluoride intakes and possibly suffering more dental fluorosis. To quell this clamor, the PHS had set up a sliding scale of recommended optimum fluoridation concentrations as a function of temperature. For southern states with the highest mean annual temperatures the optimal value was set at 0.7 ppm; for northern states with the lowest mean annual temperatures the optimal value was set at 1.2 ppm. The RMCL for fluoride that was incorporated into the 1975 EPA interim standards (and now finalized under the 1986 SDWA reauthorization as a MCLG) used this temperature-dependent scale. The MCLG for fluoride, set at twice the optimum, thus varied from state to state, taking on values from 1.4 to 2.4 ppm depending on the mean annual temperature of the state.

Very few substances have an MCLG that is so close to commonly observed (and in this case purposely generated) concentrations. The anti-fluoridation movement bridled at the "dubious brinksmanship" involved in the standard-setting process, noting that "the thin line between benefit and danger is an extremely narrow one."[7] On the other side of the fence, proponents of fluoridation noted that fluoride was not even listed as a priority pollutant. The EPA was under intense pressure from many quarters to *raise* the fluoride standard. The pro-fluoridation lobby felt that the low value of the MCLG gave the incorrect impression that there were hazards associated with the fluoridation process that did not exist. Fluoridated municipal water utilities worried that they were too often out of compliance with the law. Several states complained that the standard was too difficult to enforce. In 1981, the state of South Carolina took the EPA to court over the fluoride standard. They claimed that many municipal water supplies in South Carolina utilized natural sources that exceeded the standard and that it was too expensive to defluoridate such supplies.

EPA was sympathetic to the idea of raising the MCLG for fluoride to 4 ppm. In 1983, they requested guidance on this issue from the Public Health Service. The head of the PHS, Surgeon General C. Everett Koop, set up two ad hoc committees, one to review the *dental effects* of fluoride exposure and one to review the *nondental effects*. Anti-fluoridationists howled that asking the PHS to give advice on fluoride was like inviting the fox into the henhouse. They also raised their standard complaint that membership on the committees was heavily biased in favor of fluoridation supporters. They claimed that there was not one identifiable critic of fluoridation on either committee.

The two committees met in April 1983, and the EPA released the final report of their deliberations in September of the same year. The committee that reviewed the *nondental effects* of fluoride exposure found that the only credible adverse medical effect was that of crippling skeletal fluorosis and that there was "no scientific documentation of adverse medical effects below 8 ppm." The report stated further that a drinking water standard for fluoride that is four times the optimum value (i.e., 4 ppm) is a level that would provide "no known or anticipated adverse effects with a margin of safety."

The recommendations of the committee that reviewed the *dental effects* of fluoride exposure were more problematic for the EPA. The final report quotes their conclusion to the effect that "it is inadvisable for the fluoride content of drinking water to be greater than twice the current optimum level for children up to age 9 in order to avoid the uncosmetic effects of dental fluorosis."

Despite the latter recommendation, the EPA decided to go ahead with the 4-ppm MCLG for fluoride. They did so on the basis that an "uncosmetic effect" is not an "adverse health effect." In April 1986, the MCLG was officially promulgated at 4 ppm.[8] The EPA tried to appease the opponents of this move by setting a secondary MCL (a nonenforceable standard established for aesthetic reasons) of 2 ppm. This SMCL was defended on the grounds that it would prevent "the majority of cases of water-related cosmetically objectionable dental fluorosis while still allowing for the beneficial effects of fluoride through the prevention of dental caries." Under the rules associated with an SMCL, suppliers of fluoridated water must notify consumers if fluoride concentrations exceed the secondary standard. The EPA states that "the SMCL is intended to alert families that regular consumption of water with levels of fluoride greater than 2 ppm by young children may cause dental fluorosis in the developing permanent teeth."[9] Managers of municipal water utilities hate this requirement, not least because of the prominent appearance of the word *contaminant* in the letters of notification that must be sent out. They feel that this wording unfairly implies that the fluoridation process introduces a "contaminant" into the water rather than the "essential nutrient" that they believe they are providing.

With the MCLG in place and an SMCL established to assuage the ruffled feathers of opponents, EPA management had reason to hope that they could move briskly toward the finalization of an enforceable MCL for fluoride. But as fate would have it, that was not to happen for another 11 years. Among other things, they had failed to realize that among the most ruffled of all the feathers were those of their own scientific and technical staff.

AMICUS CURIAE

The Environmental Protection Agency exists in a peculiar borderland between science and politics. It is EPA's mandate to recommend legislation to Congress to preserve the environment and protect human health. They are expected to base this legislation on sound science that takes into account the latest developments in medical and scientific research. Yet they are buffeted at every turn by political pressures, and final EPA decisions are often more heavily influenced by politics than by science. It is a difficult milieu for in-house EPA technical staff, who are torn between their ethical mandate as scientists to tell the truth as clearly as it is known and their practical mandate as employees to serve the needs of management. This issue has led to ongoing conflict between EPA management and professional staff since the earliest days of the agency's existence. The fluoride question has been one of the sources of this conflict.

There are two unions representing workers at EPA headquarters in Washington. The American Federation of Government Employees Local 3331 represents nonprofessional staff, and the National Treasury Employees Union Chapter 280 represents professional staff. There are currently about 1600 professionals on the rolls of Chapter 280. The professional staff had originally voted against joining a union when the AFGE local was created, but in 1982, under the perceived hostility of the incoming Reagan administration, they changed their minds. They were for many years a local of the National Federation of Federal Employees, but switched to the NTEU in 1998. Although the union does address traditional labor interests such as working hours and job security, their emphasis from the beginning has been on "defending their freedom to practice their professions in pursuit of environmental and public health protection, and to do so in conformity with high ethical standards of professionalism."[10] The official history of NTEU Chapter 280, which is available on their website, makes it clear that in union eyes, the EPA has not provided an environment of scientific integrity for their technical staff.[11] In union eyes, EPA history is replete with cases where political expedience has overruled scientific facts. Of course, the management viewpoint is that NTEU Chapter 280 has been taken over by professional agitators who are out of touch with political realities and disgruntled over the policy choices made in good faith by EPA management. They accuse the union of laboring under the mistaken impression that it is the scientists' job to set environmental policy rather than that of management. It is not clear who is most at fault, but it will be very clear from what follows that there has been a massive breakdown in communication between staff and management that is anathema to the efficient working of a large government agency that is supposedly serving the public interest.

William Hirzy and Robert Carton have been the longtime spokesmen for NTEU Chapter 280. Both were founding members of the local, and both have served several terms as president. The collective agreement between the EPA and the NTEU allows for several full-time union officers and Hirzy and Carton held one or other of these posts for many years. Hirzy is the editor of the Local newsletter *Inside the Fishbowl*, and he is the author of the Official History of NTEU Chapter 280. On the technical side, both are Ph.D. scientists who worked for many years as risk assessment experts at EPA. Hirzy attained the rank of senior scientist in the Office of Pollution Prevention and Toxics. Carton performed some of the earliest EPA risk assessments for asbestos, polychlorinated biphenyls (PCBs), arsenic, and hexachlorobenzene. He wrote the first regulations controlling asbestos discharges from manufacturing plants. He left the EPA in the early 1990s and became the environmental coordinator for the U.S. Army Medical Research and Materiel Command at Fort Detrick, Maryland. Hirzy remains with the EPA union.

Hirzy claims that the union first became interested in the fluoride issue "rather by accident."[12] It was apparently the result of a chance meeting in 1985 in the hallway of the Waterside Mall at EPA headquarters between Carton and a professional staff member from the Office of Drinking Water who had been asked to write the new fluoride regulation in support of the 4-ppm MCLG. He told Carton that he was being forced to write a statement into the regulation that offended his sense of professional ethics. The statement was to the effect that even severe dental fluorosis could be considered a "cosmetic effect" and not an "adverse health effect." He felt that the proposed 4-ppm standard did not reflect the recommendations put forward by Surgeon General Koop's ad hoc committees, and that it was solely the result of political pressure on the EPA from the pro-fluoridation movement. He pointed out that the standard under consideration was a nonenforceable MCLG, not an MCL, and as such it should be set at a level below which there is *no* adverse health impact. After all, if they so desired, EPA management could still set the enforceable MCL at the higher level on the basis of reaching an acceptable trade-off between the increase in dental fluorosis and the reduction of dental caries.

The union took the professional's complaint to EPA management as an "ethics issue." Hirzy claims that they tried to settle the issue quietly in-house. In a letter to Lee Thomas, the administrator of the EPA, Carton wrote: "We do not believe that it is in the interests of the agency or its professionals to wash dirty laundry in public."[13] However, the union claims that management was not receptive to any of its overtures on this case, or ethics issues in general, refusing even to organize a timely review of the situation by the EPA Science Advisory Board.

In early 1986, the Natural Resources Defense Council filed a lawsuit against the EPA over the MCLG for fluoride. The NRDC is one of the preeminent environmental advocacy groups in the United States with over 500,000 members nationwide. It is exactly as old as the EPA, having been formed in 1970 as a partnership between a group of young idealistic Yale Law school students and older New York establishment attorneys of the Scenic Hudson Preservation Conference. Its mission is to "ensure a safe and healthy environment for all living things" and to "establish sustainability and good stewardship of the Earth as central ethical imperatives of human society."[14]

In their lawsuit, the NRDC sought to prevent the EPA from relaxing the MCLG for fluoride from the interim standard of 1.4 to 2.4 ppm to the new standard of 4 ppm. They cited the use of "fraudulent alterations of data and negligent omissions of fact to arrive at the predetermined agency political position regarding fluoride." EPA management responded to the NRDC charges by asserting that the court should defer to the agency position because of "agency expertise." The union leadership was insulted by this tactic, knowing full well that the agency "experts" closest to the case were not at all supportive of the new fluoride standard. The union then took an unprecedented step. They filed an *amicus curiae* brief in support of the NRDC position in the court case against their own employer. They state that their brief was filed "to assist the court in making an informed determination ... and to safeguard the professional reputations of union members." In their brief, they charge that EPA management "ignored important scientific and technical considerations when setting the MCLG for fluoride" and "disregarded the statutory requirement that MCLGs be based solely on considerations of public health." They accuse the agency of abusing its discretion in the process of setting the fluoride MCLG. They state that "the final MCLG does not represent a determination made on the basis of scientific and technical expertise. Instead, it represents an administrative process replete with inaccurate interpretations of the requirements of the act, inappropriate applications of political and budgetary considerations, and unprofessional scientific support documentation."[15]

These are strong words for employees to raise against their employer. The very act of going on public record with such serious charges against one's employer raises ethical issues of its own. To whom do EPA professionals owe their allegiance: to the public or to their employer? What role should salaried government employees play in the setting of public policy? Did the union position truly represent the views of all its members or only of a small cadre of labor agitators and anti-fluoridation activists? Keep these thoughts in mind while we continue the tale, because it is the next part of the story that really blew the lid off any last bits of goodwill that might have still remained between the EPA professionals and their management superiors.

THE MARCUS AFFAIR

The question of fluoride and cancer has always been an extraordinarily touchy topic. As we have seen in Chapter 8, the links between the two are incredibly tenuous. It would seem to most that there is no link at all, and in review after review that is what the many panels of medical experts have concluded. Still the idea lingers, especially in the minds of those who distrust authoritative proclamations from the medical establishment. Historically, the Public Health Service looked askance at these doubters and gave their concerns little weight, as did the Environmental Protection Agency when it came their turn to protect public health. The last thing the EPA wanted or needed was an internal doubter, but with William L. Marcus, that is what they got.

You may recall from Chapter 8 that a subcommittee of the U.S. Congress made a recommendation to the Public Health Service in 1977 to carry out toxicological and epidemiological studies on the possible carcinogenic effects of fluoride. Recall also that it took 13 years for the PHS to meet this mandate, finally doing so on the basis of work carried out at the Battelle Memorial Institute under the auspices of the National Toxicology Program. In 1990, as part of the final publication process, the PHS struck another panel of fluoride experts to review the NTP findings, and their report became a more widely quoted source of information on the results of the Battelle experiments than the NTP report that they set out to review.

William Marcus was the chief toxicologist in EPA's Office of Drinking Water during this period. In April 1990 he was asked to attend a meeting of this newly organized PHS review panel at Research Triangle Park, North Carolina, to listen to a presentation by officials from the National Toxicology Program describing the results of Battelle's animal studies. He was surprised and impressed by the experiments that indicated occurrences of the bone cancer, osteosarcoma, in male rats (which we reviewed in Chapter 8). Despite the strong negative evidence of any relationship between fluoride and cancer from the great majority of Battelle's work, he was confused as to why the final NTP report referred to these positive results as "equivocal." When he got home, he carefully reviewed the original Battelle reports and compared them with the final NTP report. On doing so, he found evidence of what he felt was skulduggery. In his opinion, *clear* occurrences of cancer in the laboratory animals, as reported by Battelle, had been systematically downgraded by NTP to the level of *equivocal*, through reclassification, deletion, and editing of the original data. When the report of the PHS panel, *Review of Fluoride: Benefits and Risks*, appeared later in the year, it further downgraded the Battelle findings, especially in the executive summary, where it was stated that the panel could find "no evidence establishing an association between fluoride and cancer *in humans*" (italics added).[16]

As Marcus recounts the experience: "I've been in the toxicology business looking at studies of this nature for nearly 25 years and I've never seen that; never ever seen where every single endpoint that was a cancer endpoint had been downgraded. I'd seen one or two endpoints argued over, usually on the definition of what is a cancer in that particular tissue. But I've never seen every one of them downgraded."[17]

Now it must be admitted here that Marcus was not a naive innocent in the fluoride battles. Like Hirzy and Carton, he was active in the union, serving as treasurer during much of this period. He was very much a part of the union's strong stand against the new 4-ppm fluoride MCLG and the filing of the *amicus curiae* brief in the NRDC lawsuit in 1986. Not only that, but he may have been especially alert to the possibility of management reworking of scientific results at this time. In 1988, a woman named Martha Bevis, working under the auspices of an anti-fluoridation group known as the Safe Water Foundation of Texas, used the Freedom of Information Act to obtain a transcript of the deliberations of the two ad hoc committees set up in 1983 by Surgeon General Koop to advise the EPA on the fluoride standard. It turns out that the members of these committees expressed many doubts and uncertainties about the safety of fluoride in their discussions, and were quite worried about the lack of available information on several health effects, including cancer. More tellingly, according to Bevis, a comparison of the draft reports that they submitted to the EPA with the final reports released by the EPA to the public showed important discrepancies. This story was confirmed, and broken in the lay press, by Joel Griffiths, the same investigative reporter whose articles on Donora and the Manhattan project are so beloved in anti-fluoridation circles. He claimed in an article published in the highly regarded medical newsletter *Medical Tribune* that the EPA had added material helpful to their case in the final report, material that was not in the draft report submitted by the experts. In particular, he claims that the draft report always referred to dental fluorosis as an "adverse health effect," never as a "cosmetic effect." Nor, he claims, was there any recommendation in the draft report for a drinking water standard at four times the optimum concentration that appears in the final report.[18]

Marcus did not want to see the scientific community flimflammed by management yet again as he now felt they had been back in 1983. He delved further into the cancer issue and familiarized himself with the other health issues raised by the anti-fluoridation camp. He wrote a letter to EPA management in May 1990 that was strongly critical of what he saw as the emasculation of the Battelle work by NTP and EPA management. He called for a full review of the fluoride cancer data. When the EPA failed to respond to his concerns, he went public with his charges. He felt that fluoride was receiving favored treatment; that for any chemical constituent other than fluoride, the Battelle work would have been sufficient to raise the flag on that constituent as a possible carcinogen. In later years he would harden his stand even further. "Fluoride is a carcinogen by any standard we use," he has said. "I believe EPA should act immediately to protect the public, not just on the cancer data, but on the evidence of bone fractures, arthritis, mutagenicity, and other effects."[19]

Marcus became a committed anti-fluoridation activist. He wrote letters to anti-fluoridation groups providing toxicological ammunition for their battles. He began accepting invitations to testify in court cases about the harmful effects of fluoride and other chemicals. He worked diligently both internally and externally to overturn the EPA's fluoride policies.

In the fall of 1990, EPA management fired William Marcus. They accused him of stealing time from the government by working as a consultant while on the EPA payroll. They proffered time records as proof. Marcus immediately went to Hirzy and Carton at the union offices, and together with their lawyers they launched a wrongful dismissal suit against the EPA over the firing. EPA inspector general John Martin prepared a summary of the case for the court on management's behalf, emphasizing the alleged time violations. In response, Marcus claimed that the inspector general's report "contained slanderous, false, and derogatory information." He charged that management had sent out memos to EPA staff identifying him as a "threat" and falsely accusing him of carrying a gun to work. He claimed that the EPA had falsified the time records and shredded documents that would have exonerated him.[20]

Two years later, on December 3, 1992, a decision on the lawsuit was finally rendered. Administrative Law Judge David Clarke ruled that EPA's firing of William Marcus was inappropriate. Judge Clarke concluded that "the reasons given for Dr. Marcus' firing were a pretext," and that "his employment was terminated because he publicly questioned and opposed EPA's fluoride policy." Clarke ordered the EPA to give Marcus back his job with full back pay, legal expenses, and $50,000 in damages.

EPA management appealed the decision. Under federal law, appeals that arise from lawsuits involving employer–employee relations are heard by the Department of Labor. In December 1994, four years after Marcus's termination, Secretary of Labor Robert Reich upheld Judge Clarke's decision. Reich concluded that the Marcus firing was "retaliatory" and based on charges that were "unsubstantiated." In early 1995, Marcus was reinstated at the EPA as a senior scientific adviser in the Office of Science and Technology.

A QUESTION OF ALLEGIANCE

There are many who are reading this who will feel that William Marcus received very favorable treatment through the courts. Most of us would expect to get sacked if we took a stand against our employer as strongly as Marcus did. Most of us would probably choose to resign rather than tilt at windmills from within if we suspected ethical malfeasance on the part of our employer or if we were as disgusted with their policies as Marcus was. There are two ways in which Marcus's situation differs from that of most of us. First, he is a government employee in a politically sensitive agency, and second, he is a scientist. Perhaps it can be argued that he had obligations that transcended those of most of us in either or both of these roles.

In his first role, the question arises as to whether a civil servant owes greater allegiance to his superiors within a government agency or to the public at large. Certainly, the primary role of the professional staff in a government agency is to provide advice to management in matters that fall within their professional competence. Management is free to take the advice or not as they choose and to set policy in the best interest of the country as they perceive it. If government policy is set in good faith, any staff member who feels that he or she cannot work in support of that policy in equally good faith has little recourse but to resign. The question at hand is what constitutes good faith for each party? In setting the fluoride MCLG at 4 ppm, the EPA downplayed cancer data that almost all reputable medical experts felt was suspect. They did so, at least in part, so as not to throw a wrench into the fluoridation movement, a public health program that had almost universal support from the medical establishment. In this light, their actions could be viewed as good faith actions on behalf of the public interest. In a contrary light, however, it is hard to defend the suppression or misrepresentation of hard data when it comes to issues of public health, as EPA staff apparently did with the Battelle data. As William Hirzy has written on behalf of the NTEU Chapter 280 position: "The people must be able to access the information necessary to decide whether the government is acting as their servant or their master. The people must be able to learn whether government decisions are being made for their benefit or the benefit of other interests."[21]

Having said this, it is difficult to defend all the actions of William Marcus. His involvement with anti-fluoridation groups during the period between his firing and reinstatement may be seen by some as inappropriate. As of 1994, he had provided testimony about the supposed links between fluoride and cancer in 38 court cases.[22] He also become a regular on the alternative medicine circuit. In 1995 he was interviewed on national radio by Gary Null, a self-appointed health and fitness guru, vociferous opponent of fluoridation, and successful marketer of nutritional products such as bee-pollen extract.[23] In the same year, Marcus gave the keynote address at a meeting of the International Academy of Detoxification Specialists, a group of devotees of L. Ron Hubbard's "purification program" to flush residual toxins from the human body.[24] L. Ron Hubbard is the controversial founder of the Church of Scientology, the prime mover behind the Narconon drug rehabilitation program and the originator of the Dianetic approach to mental health treatment. (He is also the author of hundreds of science fiction stories and novels including the classic futuristic adventure fantasy *Battlefield Earth*.) Hubbard's purification program is standard practice for adherents of the Church of Scientology. By taking part in a conference on this topic, Marcus seemed to be implying that fluoride is a "residual toxin" and that detoxification can be achieved through the academy's proscribed regimen of aerobic exercise, sauna-induced sweating, oil supplements, and vitamins.[25] Marcus must surely have known that activities of this type would bring great embarrassment to his former employer.

Marcus, Hirzy, and Carton are all scientists by training, and in this role one might also raise the question of allegiance. One could perhaps make the argument that they owe greater allegiance to the public, the courts, and Congress than they do to their own in-house superiors. This is the case made by Hirzy in one of his many discourses on scientific ethics in government service. "Scientists have no clients," he writes. "They ask Mother Nature questions and try to make sense of the answers." He argues that EPA scientists "have a duty and a right to perform our work in an ethical environment, and to see that our work is not distorted, misrepresented, stolen, or lied about, in devising false cover for agency policies." More provocatively: "In confronting our consciences, we choose not to rely on the defense that failed at Nuremberg."[26] EPA scientists will refuse to follow orders, he seems to be saying, if in their own eyes those orders are not ethical.

This is all well and good, but the reader may be excused if he finds the Chapter 280 leaders just a little bit shrill. The questions on the table, while they do have public health significance and may have been viewed as precedent setting by the union scientists, are not so black and white that there is no room for honest disagreement. The question of whether the fluoride MCLG should be set at 2 ppm or 4 ppm is only marginally an ethical issue. To a much greater degree, it is a policy issue. Setting the MCLG at 4 ppm is not unethical in principle (although finagling the reports, if indeed they did so, certainly is). When faced with the groundswell of opposition against the lower MCLG, and being advised at every turn by expert panels that there are no connections between fluoride and cancer, it doesn't seem all that unethical to make a rational trade-off and then try to sell it to the public. In the rough hurly-burly of public policy making, the EPA scientists at times appear somewhat naive and arrogant.

However, they do have one strong point. Their best argument by far is the one that charges EPA with using economic and political criteria in setting the MCLG, rather than health criteria alone as specified in the Safe Drinking Water Act. Economic and political criteria can rightly be invoked in setting the enforceable MCL, but should not have played any role in setting the health-based target that the MCLG is supposed to represent. Given their growing disillusionment with fluoridation, one wonders whether the Chapter 280 scientists would have toed the line had EPA management set the MCLG at 2 ppm and the MCL at 4 ppm as they probably should have done?

A QUESTION OF MOTIVE

In 1993, the Board on Environmental Studies and Toxicology of the National Academy of Sciences put together yet another panel of experts to look at the fluoride question. Their report, *Health Effects of Ingested Fluoride*,[27] concluded that an MCL of 4 ppm for fluoride is "an appropriate standard to protect public health." Using this recommendation as ammunition, the EPA published a Notice of Intent in the *Federal Register* on December 29, 1993, to set the enforceable MCL for fluoride equal to the MCLG of 4 ppm.[28] As usual, intent did not translate into action for some time. It took four more years, but on December 5, 1997, the Final Rule was promulgated in the *Federal Register*, setting the MCL for fluoride at 4 ppm as an enforceable federal standard.[29]

In the years since the Marcus affair and the battle over the final rule for fluoride, the stand on fluoridation of the union of EPA scientists has hardened into rock-solid opposition. They have become one of the most outspoken foes of public water fluoridation in the nation. In 1997, they endorsed the California Safe Drinking Water Initiative sponsored by the anti-fluoridation group California Citizens for Safe Drinking Water. This initiative attempted unsuccessfully to place a measure on the June 1998 statewide ballot to reverse Jackie Spier's 1995 law making fluoridation mandatory throughout the state of California. In 1999, the union published a white paper entitled *Why EPA's Headquarters Union of Scientists Opposes Fluoridation*.[30] It panders to all of the usual health fears that surface in every anti-fluoridation document: cancer, osteosarcoma, kidney damage, hip fractures, and reduction in childhood IQ. Like most other anti-fluoridation tracts, it references only the few articles that support these fears and provides no mention of the wealth of countervailing evidence. It is a natural descendant of the early style of presentation by John Yiamouyiannis in his 1982 treatise *The Lifesaver's Guide to Fluoridation*.[31] Both were prepared by scientists, but they do not follow the rules or traditions of science. There is almost no difference between the Union's white paper and similar documents prepared by lay anti-fluoridation groups with no scientific background.

It is natural to wonder whether Hirzy, Carton, and Marcus might have had a hidden agenda all along. Did they happen on fluoridation "by accident" as they claim, or did they wrest control of the union in order to turn it into an agent of their anti-fluoridation beliefs? The best evidence on this point seems to support Hirzy's version of events. It appears that Hirzy and Carton saw the issue initially as an ethical impropriety on the part of EPA management, and only later came to their anti-fluoridation position. Having said this, given the intense antagonism that developed between the Union and management over a wide variety of issues, it seems likely that the Union's anti-fluoride position may have been fueled at least in part by this antagonism.

More to the point, perhaps, one wonders whether the union membership fully supports their executive on this issue, or is it a price they are willing to pay to have such diligent leadership on their behalf in other matters? The Chapter 280 history claims that support for the California Safe Drinking Water Initiative was "unanimous."[32] Could this possibly mean that not one of the 1500 scientists at EPA headquarters favors fluoridation?

A possible measure of the cohesiveness of the EPA staff on the fluoride issue can be gleaned from the almost universal glee that accompanied the circulation of a tongue-in-cheek "press release" among staff after the promulgation of the fluoride regulation. "The Office of Drinking Water," it read, "proudly presents their new and improved Fluoride Regulation, or 'How we stopped worrying and learned to love funky teeth.' Up to now EPA, under the Safe Drinking Water Act, has regulated fluoride in order to prevent children from having teeth which looked like they had been chewing brown shoe polish and rocks. The old standard which was based upon the consumer's average shoe size and the phase of the moon generally kept fluoride levels below 2.3 ppm. EPA in response to new studies which only confirmed the old studies, and some flat out political pressure, has decided to raise the standard to 4 ppm. This increase will allow 40% of all children to have teeth gross enough to gag a maggot. EPA selected this level based upon a cost effectiveness study which showed that it is cheaper for people to keep their mouths shut than to remove the fluoride."[33]

When looking for motive, one might also turn to the strong environmental ethic among many EPA scientists. While the environmental movement has never presented a unified front on the fluoridation question, it has leaned toward opposition, often lumping fluoride together with other chemical contaminants that threaten the environment. Among the environmental groups that are on record as opposing fluoridation are Friends of the Earth, Earth Island Institute, the Pennsylvania Environmental Network, the Green Party, the Leading Edge International Research Group, some (but not all) branches of the Sierra Club, and of course the Natural Resources Defense Council, whose suit against the EPA first brought the EPA headquarters union out of the woodwork.[34] While relations between the environmental movement and EPA management have often been rocky, this antagonism does not extend to EPA staff, many of whom are environmentally active and privately support the aims of these organizations. After all, the scientists who joined the EPA in the early years often did so despite the availability of better-paying jobs from industry. It was not just a job to them, it was a mission, and they chose to do it out of a true concern for the environment and a desire to do something worthwhile for society. They were not ready for the environmental backlash of the Reagan years, and they certainly did not expect it to so politicize their agency. The fluoride question gave them a cause through which they could vent their private frustrations.

Throughout much of the early going, the EPA headquarters union treated the fluoride issue as a matter of ethics, not as a matter of scientific dispute. It was the fluoride issue that galvanized the union into trying to incorporate a code of ethics into its collective bargaining agreement with the EPA. As early as 1988 they proposed to include a set of statements in the agreement to the effect that (1) professionals must honestly represent the quality and uncertainty of their analyses, and managers must accurately represent these statements in regulatory decisions; (2) both professionals and managers must refuse to cover up or suppress information germane to the protection of public health or the environment; (3) both professionals and managers must accurately present the data and opinion of others; (4) both professionals and managers must assure that the work for which they are responsible does not involve dishonesty, fraud, or deceit; (5) both professionals and managers must assure that there is adequate quality control of the work done for them by contractors; and (6) managers must not threaten or intimidate professionals to tailor professional judgment for political, social, or economic reasons.[35] EPA management claimed to support these ideas in principle but resisted establishing a formal code. It was not until nine years later, in 1997, after much antagonism and many breakdowns in communication, that the agency finally agreed to include a code of professional ethics in the bargaining agreement. Moreover, a labor management committee was established within EPA to discuss problems and resolve disputes growing out of differences in professional judgment. In many cases, the role of this committee comes down to a decision as to whether an issue is truly an ethical one and hence a violation of the code, or simply a difference of opinion. In March 2000, EPA management published a professional ethics document entitled *Principles of Scientific Integrity*.

Whatever strictures the code of ethics may have placed on EPA management, it apparently did not prevent the union from continuing to speak out in public against water fluoridation. On June 29, 2000, William Hirzy made the congressional presentation mentioned in the opening sentence of this chapter before the Subcommittee on Wildlife, Fisheries, and Drinking Water of the Committee on Environment and Public Works of the U.S. Senate. In his presentation, Hirzy recommended an independent review of the cancer studies carried out by the Battelle Memorial Institute in 1983, an epidemiological study of dental fluorosis, a full hearing on the fluoride issue by a joint congressional committee, and a national moratorium on water fluoridation until the results of these various studies were completed.[36] Robert Carton continued to oppose fluridation long after leaving the EPA. In 2003, he co-authored a paper published in a technical journal entitled "Fluoridation: A Violation of Medical Ethics and Human Rights."[37]

When all is said and done, it is hard not to cast a pox on all their houses. EPA management has much to answer for. In the Reagan era they clearly allowed the agency to become far too politicized. EPA staff members were essentially being asked to work *against* the environmental ethic which had brought them to the agency. To the degree that management's finagling of the scientific books between draft and final reports can be substantiated, they are guilty of unacceptable ethical behavior and suppression of information that rightfully belongs in the public domain. Moreover, they failed to follow the letter or the spirit of the law as set out in the Safe Drinking Water Act in setting the MCLG for fluoride. On the flip side of the coin, it appears that the headquarters union crossed a line when they moved from grievances over management's ethical transgressions to full-scale opposition of management policies. In the latter role, they took many actions that were designed to embarrass their employer in the public eye, and in so doing, they broke the bonds of respect that must remain in place for successful employee–employer relations.

In 2002, the EPA asked the National Academy of Sciences once again to review the fluoride standards. They reported back in 2006, recommending that the EPA lower the MCLG from 4 ppm to some lower value, although they did not suggest a specific figure.[38] As for the MCL itself, it's your call. Some will find the 4-ppm value alarmingly close to concentrations that are known to cause harm. Others will see the wisdom of setting a standard that allows society to continue to reap the seemingly undeniable dental benefits of fluoridation.

REFERENCES

1. Statement of J. William Hirzy before the Subcommittee on Wildlife, Fisheries and Drinking Water, Committee on Environment and Public Works, U.S. Senate, June 29, 2000, http://www.penweb.org/issues/fluoride/hirzy.html.

2. Food and Nutrition Board, http://www.iom.edu.

3. U.S. National Academy of Sciences, National Research Council, Food and Nutrition Board, *Recommended Dietary Allowances*, 10th ed., National Academies Press, Washington, DC, 1989.

4. American Dietetic Association, Impact of fluoride on dental health: position of ADA, *J. Am. Diet. Assoc.*, 94, 1428–1431, 1994.

5. U.S. Department of Health, Education and Welfare, *Public Health Service Drinking Water Standards*, Publication 956, U.S. Public Health Service, Washington, DC, reprinted 1969.

6. As noted later, in 1986 the EPA changed the terminology for their nonenforceable standard from recommended maximum contaminant level (RMCL) to maximum contaminant level goal (MCLG).

7. A. L. Gotzsche, *The Fluoride Question: Panacea or Poison*, Davis-Poynter, London, 1975.

8. The intention to set the fluoride MCLG at 4 ppm was announced by the EPA in the *Federal Register* on May 14, 1985 (50 FR 20164-20175) and November 14, 1985 (50 FR 47142-47171. The final decision appeared on April 18, 1986 (51 FR 11396-11412).

9. American Dental Association, *Fluoridation Facts*, http://www.ada.org.

10. National Treasury Employees Union Chapter 280, *Who We Are*, http://www.nteu280.org.

11. J. W. Hirzy, for National Treasury Employees Union Chapter 280, *Official History of NTEU Chapter 280: 17 Years of Public Service at EPA Headquarters*, undated, http://www.nteu280.org.

12. J. W. Hirzy, *Why EPA's Headquarters Union of Scientists Opposes Fluoridation*, May 1, 1999, http://www.nteu280.org; connected by link to almost every anti-fluoridation website on the Internet.

13. Letter from Robert J. Carton To Lee M. Thomas, August 26, 1986. Included as Exhibit A to National Federation of Federal Employees Chapter 280 *amicus curiae* brief in support of Natural Resources Defense Council lawsuit against the EPA (see note 15).

14. Natural Resources Defense Counci, http://www.nrdc.org.

15. National Federation of Federal Employees Chapter 280 *amicus curiae* brief filed in support of *Natural Resources Defense Council, Inc., petitioner* v. *Environmental Protection Agency, respondent*, Civ. No. 85-1839, in the U.S. Court of Appeals for the District of Columbia Circuit, September 3, 1986.

16. U.S. Public Health Service, *Review of Fluoride: Benefits and Risks*, U.S. PHS, Washington, DC, 1991. The results of this study are summarized in *J. Am. Med. Assoc.*, 266, 1061–1062 and 1066–1067, 1991.

17. W. L. Marcus, radio interview with Gary Null, March 10, 1995.

18. J. Griffiths, *Med. Tribune*, 30(11), April 20, 1989.

19. Ibid.

20. *Frederick Post*, February 14, 1994. This news article, which is widely reproduced on anti-fluoridation websites, is the source of quotes in this and succeeding paragraphs on the Marcus lawsuit and appeal.

21. Hirzy, undated, op. cit.

22. *Frederick Post*, 1994, op. cit.

23. Marcus, 1995 radio interview, op. cit.

24. W. L. Marcus, Keynote Address, First International Conference on Chemical Contamination and Human Detoxification, International Academy of Detoxification Specialists, Los Angeles, 1995, http://www.detoxacademy.org.

25. L. R. Hubbard, *Clear Body, Clear Mind*, Bridge Publication, Los Angeles, 1990.

26. Hirzy, undated, op. cit.

27. National Academy of Sciences, National Research Council, Board on Environmental Studies and Toxicology, *Health Effects of Ingested Fluoride*, National Academies Press, Washington, DC, 1993.

28. *Federal Register*, December 29, 1993 (58 FR 68826-68827).

29. *Federal Register*, December 5, 1997 (62 FR 64297).

30. Hirzy, 1999, op. cit.

31. J. Yiamouyiannis, *Lifesaver's Guide to Fluoridation*, Safe Water Foundation, Delaware, OH, 1982.

32. Hirzy, undated, op. cit.

33. R. J. Carton and J. W. Hirzy, Applying the NAEP Code of Ethics to the Environmental Protection Agency and the Fluoride in Drinking Water Standard, *Proc.*

23rd Annual Conference of the National Association of Environmental Professionals, San Diego, CA, June 1998.

34. This list is taken in part from the Fluoride Action Network, http://www.fluoridealert.org.

35. Carton and Hirzy, 1998, op. cit.

36. Hirzy, 2000, op. cit.

37. D. W. Cross and R. J. Carton, Fluoridation: a violation of medical ethics and human rights, *Int. J. Occup. Environ. Health*, 9(1), 24–29, 2003.

38. National Research Council, *Fluoride in Drinking Water: A Scientific Review of EPA's Standards*, National Academies Press, Washington, DC, 2006.

CHAPTER 10

RIDING THE TIGER: THE DOSAGE ISSUE

By now it should be clear that fluoride is both savior and devil. A little bit of it is very good for you. A lot of it can do you harm. The question that stands at the heart of the fluoride controversy is where the boundary lies between the good and the bad.

Fluoride is ingested into the human body from many sources. There are traces of fluoride in the air we breathe, the water we drink, and the food we eat. Some of it is natural and some of it is placed there by humans. Since the first confirmed evidence of fluoride's beneficial impact on tooth decay over 50 years ago, there has been a large increase in the amount of fluoride ingested by most Americans. This increase in fluoride intake comes from fluoridated drinking water, increased fluoride content in foods that are processed with fluoridated water, inadvertent ingestion of fluoridated toothpastes, and the increased prescription by dental practitioners of fluoride supplements and mouthwashes.

When the optimal concentration of fluoride in drinking water was set at 1.0 ppm in the late 1940s and early 1950s, background concentrations were minimal, and it was assumed that the great majority of a person's total fluoride intake would come from fluoridated drinking water. The feedback loop that results from processing food with fluoridated water was not anticipated, nor was the associated "halo effect" that imports the effects of fluoridation into nonfluoridated communities. Given these unanticipated developments, a question arises as to whether current fluoridation practices are putting too much fluoride into the human environment. Is it time, as some have suggested, to reexamine the "optimal" concentration and perhaps cut it back to a lower value? Is it possible that community water fluoridation is no longer even needed?

The Fluoride Wars: How a Modest Public Health Measure Became America's Longest-Running Political Melodrama   By R. Allan Freeze and Jay H. Lehr
Copyright © 2009 John Wiley & Sons, Inc.

The anti-fluoridation movement has been claiming for years that fluoride dosage is out of control, but given their proclivity for exaggeration, neither the public nor the medical establishment has paid much attention. However, in recent years there has been growing concern within the dental community itself that current fluoride intake may be approaching a level that could lead to undesirable health impacts. The growing prevalence of dental fluorosis among children in America has already been documented in Chapter 7, and the reality of crippling skeletal fluorosis in other countries, in Chapter 8. The fight over the fluoride MCL within the ranks of EPA scientists described in Chapter 9 provides further evidence that current fluoridation policies may be pushing things very close to that elusive boundary that separates the good from the bad. It is one thing when ideologically committed fluoride-haters warn of danger; it is quite another when objective medical observers begin to sound the alarm.

In this chapter we look at the concept of a maximum acceptable daily dose, and then try to assess whether current intake rates could be breaching this bound. To do so, we will have to look at drinking water and beverage habits in the United States (including the increased dependence on bottled water by some segments of the population), the level of fluoride in certain foods (especially those favored by young children), and the role of fluoride toothpastes and supplements in total fluoride intake. There are a lot of numbers coming up, and one can easily get lost in the swirl of competing claims and counterclaims. We will do our best to make it all palatable.

THE CONCEPT OF A MAXIMUM ACCEPTABLE DAILY DOSE

To this point in our story, the two numbers that are most likely to be burned into the reader's mind are the *optimal fluoride level* of 1.0 ppm established by the Public Health Service many years ago, and the *maximum contaminant level* (MCL) of 4.0 ppm established fairly recently, after much wrangling, by the Environmental Protection Agency. Both of these values represent *concentrations* of fluoride in water. A concentration of 1.0 ppm by weight means that there is 1 gram of fluoride dissolved in 1 million grams of water, or equivalently, 1 milligram of fluoride dissolved in 1 million milligrams of water. Because a 1-liter volume of water weighs exactly 1 million milligrams, it is common to express concentrations in water in units of milligrams per liter (mg/L). A concentration of 1.0 mg/L is numerically equivalent to a concentration of 1.0 ppm.

It is necessary to get these units clear in one's mind, because we are going to use them to calculate fluoride *intake*. One must recognize that it is not the concentration of fluoride in drinking water per se that controls whether good or harm is done. Fluoride is not like sulfuric acid, where ingestion of a highly concentrated solution would burn your throat whereas a mild solution would not. One could drink water with a fluoride concentration many times the 4.0 mg/L MCL without suffering any acute ill effects. Adverse health impacts of fluoride, if they occur at all, are chronic in nature and arise from long-term intake.

So how is fluoride intake calculated? Well, take as an example an adult male who drinks 2 liters of water per day at the optimal fluoride concentration of 1.0 mg/L. His fluoride intake from this source is 2 mg/day (2 L/day × 1.0 mg/L). If he drinks water that contains a fluoride concentration equal to the MCL of 4.0 mg/L, his intake is 8 mg/day. The first intake ought to be ideal; the second, as we shall see below, pushes the limits of an acceptable intake.

Recall from Chapter 8 that the *dose* is defined as the rate of intake per kilogram of body weight. Chronic fluoride dose therefore has units of milligrams of fluoride per kilogram body weight (mg/kg) per day. An adult male who weighs 80 kg (about 180 pounds) and has a fluoride intake of 2 mg/day is receiving a dose of 0.025 mg/kg per day. At 8 mg/day, his dose is 0.10 mg/kg per day. A young female toddler who weighs 20 kg (45 pounds) weighs only one-fourth as much as the adult male, but it is also likely that she drinks only one-fourth as much water (0.5 L/day). If so, her fluoride dose would be identical to that of the adult male. It is the dose, continued over many years, that controls whether a person enjoys enhanced dental health without undesirable side effects or whether the enhanced dental health is accompanied by increased dental fluorosis, problems with bone health, or in the worst-case scenario, the development of crippling skeletal fluorosis.

In the opinion of some, the inclusion of a person's weight in these dosage calculations makes the issue more complicated than it need be. In point of fact, it is necessary only if one is trying to compare apples with oranges. As long as one keeps the statistical population fairly homogeneous (say, adult males, 6- to 7-year-old children, or infants less than 6 months old), one can dismiss the need for weight correction and provide dosage statistics and guidelines in the simpler units of milligrams per day. In the sections that follow we see examples of both sets of dosage units in play (mg/day and mg/kg per day).

The maximum acceptable daily dose of fluoride is one that produces no observable adverse effects of any kind over a long period of use. There have been many estimates of this value over the years, but most of them can be traced back to the work of Kaj Roholm's 1937 book on *Fluorine Intoxication*.[1] Unfortunately, as we learned in Chapter 4, the interpretation of Roholm's data that became most widely quoted in the United States was in error.

Harold Hodge, America's preeminent fluoride toxicologist in the early years of the fluoridation movement, incorrectly calculated a range of 20 to 80 mg/day (depending on body weight) for the maximum acceptable daily dose. He presented this recommendation to a 1953 National Academy of Sciences meeting and repeated it for many years in several publications.[2] Hodge publicly recognized his error in 1979, but the incorrect values continued to appear in publications of the Public Health Service and the American Dental Association as late as 1993. All during this period the World Health Organization published a range of values for the maximum acceptable daily dose that was calculated correctly from Roholm's data, albeit rather conservatively, at 2.5 to 5.0 mg/day. The WHO still uses these figures as their recommended guideline. The Hodge-based PHS and ADA guidelines of 20 to 80 mg/day were at least three times too high and perhaps more.

In the United States, the specification of an official dosage recommendation falls to the Food and Nutrition Board (who we first met in Chapter 8, then again in Chapter 9, during their struggle over whether fluoride is an "essential nutrient" or merely a "beneficial nutrient" for human health). In 1997, the FNB published a revised set of *dietary reference intakes*. For all nutrients, they specified both an *adequate intake* (AI), which is defined as the "requirement to optimize health," and a *tolerable upper intake level* (UL), which is defined as the "maximum level that reduces the risk of adverse effects of excessive consumption."[3] The recommended AI value for fluoride is 0.05 mg/kg per day, and the recommended UL value is 0.10 mg/kg per day. If some assumptions are made about average body weights for people in various age ranges, it is possible to convert these values into the more easily grasped units of mg/day. The FNB has done so in the form of Table 10.1, which provides age-specific recommendations for AI and UL values.

The UL values in Table 10.1 can be taken as the current federal position on the maximum acceptable daily dose for fluoride. The limits recommended vary from less than 1 mg/day for infants to 10 mg/day for adults. The value for adults is much less than the erroneous range of Harold Hodge (20 to 80 mg/day) that was promoted by U.S. fluoridation agencies for so many years, and slightly higher than the very conservative range currently published by the World Health Organization (2.5 to 5.0 mg/day). The UL values in Table 10.1 are presumably designed to be protective against both skeletal fluorosis and dental fluorosis. From the earlier discussions of these issues, it seems likely that adherence to these limits would provide complete protection against the onset of skeletal fluorosis, with a suitable (although not overly large) margin of safety and considerable protection against the occurrence of moderate-to-severe dental fluorosis, but possibly not against the milder "cosmetic" forms.

TABLE 10.1   Dietary Reference Intakes for Fluoride Established by the Food and Nutrition Board[3]

Age	Adequate Intake (AI)[a] (mg/day)	Tolerable Upper Intake Levels (UL)[b] (mg/day)
0–6 months	0.01	0.7
7–12 months	0.5	0.9
1–3 years	0.7	1.3
4–8 years	1.0	2.2
9–13 years	2.0	10.0
14–18 years	3.0	10.0
>19 years	Female: 3.0	10.0
	Male: 4.0	

[a]AI values are based on a weight-dependent optimal daily dose of 0.05 mg fluoride per kg body weight per day.
[b]UL values are based on a weight-dependent maximum acceptable daily dose of 0.10 mg fluoride per kg body weight per day.

Anti-fluoridation arguments about dosage take two forms. First, they argue that the values currently recommended for the maximum acceptable daily dose are too high. It is their contention that lower values are needed to provide a greater margin of safety against crippling skeletal fluorosis and more complete protection against all forms of dental fluorosis. Earlier discussions of the current status of dental fluorosis in Chapter 7 and of skeletal fluorosis in Chapter 8 should give the reader sufficient information to come to his or her own conclusion on this issue.

Second, they argue that current fluoride intake by many people in society already exceeds the recommended maximum values, and that under current fluoridation policy and practice, such intakes are likely to increase even more. They see a future of uncontrolled dental fluorosis, and the emergence of crippling skeletal fluorosis as a serious problem in the United States as it is in many other countries. Of all the issues raised by the anti-fluoridation movement, the question of excessive fluoride intake is the most provocative, and it deserves our attention. The remainder of this chapter is concerned largely with this issue.

FLUORIDE INTAKE IN OUR DIET

The most obvious source of fluoride in our diet is from fluoridated drinking water. Surveys of drinking water habits by the Environmental Protection Agency suggest that an average American adult drinks about 1.0 liter of water per day (about four 8-ounce glasses). However, 10% of the population drink more than 2 liters per day, 5% more than 4 liters per day, and upward of 1% (on the order of 2 million people) drink more than 5 liters per day.[4] For those living in communities that are fluoridated at 1.0 mg/L, fluoride intake from drinking water averages 1.0 mg/day, but for heavy water drinkers it can run as high as 5 mg/day or more. In nonfluoridated communities, fluoride intake from drinking water is, of course, much less. However, one cannot forget those naturally fluoridated communities where fluoride is *removed* from public water supplies rather than *added*. The EPA recommends removal to the secondary MCL value of 2 mg/L (see Chapter 9), but if removal leaves fluoride concentrations anywhere near the primary MCL value of 4.0 mg/L, average water drinkers would ingest 4.0 mg/day, and heavy water drinkers even more. Such intake levels can approach or exceed the FNB's tolerable upper intake level for adults of 10 mg/day. If you want to know the fluouride levels in your drinking water, the CDC maintains a website, "My Water's Fluoride," that provides this information.[5]

Water intake for the average American is about one-third of total fluid intake. Fluid intake from beverages other than water provides an additional source of fluoride in the diet. Soft drinks account for 30% of the nonwater fluid intake, with milk, beer, coffee, fruit juices, and bottled water accounting for another 8 to 12% each.[6] When these beverages are processed with fluoridated water, they too will have elevated fluoride concentrations. One study found the majority of soft drinks on the market to have fluoride concentrations greater than 0.6 ppm (about two-thirds that of "optimally fluoridated" water). Most studies indicate a wide variation in the fluoride content of off-the-shelf beverages. Analysis of 175 ready-to-drink juices in Iowa indicated fluoride concentrations from 0.03 to 2.80 ppm. An assay of 275 beverages available in North Carolina exhibited a range from 0.1 to 6.7 ppm.[7] The highest concentrations are found in grape juice and tea. This odd finding is apparently explained by the ready absorption of fluoride-containing pesticides by grape skins and tea leaves. The average fluoride intake from beverages other than water is generally thought to be less than half that from direct water intake.

Many consumers who are disenchanted with the quality of their tap water have turned to bottled water for solace. This group includes many anti-fluoridationists who hope to reduce their fluoride intake by switching from fluoridated public water supplies to bottled water. Per capita consumption of bottled water has increased from 5.7 gallons per year in 1987 to 23.8 gallons per year in 2004.[8] There are now almost 900 brands on the market (including one designed especially for dogs!). The bottled water industry has seen a 9.5% growth since 1997, and it now rings up $5 billion per year in business.[9]

Unfortunately, consumers may not always get what they are seeking. As one industry watchdog commented: "Bottled water is vastly more expensive, and not necessarily safer than its municipal counterpart."[10] Bottled water users are protected by FDA guidelines rather than by EPA drinking water standards. The FDA's rules are weaker than EPA's with respect to standards, testing frequency, violation triggers, operator training, and nature of reporting. In addition, the FDA rules cover only water that is *not* packaged and sold in the same state (30 to 40% of all bottled water). "In-state" water is regulated by 40 of the 50 states, but neither the FDA nor the states have significant resources for enforcement.[11] In any case, those seeking lower fluoride intake ought to look carefully at the label. One study of 328 bottled waters found that 67 of them had fluoride concentrations greater than 1.0 ppm.[12] One anecdote posted on a healthy-living website tells of a health food store exhibiting a colorful anti-fluoride petition on the wall, side-by-side with racks of bottled water at 3.6 ppm fluoride.[13]

Having issued this warning about bottled waters, it is only fair to note that the 328-brand test took place in Europe. A study of 103 North American brands found only two bottled waters with excessive fluoride.[14] Perhaps concerns expressed in the other direction may be more germane. Many in the dental community fear that a widespread abandonment of fluoridated public water supplies in favor of low-fluoride bottled waters may auger a return of the dental caries epidemic that they thought was beaten.[15]

The use of a body-weight correction in dose calculations implies that infants and children consume less fluids than adults, and studies confirm this. Fluid intake increases yearly from birth to adulthood, reaching 1 liter or so per day by 8 years of age.[16] In the 1980s, over half of the average childhood intake was milk and water, but in recent years there has been a trend in children's beverage selection toward more juices and soft drinks. The total fluoride intake derived from fluids depends on the fluoride content of both the drinking water and the other beverages, but studies show that it seldom exceeds 2.0 mg/day for young children, even in fluoridated communities. There was some concern in past years that the fluoride content of infant formula might be leading to inappropriate dosages for very young children, but recent studies show that manufacturers are now controlling fluoride content more carefully.[17]

It is estimated that about 75% of our dietary fluoride intake comes from drinking water and other beverages. The other 25% comes from food. Some foods, including fish, seafood, and chicken products, can be naturally high in fluoride, but most foods get their fluoride content through processing with fluoridated water. Foods processed with fluoridated water may have up to three times the fluoride content of those processed with nonfluoridated water.[18] Even under these circumstances, however, fluoride intake from food is generally less than 1.0 mg/day. The U.S. Department of Agriculture maintains a database of fluoride contents of selected beverages and foods, and it is available on the web.[19]

There have been many estimates of total dietary fluoride intake (from food, water, and beverages) for both adults and children. All of them show that intakes in fluoridated communities exceed those in nonfluoridated communities by two to three times. Adult intake generally falls in the range of 1.4 to 3.4 mg/day in fluoridated communities and 0.3 to 1.0 mg/day in nonfluoridated communities.[20] Intake for 2- to 3-year-old children falls in the range 0.4 to 1.0 mg/day in fluoridated communities and less than 0.5 mg/day in nonfluoridated communities.[21]

Comparison of these values with the numbers in the right-hand column of Table 10.1 indicates that even at the high end of these dietary intake ranges, the values fall well below the maximum acceptable daily doses. Unfortunately, this is not the entire story. We must still look at the additional fluoride intake generated by the use of fluoridated toothpastes and from fluoride supplements and mouthwashes.

DO NOT SWALLOW

The first successful clinical trials of a fluoridated toothpaste were reported in 1955 by J. C. Muhler of the School of Dentistry at the University of Indiana. These studies involved 1200 public school students in Bloomington, Indiana, who used a toothpaste containing a stannous-fluoride additive for a three-year study period.[22] The results indicated a reduction in dental caries of 15 to 30% in the study group after two to three years of use. The Indiana studies were sponsored by Proctor & Gamble, and they soon led to the appearance on drugstore shelves of Crest toothpaste "with fluoristan." Few people old enough to remember will forget the original "Look Ma. No Cavities" ads that saturated the airwaves at that time. Crest quickly built up a significant market share in the budding toothpaste wars.

In 1960, Proctor & Gamble approached the American Dental Association and asked if they would endorse Crest as "an effective decay-reducing agent." In August of that year the ADA Council on Dental Therapeutics acceded to Crest's request,[23] and Crest advertisements immediately ballyhooed this professional endorsement. Proctor & Gamble's stock rose by $8 a share, and sales of Crest doubled within the year. In October 1960 at the annual conference of the ADA in Los Angeles, the ADA leadership took considerable flak from the membership over the Crest endorsement,[24] and it was publicly suggested that some of the ADA leadership might have profited from the rise in Procter & Gamble's stock. The ADA also came in for much criticism from competitive toothpaste manufacturers. In January 1961, ADA officials tried to calm the waters by claiming that they had merely given their "approval" to Crest, not their "endorsement," but this clarification didn't cut much ice with opponents.[25] Despite the furore, a move to rescind the approval did not succeed. Crest went on to become the best-selling toothpaste in the United States for three decades. In fiscal year 2000, annual sales of Crest toothpaste reached $463.7 million, and sales of all Crest products (which include such items as teeth-whitening strips and battery-operated spin brushes) were greater than $1 billion per year. In 1990, Procter & Gamble gave the American Dental Association a gift of $100,000 "to commemorate the 30th anniversary of ADA's recognition of Crest."[26]

Meanwhile, Colgate, which had been the best-selling brand prior to the appearance of Crest, entered the market with a fluoridated toothpaste of its own in 1961. Their additive was sodium monofluorophosphate (marketed as "Colgate with MFP"). It, too, was approved by the ADA, as were three other toothpastes by 1980. In 1985, the ADA set up its Seal of Approval program, which applied to all dental products, including toothpaste. Careful guidelines were promulgated for acceptance of fluoride-containing dentifrices.[27] In 1981, Crest quietly switched from stannous fluoride to sodium fluoride, and since that time no American toothpaste has used stannous fluoride, the original additive that changed the toothpaste game. By 1990, fluoride dentifrices accounted for over 90% of the toothpaste market in the United States and Canada. It can safely be assumed that almost every child who brushes his or her teeth regularly does so with a fluoride toothpaste.

This, then, is the background that leads to concern about the level of fluoride intake that might accompany toothbrushing with fluoridated toothpastes, especially by small children. Fluoride concentrations in toothpaste are very high, generally running about 1000 ppm. A large tube of toothpaste contains as much as 2 grams of fluoride (or 2000 mg). A ribbon of toothpaste of the type that appears regularly in toothpaste ads can contain several milligrams of fluoride. In the worst-case scenario, it has been claimed that small children might swallow up to a third of the toothpaste that goes on their brush at each brushing.[28] A daily fluoride intake of this amount would exceed that received from all other sources put together. A more likely intake from swallowed toothpaste, determined from studies of actual children's habits, is about 0.3 mg per brushing, or 0.6 mg/day.[29] Comparison of this value with the figures in Table 10.1 show that this fluoride source alone far exceeds the adequate intake recommendations for small children and approaches the tolerable upper intake levels.

When Crest toothpaste first came onto the market in 1955, it carried a government warning that fluoride toothpastes should not be used in areas where the water supply is fluoridated. Later in the 1950s, a further caution was added that children under 6 should not use Crest. These warnings disappeared in 1958, but in 1960, when the American Dental Association began endorsing fluoride toothpastes, they coupled their endorsement with a requirement that the manufacturers place a warning label on the tube. A sample warning reads: "Do not swallow. Use only a pea-sized amount for children under 6. To prevent swallowing, children under 6 years of age should be supervised in the use of toothpaste."

There is no question that fluoride toothpastes are used widely in fluoridated as well as nonfluoridated areas. It is also unlikely that parents pay much heed to the various warnings that appear on toothpaste tubes. One must conclude that fluoride ingestion from fluoridated toothpaste represents a significant component of overall intake for young children.

CONTESTING CONVENTIONAL WISDOM

When the value of fluoride became clear in the early 1950s as a preventive agent against dental caries, pharmaceutical companies were quick to see the market possibilities of fluoride supplements for children and adolescents. Fluoride tablets at 0.25, 0.5, and 1.0 mg strength were soon available on drugstore shelves. They remain available today, although only by prescription, and their role in the prevention of decay remains controversial.

Fluoride supplements first came onto the market when the impact of fluoridation was thought to be systemic. With the emerging consensus that topical effects trump systemic, the value of ingesting supplemental fluoride in the form of tablets has been called into question. The pharmaceutical companies have tried to keep up with the times by marketing chewable tablets and lozenges that are designed to be sucked for a minute or two in order to get the topical effect, but it is highly questionable whether small children understand the concept, or whether parents are willing to be vigilant enough to ensure effective topical contact.

Early studies did find that if a regimen of supplementation is carefully followed, significant caries reduction can be achieved.[30] However, these studies were carried out during the years of increasing water fluoridation and increased use of fluoride toothpastes, and critics argue that it is "impossible to separate out the effects specifically attributable to fluoride tablets."[31] Furthermore, as noted by almost all creditable observers, home-based supplemental programs are "notorious for their lack of long-term compliance."[32] Children simply don't take their pills regularly enough, and parents are unlikely to monitor the regimen vigorously. A workshop on the effectiveness of the various approaches to fluoride delivery found the use of supplements to be much more expensive and much less effective than community water fluoridation.[33] Given that caries is declining, fluorosis is increasing, and cariostatic effects are topical, one study concluded that "the continued use of dietary fluoride supplements is not warranted as a routine public health measure."[34] The American Dental Association states that the compliance difficulties make supplementation "impractical as an alternative to water fluoridation as a public health measure."[35]

According to the Food and Nutrition Board, "dietary fluoride supplements are only intended for use by children living in non-fluoridated areas, to increase their fluoride exposure so it is similar to that by children living in optimally fluoridated areas."[36] This advice would limit supplement intake to the one-third of the U.S. population who do not have access to community water fluoridation. However, a 1980 study found that 20% of family pediatricians prescribed fluoride supplements for children who lived in fluoridated communities.[37] The practice may still be more common than it should be.

The ADA introduced guidelines for fluoride supplementation in 1958, then revised them downward in 1979, and again in 1994. For children in non-fluoridated communities (less than 0.3 ppm fluoride in their water supply), the ADA currently recommends no supplements before 6 months of age, 0.25 mg/day from 6 months to 3 years, 0.50 mg/day from 3 to 6 years, and 1.0 mg/day from 6 to 16 years. For mildly fluoridated communities (0.3 to 0.6 ppm fluoride in the water supply), the limits recommended for the four age groups are 0, 0, 0.25, and 0.5 mg/day, respectively. For communities with greater than 0.6 ppm fluoride in their water supply, no supplements should be taken at any age.[38]

The Public Health Service has always supported the judicious use of fluoride supplements as an alternative method of fluoride delivery, but it has never been their method of choice. Since the early years of the fluoridation crusade, their favored alternate delivery vehicle has been regular oral rinsing with fluoride. For years, the PHS developed and supported school-based mouth-rinsing programs across the United States. By 1988, 24% of all U.S. school districts had initiated such a program, and there were 3.25 million schoolchildren rinsing regularly in the classroom (about 14% of all school-aged children).[39] However, popularity within the PHS never translated into strong support across the dental research fraternity. School mouth-rinsing programs have come under even more internal fire than have programs that promote the use of fluoride supplements.

The most common recommended mouth-washing regimen is for one 10-milliliter rinse for 1 minute once a week. Fluoride oral rinses are highly concentrated solutions of sodium fluoride, containing up to 1000 ppm fluoride. This means that there are 10 milligrams of fluoride in each 10-mL rinse, so the potential for significant inadvertent fluoride intake is considerable, especially by small children. Two independent studies of this problem found that most regular childhood users of oral rinses swallowed between 22% and 35% of the rinse, and a few subjects swallowed it all. Individual fluoride intakes from mouthwash by children under school age probably run in the range 0.9 to 4.6 mg per rinse (or 0.1 to 0.7 mg/day assuming a weekly rinse schedule).[40] The higher end of this range represents a third to a half of the maximum total acceptable daily dose for young children aged 1 to 8 (Table 10.1).

Surprisingly, the main criticism of mouth-rinsing programs has not been against their safety, but rather, their effectiveness. The original assessment of these programs,[41] carried out by the National Institute of Dental Research (an arm of the Public Health Service) in the mid-1970s, claimed that caries reductions of 20 to 50% could be achieved at a cost of less than $1 a year per child. As with similar studies of fluoride supplements, critics noted that the NIDR study was carried out during a period of declining national caries rates, and because there were no control groups in the study, it was impossible to know what contribution to ascribe to oral rinsing relative to the growth of community water fluoridation and increased use of fluoridated toothpastes. A second study carried out by others in the mid-1980s called the earlier results into question.

This study, termed the National Preventive Dentistry Demonstration Program (NPDDP), was a truly independent assessment. It was funded by the private sector (through the Robert Wood Johnson Foundation), managed by the dental research community (through the American Fund for Dental Health), supervised by a National Advisory Committee, and carried out by independent data gatherers (from the Rand Corporation).[42] The results found the school-based mouth-rinsing program to be of marginal value and suggested that such programs are unlikely to add any effectiveness to the already effective mix of community water fluoridation and fluoridated toothpaste.[43] They also questioned NIDR's cost estimates, dismissing the issue by stating that whatever the cost, it was money wasted.

The NPDDP findings challenged prevailing national policy and public health practice. Not surprisingly, there was an outcry from the NIDR. Scientists from the NPDDP claim that NIDR staff sent out letters to a lengthy list of correspondents in the dental research community attempting to discredit the NPDDP program. Furious debates ensued at dental conventions. Lifelong friendships were fractured. A few years later, the NPDDP team wrote an article that traced the history of the controversy. They called it *A*

Case Study in Contesting the Conventional Wisdom.[44] They speculated that their results may have been seen as an attack on the integrity of the NIDR, which they did not intend. But intended or not, their study certainly attempted to discredit the earlier study, and in so doing it represented a threat to the scientific standing of many highly regarded dental researchers and administrators at NIDR. When the Association of Public Health Dentistry decided to have a workshop in 1989 on preventive strategies, they chose Dennis Leverett, a respected researcher from the Eastman Dental Center in Rochester, New York, and not a member of either the NIDR or NPDDP camp, to review the evidence on mouthrinsing. He reported carefully that there was "no justification for recommending use of a mouthrinse by a person known to use a fluoride dentifrice regularly," but that there still might be opportunities for use with people of "known high risk" for dental caries.[45]

In several European countries where community water fluoridation has not proven popular enough or practicable enough for implementation, governments have approved the delivery of fluoride to the populace through alternative distribution vehicles. Among those that have been available at one time or another are fluoridated milk, salt, flour, and sugar. The products are provided to grocer's shelves in both fluoridated and unfluoridated form, and people are free to choose whichever variety they wish. The main arguments against this approach revolve around the likely ineffectiveness of delivery methods based on voluntary intake and the difficulty in maintaining quality control over the manufacture and distribution of fluoridated products.

The most widely used alternative delivery vehicle has been salt. Studies show that salt fluoridation produces reductions in tooth decay that are similar to those of fluoridated water.[46] The approach has been particularly successful in Switzerland, in large part because the Swiss Cantons have an exclusive monopoly on the centralized manufacture and distribution of salt. Fluoridated salt is also available in several other European countries, including France, Germany, Spain, and Hungary (as well as several Latin American countries, including Mexico, Costa Rica, and Colombia).[47] The idea has never caught on in North America, and is unlikely to do so now, given the contributing role of salt in the development of hypertension, and the resulting trend toward cutbacks in salt consumption.

TOO MUCH OF A GOOD THING?

All these estimates of fluoride intakes (in mg/day) and dose rates (in mg/kg per day) are probably enough to make a faithful reader's eyes glaze over, but there are a couple of points that might have come clear. First, it is not a simple matter to calculate the total fluoride intake or dose for a particular person. Second, there is the potential for a very wide variability in total fluoride intake and/or dose from one person to another.

Total fluoride intake includes all the fluoride taken in from drinking water, other beverages, food, and fluoride supplements. It also includes the inadvertent ingestion of fluoride toothpastes and oral rinses. The lowest levels of intake are experienced by light-drinking persons in nonfluoridated communities who do not partake of fluoride supplements, toothpastes, or oral rinses. The highest levels of intake are experienced by heavy drinkers in fluoridated communities who also receive fluoride from supplements, toothpastes, and oral rinses. Within a given intake bracket, the highest dose rates (i.e., the intake, corrected for body weight) accrue to infants and small children; the lowest dose rates to older adolescents and adults. Among adults with similar intakes, women are more likely to receive a higher dose than men.

If we look at the figures quoted earlier in this chapter and at the few estimates of total fluoride intake that have appeared in the literature,[48] it appears that an average adult (one who lives in a fluoridated community, drinks a liter of water a day, uses fluoridated toothpaste, but doesn't take fluoride supplements or use mouthwash) will receive a total fluoride intake in the range of 2.0 to 5.0 mg/day. Those who live in nonfluoridated communities, or who avoid fluoride toothpastes, will probably have intakes that are less than half this range. All these values are considerably less than the maximum tolerable UL values quoted on Table 10.1.

The use of supplements adds 0.5 to 1.0 mg/day to these figures. Heavy water drinkers have to add 1.0 mg/day for each additional liter ingested over the average. If you are one of those 2 million people who drink more than 5 liters of water a day, and if you also use fluoride toothpaste and fluoride supplements, your daily intake could be approaching (or perhaps even exceeding) the 10.0-mg/day tolerable upper intake level recommended by the Food and Nutrition Board.

Even more disturbing to some observers is the documented increase in fluoride intake levels over the years. In the 1940s, when the optimal fluoridation concentration of 1.0 ppm was set, fluoride intake levels were probably less than 0.5 mg/day across the board. By the 1970s, total dietary intake by heavy water consumers had reached 3.5 mg/day, and by 1991, 6.5 mg/day. Some anti-fluoridation activists claim that current intake rates by this high-risk group may reach 12 mg/day.[49] There is no evidence of a slowdown in the rate of increase. If it were to continue unabated, even lower-risk segments of society might soon begin to receive more fluoride than is good for them.

Anti-fluoridationists claim that this has already come to pass with respect to dose rates for infants and young children. They point to studies by establishment research teams that indicate dose rates approaching or exceeding the maximum acceptable daily dose of 0.10 mg/kg for this vulnerable segment of society.[50] Paul Connett, the much-traveled feature speaker at many a fluoride debate, makes this a central point of his presentations. "Right now," he says, "American children are being overdosed."[51] Hardy Limeback, the University of Toronto dental researcher who has turned against fluoridation, says: "Kids exposed to all these sources are getting too much. They are way past the optimum."[52]

Of course, it is not that surprising to find anti-fluoride activists railing against fluoride dosage. It is perhaps more surprising to find that there is a long history of doubt among pro-fluoride dental researchers. The first establishment call for a reexamination of fluoride dosage came as early as 1982, when Dennis Leverett published an article in the journal *Science* claiming that "the widespread use of fluorides may have created a situation in which we are approaching a critical mass of fluoride in the environment." He suggested that "the definition of the optimum concentration of fluoride in community water supplies needs to be reassessed."[53]

Leverett's article generated much discussion but little action. In the years that followed, several articles appeared, written by others, making similar arguments. Geoffrey Smith, an Australian dental surgeon, published a paper in 1985 whose title asked whether we were now suffering under "A Surfeit of Fluoride?"[54] In 1987, A. S. Gray, director of the Division of Dental Health Services for the province of British Columbia, wrote a paper titled "Time for a New Baseline."[55] A 1995 article in the journal *Community Dental and Oral Epidemiology* argued that a new lower fluoride guideline was needed.[56] A paper accepted for publication in the *Journal of Public Health Dentistry* in the same year suggested that a reassessment of fluoride dosage was necessary in light of "total fluoride exposure, its safety margin, and the distribution and severity of fluorosis."[57] B. A. Burt and S. A. Eklund, coauthors of one of the most widely used textbooks in American dental schools, joined the growing list of concerned fluoride supporters in a paper published in 1997. They noted that "current standards for water fluoridation in the United States have stood since 1962. Many things have changed since then, however, and data suggest that perhaps it is time to reconsider these standards." Based on their data, they recommended 0.7 ppm fluoride as a suitable trade-off point between fluorosis and caries rather than the 1.0 ppm traditionally used.[58]

The arguments put forward in these papers for a lower level of fluoride in community water supplies emphasize the increased exposure to fluoride in the modern world, the increase in observed levels of dental fluorosis, the broader choice of possible intervention points for fluoride therapy, and the increase in cost relative to effectiveness. Several authors quote Leverett's original exhortation that the dental community should "strive to maintain the lowest fluoride levels capable of producing the desired therapeutic effect."[59] David Locker, in his assessment of fluoride safety for the Ontario Ministry of Health, suggests that under current levels of exposure from other sources, fluoride concentrations as low as 0.5 ppm may be optimal for many community water supplies.[60]

In October 1994, the American Association of Public Health Dentistry held a symposium at their annual meeting in New Orleans, Louisiana entitled "Fluoride: How Much of a Good Thing?" Most of the speakers at the symposium, all of whom came from the dental research establishment, attested to the increased exposure to fluoride in the modern world and the unwelcome increase in dental fluorosis. A few raised the question of the role of fluoride in bone strength among older people and were willing to admit that it was not well defined. Most spoke of the need to maximize the benefits of fluoride while minimizing undesirable side effects.[61] The need for a reduction in overall fluoride levels was in the air.

One group that is conspicuous by their silence on this issue is the U.S. Public Health Service. Throughout this period of reassessment among their peers, the PHS (and its research arm, the National Institute of Dental Research) continued its call for community water fluoridation at current levels and increased delivery at these levels to those segments of the population not yet served. At the New Orleans "How Much of a Good Thing?" meeting, Herschel Horowitz, a retired NIDR scientist and longtime supporter of public health fluoridation, was the only speaker to buck the trend toward concerns over dosage. He publicly disagreed with the apparent view of most conference attendees that fluoride availability and use is getting out of control. In his emotional presentation, he lamented the fact that the dentistry profession could so soon have forgotten the horrible trauma of tooth decay.[62]

Anti-fluoridationists are not surprised at the intransigence of the government agencies that originally sponsored the fluoride revolution. Brian Martin, in his book on the social dynamics of fluoridation, feels that the health and safety issue lurks ominously in the background—and not just the observed increase in dental fluorosis, but also the possibility of chronic toxicological impact. "Once the dental profession made such a strong commitment to fluoride," he suggests, "it staked its reputation on the measure. It became very difficult to reverse or even modify the policy, because this would be tantamount to admitting that the dental experts were wrong—both scientifically and ethically—in promoting an insufficiently tested procedure." He argues that the dental profession has an investment in its own credibility. Rejecting fluoride would mean losing face and admitting culpability for imposing an unnecessary risk on the public.[63] William Hirzy of the renegade EPA union agrees. In his view, the government and certain elements in the private sector, including the American Dental Association, have a vested interest in keeping up the pronouncement that fluoride is good for you. As he puts it: "They're riding a tiger that's hard to get off."[64]

A few communities have actually reduced the fluoride concentrations in their community water supplies, but by and large there has been little action, despite concerns over fluoride dosage that go back over 20 years now. It seems likely that the word will soon filter down to the local water authorities and that over the next decade we will see further reductions. Perhaps we will even see a tacit acceptance from fluoridation-promoting agencies that the "optimal" fluoride concentration for the new reality lies closer to 0.5 ppm than the traditional 1.0 ppm.

Of course, the pro-fluoridation movement is sick with fear that this backing off will be interpreted by the public as a signal that fluoridation is no longer needed at all. Such an interpretation would be a sad mistake. There is no question that fluoride is responsible for the near-eradication of dental caries. There also seems little question that community water fluoridation is the most reliable and cost-effective method of fluoride delivery. What is needed is simply a slight dialing back of the knob that controls fluoride input to public water systems: a recalibration, not a shutdown. Continued vigilance by the dental and medical communities is of course in order, but it seems likely that lower fluoride concentrations, coupled with the widespread use of fluoride toothpastes, should be sufficient to ensure the continued caries miracle, while protecting against the possibility of deteriorating bone health and the unwelcome increase in dental fluorosis. The search should continue, in Leverett's words, for "the lowest fluoride levels capable of producing the desired therapeutic effect."

REFERENCES

1. K. Roholm, *Fluorine Intoxication*, H. K. Lewis, London, 1937.

2. H. C. Hodge and F. A. Smith, Some public health aspects of water fluoridation, in *Fluoridation as a Public Health Measure*, edited by J. H. Shaw, American Association for the Advancement Science, Washington, DC, 1954; H. C. Hodge and F. A. Smith, Metabolism of inorganic fluoride, in *Fluorine Chemistry*, edited by J. H. Simons, Academic Press, New York, 1965.

3. Food and Nutrition Board, http://www.iom.edu.

4. See http://www.epa.gov/waterscience/drinking/percapita/; K. E. Heller, W. Sohn, B. A. Burt, and S. A. Eklund, Water consumption in the U.S. in 1994–96 and implications for water fluoridation policy, *J. Publ. Health Dent.*, 59, 3–11, 1999.

5. http//:apps.nccd.cdc.gov/MWF/Index.asp.

6. *What America drinks, USA Today*, April 18, 2001.

7. S. M. Levy, M. C. Kiritsy, and J. J. Warren, Sources of fluoride intake in children, *J. Publ. Health Dent.*, 55, 39–51, 1995.

8. American Dental Association, *Fluoridation Facts*, http://www.ada.org.

9. H. Mayell and P. Murphy, The bottled water craze, *Environmental Newsnet*, http://www.enn.com, November 13, 1999.

10. N. Bailey, *Bottled water not subject to strict safety rules, Vancouver Sun*, October 20, 2001.

11. K. L. Bryan, In search of a uniform standard for bottled water, in *Springs and Bottled Waters of the World*, edited by P. E. LaMoreaux and J. T. Tanner, Springer-Verlag, New York, 2001; Natural Resources Defence Council, Bottled water: pure drink or pure hype, http://www.nrdc.org.

12. http://www.pmgeiser.ch.

13. http:/emporium.turnpike.net/P/PDHA/health.htm.

14. Natural Resources Defence Council, op. cit.

15. Mayell and Murphy, 1999, op. cit.

16. G. Nikiforuk, Fluorides and dental caries, Chapter 2 in *Understanding Dental Caries*, Vol. 2, *Prevention: Basic and Clinical Aspects*, Karger, Basel, Switzerland, 1985.

17. Levy et al., 1995, op. cit.

18. Levy et al., 1995, op. cit.; D. H. Leverett, Fluorides and the changing prevalence of dental caries, *Science*, 217, 26–30, July 2, 1982.

19. U.S. Department of Agriculture, *National Fluoride Database of Selected Beverages and Food*, 2004, http://www.nal.usda.gov/fnic/foodcomp/Data/Fluoride/Fluoride. html.

20. American Dental Association, *Fluoridation Facts*, op cit.; B. A. Burt and S. A. Eklund, *Dentistry, Dental Practice, and the Community*, W. B. Saunders, Philadelphia, 1999; J. R. Marier and D. Rose, *Environmental Fluoride*, 2nd ed., Publication 16081, National Research Council of Canada, Toronto, Ontario, Canada, 1977.

21. L. Singer and R. Ophaug, Total fluoride intake of infants, *Pediatrics*, 63, 460–466, 1979; Burt and Eklund, 1999, op. cit; ADA, *Fluoridation Facts*, op. cit.

22. J. C. Muhler, Effect of stannous fluoride dentifrice on caries reduction in children during a three-year study period, *J. Am. Dent. Assoc.*, 64, 216–224, 1962.

23. *ADA News*, August 1, 1960.

24. R. R. Harris, *Dental Science in a New Age: A History of the National Institute of Dental Research*, Montrose Press, Rockville, MD, 1989.

25. *ADA News*, January 23, 1961.

26. *ADA News*, March 5, 1990.

27. American Dental Association, Council on Dental Therapeutics, Guidelines for the acceptance of fluoride-containing dentifrices, *J. Am. Dent. Assoc.*, 110, 545–547, 1985.

28. T. McGuire, *Tooth Fitness: Your Guide to Healthy Teeth*, St. Michael's Press, Grass Valley, CA, 1994.

29. E. D. Beltran and S. M. Szpunar, Fluoride in toothpaste for children: suggestions for change, *Pediatri. Dent.*, 10, 185–188, 1988; ADA, *Fluoridation Facts*, op. cit.

30. Nikiforuk, 1985, op. cit.; W. S. Driscoll, S. B. Heifetz, and D. C. Korts, Effect of chewable fluoride tablets on dental caries in schoolchildren: results after six years of use, *J. Am. Dent. Assoc.*, 97, 820–824, 1978; H. S. Horowitz, Effectiveness of school water fluoridation and dietary fluoride supplements in school-aged children, *J. Publ. Health Dent.*, 49(5), Special Issue, 290–296, 1989.

31. L. Ripa, A half-century of community water fluoridation in the United States: review and commentary, *J. Publ. Health Dent.*, 53, 17–44,1993.

32. Ibid.

33. B. A. Burt, Introduction to the workshop, *J. Publ. Health Dent.*, 49(5)(Special Issue), 256–258, 1989.

34. S. M. Szpunar and B. A. Burt, Evaluation of appropriate use of dietary fluoride supplements in the U.S., *Comm. Dent. Oral Epidemiol.* 20, 148–154, 1992.

35. ADA, *Fluoridation Facts*, op. cit.

36. As quoted in ADA, *Fluoridation Facts*, op. cit.

37. Burt and Eklund, 1999, op. cit.

38. New fluoride schedule adopted, *ADA News*, 25(10), 12–14, May 16, 1994.

39. Burt and Eklund, 1999, op. cit.; Levy et al., 1995, op. cit.

40. Levy et al., 1995, op. cit.

41. A. J. Miller and J. A. Brunelle, A summary of the NIDR community caries prevention demonstration program, *J. Am. Dent. Assoc.*, 107, 265–269, 1983.

42. D. H. Leverett, Effectiveness of mouthrinsing with fluoride solutions in preventing coronal and root caries, *J. Publ. Health Dent.*, 49(5)(Special Issue), 310–316, 1989.

43. S. P. Klein, H. M. Bohannan, R. M. Bell, J. A. Disney, C. B. Foch, and R. C. Graves, The cost and effectiveness of school-based preventive dental care, *Am. J. Publ. Health*, 75, 382–391, 1985.

44. J. A. Disney, H. M. Bohannan, S. P. Klein, and R. M. Bell, A case-study in contesting the conventional wisdom: school-based fluoride mouthrinse programs in the USA, *Comm. Dent. Oral Epidemiol.*, 18, 48–56, 1990.

45. Leverett, 1989, op. cit.

46. T. M. Marthaler, R. Mejia, K. Toth, and J. J. Vines, Caries-preventive salt fluoridation, *Caries Res.*, 12(Suppl. 1), 15, 1978.

47. Burt and Eklund, 1999, op. cit.; R. Roemer, Legislation on fluorides and dental health, *Int. Dig. Health Legislation*, 34, 3–31, 1983.

48. Marier and Rose, 1977, op. cit.; D. W. Lewis and H. Limeback, Comparison of recommended and actual mean intakes of fluorides by Canadians, *J. Can. Dent. Assoc.*, 62, 708–715, 1996; U.S. Public Health Service, *Review of Fluoride: Benefits*

and Risks, U.S. PHS, Washington, DC, 1991. The results of this latter report are summarized in *J. Am. Med. Assoc.*, 266, 1061–1067, 1991.

49. Stop Fluoridation USA, http://www.rvi.net; R. G. Foulkes, affidavit in case of *Safe Water Assoc. Inc.* v. *City of Fond du Lac, WI*, 1994.

50. Levy et al., 1995, op. cit.; Singer and Ophaug, 1979, op. cit.

51. F. Henry, *The invisible fear, Cleveland Plain Dealer*, Sunday Supplement, March 26, 2000.

52. K. Foss, *Are we getting too much fluoride? Toronto Globe and Mail*, May 4, 1999.

53. D. H. Leverett, Fluorides and the changing prevalence of dental caries, *Science*, 217, 26–30, July 2, 1982.

54. G. E. Smith, A surfeit of fluoride? *Sci. Prog. Oxford*, 69, 429–442, 1985.

55. A. S. Gray, Time for a new baseline, *J. Can. Dent. Assoc.*, 53, 763–765, 1987.

56. A. I. Ismail, What is the effective concentration of fluoride? *Comm. Dent. Oral Epidemiol*, 23, 246–251, 1995.

57. R. G. Rozier, A new era for community water fluoridation? Achievements after one-half century and challenges ahead, *J. Publ. Health Dent.*, 55, 3–5, 1995.

58. K. E. Heller, S. A. Eklund, and B. A. Burt, Dental caries and dental fluorosis at varying water fluoride concentrations, *J. Publ. Health Dent.*, 57, 236–243, 1997.

59. Ibid.

60. D. Locker, *Benefits and Risks of Water Fluoridation*, Ontario Ministry of Health, Toronto, Ontario, Canada, 1999, http://www.gov.on.ca/health.

61. B. A. Burt, Introduction to the symposium: Fluoride: How Much of a Good Thing? *J. Publ. Health Dent.*, 55, 37–38, 1995.

62. H. S. Horowitz, Commentary on and recommendations for the proper use of fluoride, *J. Publ. Health Dent.*, 55, 57–62, 1995.

63. B. Martin, *Scientific Knowledge in Controversy: The Social Dynamics of the Fluoridation Debate*, State University of New York Press, Albany, NY, 1991.

64. As quoted in Henry, 2000, op. cit.

CHAPTER *11*

SCIENCE AND NOT SCIENCE

Most scientists hear about it first from their high school science teachers. In college, it is drummed into them in every physics class. It is called the *scientific method*, and it is the gospel on how science is supposed to work. Under the scientific method, hypotheses are put forward, experiments are carried out to test the hypotheses, and the results of the experiments are published in peer-reviewed journals for all to see. The published articles are expected to include all the methodological details and all the experimental data in sufficient detail to allow for replication of the work by any scientist who chooses to carry out such a confirmatory effort. This self-policing cycle of publication, peer review, and replication is designed to separate the scientific wheat from the chaff. Half-baked ideas that cannot survive the rigorous peer review process do not make it into the scientific literature. Experimental results that cannot be replicated independently by other laboratories are given no credibility. All published work is open for public comment and criticism by other scientists at any time. Scientists whose work continually fails to pass muster are culled from the herd. The theories, data, and interpretations that remain after this harsh distillation process become the building blocks on which further scientific progress is achieved.

Carl Sagan claims that the scientific arena is the only cultural milieu that offers an acceptable balance between "a no-holds-barred openness to new ideas" and a "rigorous skeptical scrutiny" of every idea that is put forward. "Science," he says, "thrives on the free exchange of ideas. There are no forbidden questions, no matters too sensitive or too delicate to be probed, no sacred truths." He sees the scientific method as the best template for encouraging meaningful debate by knowledgeable proponents of all points of view. Furthermore, he points out, scientific facts are in themselves value-free. Scientists are not supposed to be influenced by whether they *like* the conclusion that emerges from a line of reasoning, but only whether that conclusion logically *follows* from the available data.[1]

Unfortunately, this idealistic perception of the scientific calling is not exactly how things have come to pass in the conflicted world of fluoridation science. If it were, the quest for truth would always be paramount. Interactions between scientific researchers would always be open, collegial, and cooperative. Scientists would have no preconceived notions or pet theories, and those that do would acquiesce gracefully when their dreams were shot down in flames by their peers. In short, the scientific endeavor would be clearly divorced from human emotion. If only it were so.

JUNK SCIENCE: VALUES AND BIAS IN SCIENTIFIC RESEARCH

It turns out that scientists are human, too. Like the rest of us, they may have too much ambition or too little humility. They may be incompetent, or open to wishful thinking, or let their work slide under the weight of a stressful marriage. Most of them love to gossip, and many of them are reluctant to admit error even when such reluctance threatens their career.

It is human nature that skews the conventional portrait of science from one of logic and objectivity to one that includes jealousy and vanity and all the other original sins. In real life, most scientific endeavor bears almost no resemblance to the received gospel of the scientific method. Far from being cooperative, most science is intensely competitive. Individual scientists, famous laboratories, and top-10 universities compete with one another for fame and funding. And with so much riding on the outcome, the potential arises for unfair criticism, biased judgments, and outright skulduggery. Even greater temptations may arise out of every scientist's need to gain the respect and esteem of his or her peers. Scientists do not get rich; they measure success on a vanity scale that is based on peer recognition and status within the scientific community. The thirst for personal recognition has driven many a scientist to shave the point spread.[2]

When science goes bad, it usually takes one of two forms: either outright fraud or self-delusion. Outright fraud, in the form of fabricated results, plagiarism, and faked résumés, is usually committed by unsuccessful scientists who seek the personal recognition that they are unable to attain through honest achievement. From a psychological viewpoint, it is the less interesting of the two types of pathology, and it is not a prominent feature in the annals of the fluoridation controversy.

Self-delusion is more interesting. Sagan calls it "the confusion of hopes and facts." Such confusion often arises from a scientist's strong belief in a theory that is not widely accepted and from a vain desire to see his or her oppressors eat humble pie. It can seduce susceptible personalities into a selective choice of data points that better support their thesis, or the smoothing of raw data to produce cleaner-looking results. It can lead to the publication of "Cheshire facts," the kind of data that are "solemnly recorded, earnestly explained, vehemently defended, and then never seen again."[3]

This pathological version of the scientific method has been christened *junk science*. It is "the mirror image of real science, with much of the same form, but none of the same substance."[4] It features biased data, spurious inference, wishful thinking, and logical legerdemain. Junk science is often carried out in support of political goals. The inferences that are drawn from the scientific data are usually self-serving. Unexplained correlations of related parameters may be presented as if they were proven cause-and-effect relationships. Or it may be argued that whatever has not been proved false must be true. The junk scientist is good at "counting the hits and forgetting the misses."[5] Those who put forward shady science in support of political goals have consciously or unconsciously given priority to their doctrinaire beliefs over their scientific responsibilities. As William Broad and Nicholas Wade put it in their book *Betrayers of the Truth*, they are lying for what they think is the truth.[6]

In the fluoridation controversy, it is the pro-fluoridation movement that has been most vociferous in accusing the anti-fluoride camp of fomenting junk science. They see George Waldbott's fluoride hypersensitivity diagnoses as being driven by his powerful aversion to fluoridation. They see the results of John Yiamouyiannis's reanalysis of the 1986–1987 NIDR caries study of American schoolchildren, and his later analysis with Dean Burk of the possible links between fluoride and cancer, as examples of wishful thinking and biased interpretation of the data available.[7]

Even more, they attack the scientific work that underlies anti-fluoride claims of adverse health impacts from fluoridation. They believe that the experimental studies of Alfred Taylor that first drew a purported link between fluoride intake and tumor growth in mice were discredited completely by the National Cancer Institute (see Chapter 8). They are livid that anti-fluoride forces continued to quote the work long afterward. They point to Ionel Rapaport's studies linking the prevalence of Down's syndrome and fluoride intake, and Isabel Jansen's claim of a relationship between heart ailments and fluoridation, as examples of flawed epidemiological thinking. They see Aly Mohamed's original experiments on the mutagenic effects of fluoride on mice as highly suspect. In all of these cases, the medical and dental establishments view the scientists who published the works as mavericks. They claim that these self-serving results stand more or less alone; that establishment researchers have never been able to replicate the results.

Indeed, in many of these cases, a host of other independent studies have come to conclusions that are diametrically opposed to the studies that are held in such thrall by anti-fluoride activists.

It would certainly be helpful to know the predilections of these scientists prior to carrying out their studies. Did they undertake the work out of scientific curiosity in a truly objective fashion, or were they anti-fluoride zealots looking for ammunition? As a hint to their state of mind, pro-fluoridation scientists point to the fact that many of these scientists subsequently became active in anti-fluoridation circles. Jansen, for example, later wrote an anti-fluoridation book. Taylor gave anti-fluoridation testimony before a congressional committee. Almost all of them have accepted speaking engagements at anti-fluoride gatherings and lent their name and reputation to anti-fluoride causes. It is the suspicion of the pro-fluoride camp that these scientists undertook their studies with a strong stake in the results. They have never openly accused any of them of scientific fraud, but they clearly believe that these scientists are guilty of "confusing their hopes with the facts."

These anti-fluoridation studies all claim to have uncovered a positive relationship between the ingestion of fluoridated water and a specific adverse health impact. Pro-fluoridation scientists who wish to negate these studies are faced with the more difficult task of trying to prove a negative. They get very frustrated with anti-fluoridation charges that establishment scientists have not carried out enough studies to prove that fluoride is *not* a toxin (or a carcinogen, or a mutagen, or whatever). They point out that science cannot prove a negative. It is not possible to design an experiment that *proves* that *no harm* will come from ingesting fluoride. What *can* be done is to test experimental results against the *null hypothesis*. Under the null hypothesis it is anticipated that there will be no difference in health impact between a group of people (or laboratory animals) that ingest fluoridated water and a control group that doesn't. Of course, one would never expect absolutely no difference; there is always some random variation. So a level of statistical significance is established and the null hypothesis is accepted or rejected at that level of significance. If the experimental data lead to acceptance of the null hypothesis, it is concluded that there is no difference in health impact between the two groups. Only if the null hypothesis is *rejected*, and *at a reasonable level of significance*, can it be claimed that a meaningful health impact has been uncovered. The pro-fluoride camp claims that the anti-fluoride camp latches onto insignificant experimental or epidemiological variations and blows them out of proportion. It is proof, they say, of a lack of understanding of the scientific method.

The anti-fluoridationist response to these attacks is to turn them back on their assailants. Surely, they argue, scientists with a pro-fluoridation bent are just as committed to their cause as those with an anti-fluoridation bent, and just as likely to fall prey to wishful thinking and preordained findings. They hold up the original fluoride trials as an example of this. You will recall from Chapter 5 that anti-fluoridationists have expressed great disdain for the lack of double-blind design in these early experiments, or indeed for any significant recognition that dental examiners may have been tempted to see what they wanted to see. As with charges thrown the other way, they suspect wishful thinking and self-delusion.

Of course, as we concluded in Chapter 7, it appears that fluoride really does reduce cavities, and in that sense, anti-fluoridation carping over the original trials can now be viewed as so much whistling in the wind. Furthermore, as time has gone on, the experimental design of studies carried out by the dental research community has improved, leading to much greater credibility for the results of their recent experimental studies on the impact of fluoride on both caries and health. It is these more recent studies that have confirmed the reduction in caries, and clarified the unlikelihood of serious health impacts from the ingestion of fluoridated water supplies. Because the anti-fluoride community doesn't like these findings, they have tended to stick with their attacks on the earlier more questionable studies in their promotional material. In this sense, they are more open to the charge of misusing the scientific record than is the pro-fluoridation camp.

Having said that, the pro-fluoridation camp still has much to answer for. Their suppression of anti-fluoridation articles in establishment journals, and their shunning of reputable scientists who developed an anti-fluoridation viewpoint, make a travesty of the open dialogue that is supposed to drive scientific endeavor. These actions represent an embarrassing stain on the record of the dental research establishment. It is worth looking further at the damage done by these unhealthy developments.

SINGLE-MINDED SCIENCE: THE ISFR AND THE JOURNAL *FLUORIDE*

The first evidence that something is amiss can be found in the peculiar status of the journal *Fluoride*. In researching this book we came across hundreds of references to scientific articles in this journal. The titles of the articles were filled with the usual scientific jargon; the abstracts were similar to those that appear in other journals; and the content reflected the usual style of scientific writing. We had no reason to believe that we were dealing with anything other than a well-respected journal specializing in the very topic we were researching. It took a while before we realized that all the papers from this journal had an anti-fluoride twist. Not just some of them; *all* of them.[8] We never came across one *Fluoride* paper that had anything remotely positive to say about fluoride. We also noticed that all the papers tended to come from a relatively small stable of authors and that many of the references to articles in *Fluoride* came from other articles in the same journal. It is natural to wonder what is going on here. It is certainly not common in other branches of science to have an ostensibly reputable journal that publishes papers that support only one side of a political controversy. This is a far cry from Sagan's promise of a free exchange of value-free ideas.

It turns out that *Fluoride* is the quarterly journal of the International Society for Fluoride Research. On the homepage of the Society's website, it is stated that the ISFR was founded in 1966 "with the purpose of advancement of research and dissemination of knowledge, pertaining to the biological and other effects of fluoride on animal, plant, and human life."[9] The journal *Fluoride* invites contributions on the "biological, chemical, ecological, industrial, toxicological, and clinical aspects of inorganic and organic fluoride compounds." It all sounds very doctrinaire, but there's more to the story than meets the eye.

The International Society for Fluoride Research grew out of the deliberations at two conferences, one held in Bern, Switzerland in 1962 and another held in Detroit, Michigan in 1966. The primary organizer of these conferences was George Waldbott, who we met earlier. Although respected as a medical researcher in the field of allergic reactions, he was a man who had already got under the skin of fluoridation proponents at the Public Health Service through his perhaps-obsessive belief in the role of fluoride as a cause of allergies in hypersensitive persons. Waldbott always claimed that researchers of all stripes were welcome at the two founding conferences and in the ranks of the ISFR. However, the scientists who were responsible for the early promotion of fluoridation were suspicious of his motives. Those at the Public Health Service, and even those at other institutions who relied on PHS research funds, were encouraged to give the new organization a pass. The American Dental Association also clarified their hostility by issuing a highly critical press release that undoubtedly served to discourage their members from fraternization. A news item in *Science* was patronizingly critical of the new organization.[10]

Whatever hopes Waldbott may have had for a vibrant society of multiviewed, openminded debate, they were never realized. Forty-some years later, the ISFR is alive and well and still holds regular annual meetings, but the attendance continues to be limited to those whose research will find resonance in the anti-fluoridation movement. A perusal of the program for the 1998 annual conference in Bellingham, Washington, for example, reveals seven papers on environmental fluoride pollution, three papers on the toxic effects of dietary fluoride, and many papers on adverse health impacts, such as fluorosis, neurological disfunction, and reduced intelligence. The list of contributors reads like a reprise of the names that came to light in Chapter 8 in discussions of the possible negative impacts of fluoride on humans: Masters and Coplan, Jensen, Varner, Mullenix, and others.

So, too, with respect to the editorial board for *Fluoride*. The longtime editor-in-chief is Albert Burgstahler, who was a coauthor with George Wald-bott of the 1978 anti-fluoridation book *Fluoridation: The Great Dilemma*. The list of associate editors includes many familiar names from the scientific side of the anti-fluoride crusade, including S. P. S. Teotia and A. K. Susheela. Teotia is the author of a paper which claims that dental caries is *caused* by fluoride rather than cured by it.[11] Both Teotia and Susheela have written several papers on the threat of crippling skeletal fluorosis. Clearly, these are not topics that will attract mainstream fluoride researchers into the ranks of the ISFR or onto the pages of its journal.

So who should we blame for this segregation of anti-fluoride scientists? Although it might be more painless to chalk this development up to the anti-social tendencies of a group of maverick researchers, there is considerable evidence to suggest that they were *pushed* to the fringes by the establishment rather than choosing to light there themselves. There is a long and well-documented history of suppression of research findings that are not favorable to the mainstream pro-fluoridation paradigm. If one reviews the citations from Chapter 8 for papers by American authors that report potential adverse health impacts of fluoride, one finds that most of them were published in obscure foreign journals, not in the mainstream American scientific press. The reason that these papers appear there is not authorial choice. It is because most of them were rejected by the mainstream American press.

The experience of S. L. Manocha and Harold Warner is representative. In 1974, Manocha held an appointment at the Yerkes National Primate Research Center in Lawrenceville, Georgia, and Warner was a professor emeritus of biomedical engineering at Emory University in Atlanta. In that year they wrote a paper reporting the results of an experiment that documented enzyme changes in monkeys that drank fluoridated water. It was rejected by the American Medical Association's *Archives of Environmental Health*. They were told that the journal's reviewers felt that publication was inappropriate because the findings might be subject to misuse by anti-fluoridation groups. When the director of their research program was informed of the rejection, he suggested that they not make any further attempt to publish their findings in the United States. The paper was ultimately accepted by the reputable British publication *Histochemical Journal*.[12]

The anti-fluoridation literature abounds with such stories, most of them coming in anecdotal form from the affected scientists themselves. Even if one is suspicious of this source, there seem to be too many stories to ignore. One of the first papers to suggest that there might be a surfeit of fluoride in the environment, written by an Australian dental surgeon named Geoffrey Smith,[13] was rejected by the *New York State Dental Journal* because the editor felt it might be misused by fluoridation opponents.[14] Philip Sutton, the author of the book *Fluoridation: Errors and Omissions in Experimental Trials*, claims in a letter to the editor regarding Bette Hileman's 1988 article in *Chemical and Engineering News* that Cambridge University Press, the distributor of his book, was approached by American pro-fluoridation lobbyists in an unsuccessful attempt to prevent distribution of his book in the United States.[15]

A more objective source of information about the role of suppression in science comes from the work of Brian Martin, a professor of science, technology, and society at the University of Wollongong in New South Wales, Australia. He has taken the topic of suppression of dissent in science as his primary area of research. It seems noteworthy that one of the three topics he has highlighted in this regard is fluoridation.[16] His findings are summarized in his book *Scientific Knowledge in Controversy: The Social Dynamics of the Fluoridation Debate*. Pro-fluoridationists tend to feel that this book is a thinly veiled argument against fluoridation, but in taking this stance, they miss Martin's true target. Perusal of his wider writings make clear that his disdain is not for fluoridation itself but for the suppression of alternative viewpoints that was such a pernicious feature of the fluoridation movement.

Of course, as Martin points out, it is often difficult to distinguish suppression from commonly accepted scientific practice. Most high-quality journals reject far more papers than they accept. All the editors of these journals claim that this policy is designed to filter out half-baked ideas, not to discourage the publication of points of view that oppose those of the establishment. The question that is difficult to answer is this: Were the papers by Manocha and Warner, and Smith, for example, half-baked ideas, or were they of similar quality to many accepted papers? Did they perhaps differ from accepted papers only in the fact that their findings were antithetical to the fluoridation movement?

All reputable scientific journals make their decisions about acceptance or rejection of submitted papers on the basis of peer reviews that are provided by referees solicited by an editorial board. Scientific dogma holds that this is the only way to protect the scientific literature from the onslaught of charlatans. However, if editors and reviewers are prejudiced against the findings that are submitted, peer review can sometimes act as a barrier to new ideas. In the case of fluoridation research, the overwhelming majority of experts who are likely to be selected as referees come from the pro-fluoridation side of the fence. Scientists who carry out research that threatens the establishment paradigm may find themselves out on the doorstep.

Anti-fluoridation activists ascribe the worst possible motives to establishment scientists on this issue, especially those attached to the Public Health Service or the American Dental Association. They believe that these groups purposefully orchestrated a systemic rejection of scientific papers that threatened the political goals of fluoridation. The truth is probably more mundane. We suspect that the mainstream dental research community, especially in the early years, believed in the fluoridation paradigm so strongly and so universally that they truly felt that any research results that countered this paradigm must be flawed and should therefore be rejected for publication. In their eyes the term *anti-fluoridation science* was an oxymoron, and it was viewed in much the same way that most current scientists view "creation science." They saw the benefits of fluoridation as being so surely proven, and found the motives of anyone who floated results to the contrary so suspicious, that they were blinded to the possible worth of much sincere research.

The level of their derision can be gleaned from three independent incidents from the historical record. First, there is the fact that Sutton's book on the perceived "errors and omissions" in the original experimental trials never found its way onto the ADA's *Index of Dental Literature*, despite the fact that Sutton was a reputable university researcher and the report offers a credible scientific analysis. Second, it is noteworthy that articles from the journal *Fluoride* have never been listed by the Public Health Service in its medical indexing system, the *Index Medicus*. They *are* included in other establishment indexing services, such as *Chemical Abstracts*, *Biological Abstracts*, and the *Science Citation Index*, which implies that despite the origins and apparent one-sidedness of *Fluoride*, there must be papers of scientific merit appearing there.

Third, and most repugnantly, there is the embarrassing episode of the anti-fluoridation "dossiers" that appeared in the *Journal of the American Dental Association* in 1962 and 1965 under the title "Comments on the Opponents of Fluoridation."[17] These listings present thumbnail sketches of all the various opponents of fluoridation. Derogatory McCarthyesque write-ups of George Waldbott and other reputable scientist-opponents of fluoridation are lumped together with those for the John Birch Society, the Ku Klux Klan, and various quacks and cranks (some of whom are documented as having been patients in mental hospitals). Waldbott and Yiamouyiannis and others may have disagreed with the establishment, and they may or may not have been right in their claims, but all objective observers credit their sincerity, and they did not deserve to be treated with such disdain.

In recent years, there is evidence of a growing openness in the primary dental journals toward experimental results, epidemiological findings, and credible scientific analyses that do not toe the party line. We have seen examples of this trend in the discussion of dental fluorosis in Chapter 7 and in the handwringing over possible fluoride overdosage described in Chapter 10. However, most of the second-guessing that has appeared in the mainstream scientific press has come from the establishment itself. The authors of these papers still support fluoridation as a concept; they just want to optimize it. It is unlikely that the true mavericks, who hate fluoride like the curse, will ever be welcome. Their ostracization in the ISFR is probably permanent.

THE SHUNNING OF PHYLLIS MULLENIX

Those who speak out against fluoridation from within the ranks of science have suffered many indignities. Having the door closed to credible publication outlets is perhaps one of the lesser affronts that they have had to face. In the early years, many medical and dental societies passed resolutions publicly censuring physicians and dentists who opposed fluoridation. There are also many documented cases where dentists had their membership in state or local dental societies suspended for anti-fluoride activism. Doctors have lost hospital privileges. Dental researchers have been reprimanded by their superiors, have been denied access to research facilities, have been refused permission to attend conferences, and have lost access to their funding.[18]

The ultimate disciplinary measure for failing to toe the line on fluoridation is dismissal, and there are several notable cases. Each garners highlight coverage in the books and websites that constitute the anti-fluoridation history of the world. We have already covered the most infamous of them in Chapter 9: that of William Marcus's long battle with the Environmental Protection Agency, his firing, his suit for wrongful dismissal, and his reinstatement. A tale of almost equal renown is that of Phyllis Mullenix and the Forsythe Dental Center.

Phyllis Mullenix is a respected toxicologist with a Ph.D. in environmental medicine from the Johns Hopkins School of Hygiene and Public Health. Her speciality lies in the detection of the impacts of drugs and chemicals on the central nervous system (CNS). The Forsythe Dental Center is a highly regarded research laboratory affiliated with Harvard University in Boston. In 1983, Mullenix was invited to join the staff of the Forsythe Center by Jack Hein, the director of the laboratory. Hein was a former student of Harold Hodge, the renowned fluoride toxicologist who we met earlier in his role as leader of the fluoride safety program for the Manhattan Project in Rochester, New York. Like Hodge, Hein was a strong supporter of a role for fluoride in reducing dental caries; in fact, he carried out some of the primary research on the use of monofluorophosphate as a fluoride additive in toothpaste. But also like Hodge, he was aware of the possible health hazards of fluoride overdosage. Hein decided to set up a research program at the Forsythe Center to look at the possible health impacts of various dental products, including fluoride. He brought Mullenix on board specifically to develop a screening program to test for the neurotoxicity of these products. Mullenix was made head of a new toxicology department at the Forsythe Center, the first such lab to be established in any dental research institute. She held the position for 11 years.

In 1987, Mullenix began her first experiments to determine the CNS impact of sodium fluoride ingestion in rats. She claims that before these experiments she knew nothing of fluoridation per se and had no opinion on it. "Frankly," she says, "we expected to find nothing." In fact, she and her team were anxious "to move onto something academically more exciting."[19] Surprisingly, the experiments yielded evidence suggesting "behaviorspecific changes" in the rats that were "typical of cognitive deficits." The study team thought that the results must be wrong. They repeated the experiments with "more animals, different doses, sexes, and ages." As Mullenix describes it, "like quicksand, every effort we made sank us further into the realization that brain function was impacted by fluoride." The work went on for several years. By 1994, she was firmly convinced that the rat studies flagged the potential for fluoride-induced motor dysfunction, IQ deficits, and learning disabilities in humans.

It was then that her troubles began. Senior staff at the Forsythe Center became nervous that publication of Mullenix's results might have an adverse effect on their ability to attract funding grants to the laboratory. They encouraged her to sit on the results. Mullenix insisted on submitting them for publication. Three days after telling her superiors that her 1995 paper[20] had been accepted, she was dismissed from her position. She sued for wrongful dismissal and received an out-of-court settlement.[21] She was able to get a new position at Boston Children's Hospital, but only time will tell whether she can maintain her research career from that base. In the meantime, like so many other scientists who have been ill-treated by the establishment, she has become active in the International Society for Fluoride Research, speaking at their meetings and allowing her name to be used in the anti-fluoridation cause. It is now her opinion that "fluoride exposures are out of control" and that "the risks far exceed the hoped-for benefits."[22]

There is a bittersweet sidelight to the Mullenix story. In the late 1980s, Hein invited his old mentor, Harold Hodge, to come to Boston and act as an adviser on Mullenix's fluoride neurotoxicology studies. It turns out that back in the 1940s when Hodge was with the Manhattan Project, he observed that workers who were accidentally exposed to uranium hexafluoride exhibited symptoms of CNS impact in the form of "sluggishness, nervous tension, and silliness." He actually requested Manhattan Project funding for animal experiments to determine the CNS effects of inhalation of hydrogen fluoride gas, but the studies were never funded. Years later in Boston, as a "gently-ambling, elderly man," Hodge showed great interest in Mullenix's work, but ever faithful to the fluoridation revolution that he helped to bring about (and perhaps also to the dictates of military security), he never told her about his own concerns from those many years past.[23] He died in 1990, before Mullenix's troubles erupted. One has to wonder had he lived whether he would have supported her cause or kept his vow of silence.

Not every fluoridation flare-up ends up in a career meltdown. Edward Groth III has somehow managed to weather many storms. Groth has an undergraduate degree from Princeton and a Ph.D. from Stanford, both in biology. As a grad student in the Department of Biological Sciences at Stanford in the late 1960s, he decided to write his doctoral thesis on public policy matters, choosing fluoridation and air-pollution control as his two case histories. After interviewing a large number of pro- and anti-fluoridation enthusiasts, he came to the conclusion that the proponents had not adequately proven their claim that lifelong ingestion of fluoridated water would not lead to adverse health impacts. On learning of his developing viewpoint, one of the pro-fluoride interviewees approached the head of the department and suggested that Groth should be expelled from grad school before his maverick stance damaged the fluoridation movement. To their credit, the school rejected this request.[24]

In 1970, Groth further clarified his position by sending a letter to the editor of *Consumer Reports* complaining about pro-fluoridation bias in their 1969 article on fluoridation. Later yet, in 1974, Groth's anti-fluoride concerns were picked up and broadcast to the nation by syndicated columnist Jack Anderson. Despite all this activism, Groth landed a research fellowship at the California Institute of Technology in 1974 and spent five years as a senior staff officer with the Environmental Studies Board of the National Research Council. In 1979 he became technical director of policy and public service with the Consumers Union, the very organization that published his critical letter in *Consumer Reports*.

Perhaps Groth was able to maintain a successful career because he largely abandoned his pure science roots and became involved in the fluoridation controversy as an observer rather than as a scientist. Mullenix, on the other hand, stuck to her science and reported experimental results that threatened the existing paradigm. It seems that the scientific establishment is more likely to try to suppress maverick science from one of its own than from a dissident outsider.

JOHN COLQUHOUN FALLS OFF THE WAGON

Every once in a while, a reputable scientist announces his conversion from a position of strong support for fluoridation to one of vocal and active opposition. There have not been many to take this plunge, but those few who have done so have had considerable impact on the dynamics of the controversy. One of the most influential of these born-again dissenters was a high-profile dental administrator from Auckland, New Zealand named John Colquhoun (pronounced "Co-houn"). His attention-getter was an article published in the scientific review journal *Perspectives in Biology and Medicine* in 1997 under the title "Why I Changed My Mind about Water Fluoridation." It documented Colquhoun's loss of faith in the miracle of fluoridation.[25]

Colquhoun is not in any sense an outsider in the New Zealand dental research community. He is a former principal dental officer for Auckland, New Zealand and the former president of the New Zealand Society of Dentistry for Children. He was known as a fervent supporter of fluoridation through his role as the chairman of the Fluoridation Promotion Committee of the New Zealand Dental Health Foundation. Moreover, as an elected town councilor, he persuaded the mayor and a majority of the town council to fluoridate the water supply in his hometown. He even published a paper in the New Zealand Dental Journal reporting the declining rates of caries following the onset of fluoridation.

In 1980, Colquhoun went on a world study tour at the behest of the New Zealand Dental Health Foundation with an eye to becoming their fluoridation spokesman in those parts of New Zealand that had not already signed on. It was during this trip that he began to have doubts. On his return to New Zealand, he looked more carefully at the demography of caries rates in his home country and discovered that they were declining just as effectively in nonfluoridated areas as in fluoridated areas. He dismissed the halo effect as an explanation, claiming that the caries decline in New Zealand began before fluoride supplements or fluoride toothpastes were in common use. He critically reexamined the original data from New Zealand fluoridation trials, noting the same flaws that Philip Sutton had seen elsewhere. He became concerned about increases in dental fluorosis and the threat of declining bone health.

By the late 1980s, Colquhoun was convinced that fluoridation did more harm than good. He began questioning the procedure and was formally warned by his superiors to stick to official policy. His opposition tended to be fairminded rather than shrill. He argued that there has been misrepresentation by fluoridation proponents, but he never argued that it was deliberate. As he put it, "enthusiasts for a theory can easily fool themselves." It took him over a decade to finally put his thoughts on paper, but once he did, the simplicity of his title and the clarity of his prose have made his manifesto of conversion arguably the most effective anti-fluoridation document ever written.

Another recent defector from the fluoride cause is Hardy Limeback, the head of the Department of Preventive Dentistry at the University of Toronto. He is a former president of the Canadian Association for Dental Research, and a former consultant on fluoride to the Canadian Dental Association. He is the author of nine publications on fluoride in reputable peer-reviewed journals between 1993 and 1998. However, in May 1999 he eschewed his former support for fluoridation and announced his reversal of opinion by way of an interview reported in the *Toronto Globe and Mail*.[26] He told the reporter that careful study of the available toxicological information had convinced him that fluoridation does more harm than good. He claimed that "it now costs more money to treat fluorosis than it would cost to treat dental decay if we took the fluoride out of the water." In December 1999, Limeback addressed the faculty and students of his department, apologizing for having unintentionally misled them for over 15 years. "It was a bitter pill to swallow," he says.[27]

These stories make for a good media splash. But one must remember that Colquhoun and Limeback and the few others whose loss of faith has been noted along the way represent an incredibly small minority from the ranks of the worldwide dental research community. By far the greater majority of fluoride researchers have remained faithful to the cause. Although some of them have come around to the viewpoint that societal fluoride dosage may be a bit high (as documented in Chapter 10), only a minuscule percentage of them would join Colquhoun and Limeback in their claim that community water fluoridation does more harm than good.

One cannot help but notice that most of the scientists who have publicly turned their back on fluoridation come from countries other than the United States: Colquhoun from New Zealand; Limeback from Canada; Sutton and Smith from Australia. Anti-fluoridationists feel that this is because the scientific milieu is more conducive to vigorous open debate in those countries than in the United States. They think that the heavy hand of the Public Health Service and the American Dental Association, and the fears that are generated about loss of grants, loss of reputation, and ostracism from colleagues, have kept many American scientists from speaking out. Although there may be some truth to this charge, it may not be as important a consideration as anti-fluoride forces might wish. All indications point to the fact that a very large percentage of American doctors, dentists, and scientists fully support the goals and methods of community water fluoridation. The support is long-standing and monolithic, and those who oppose it are likely to be assigned maverick status for some time to come.

SCIENCE, FUNDING, AND SELF-INTEREST

Experimental science costs money, and every research scientist scrambles hard to get his or her fair share of the available spoils. Agency-based scientists must fight for their funding within the hurly-burly of internal agency politics. University-based researchers get most of their support from government-based granting programs or private corporate interests. The distribution of funds takes place in response to grant proposals prepared by the scientists themselves. Grant applications are subjected to peer review. Successful applicants tend to be reputable mainstream scientists with a good track record on publication.

The anti-fluoride camp has always charged that under this system, the funding sources available to American scientists are strongly biased in support of research that can be used to push the fluoridation agenda, at the expense of research that might expose evidence of harm. They see the same old-boy network at play in the acceptance or rejection of grant applications as comes into play in the acceptance or rejection of journal articles. The entire game is designed for one purpose, they claim: to protect the establishment against threats to the mainstream paradigm. They view the role of the Public Health Service as especially irksome. Here is an agency that is the leader of a political crusade, they argue, that is also asked to act as guardian of the scientific pursestrings. What could be more inappropriate than allowing the very groups that espouse the fluoridation of public water supplies to carry out the scientific studies that validate the practice?

There is some truth to these charges, especially as they pertain to the earlier years of the movement, when fluoridation proponents saw any proposal that might serve to discredit fluoridation as proof of hostile motives and scientific illiteracy. However, in recent years, with the growth of the environmental movement, the coming of age of the science of toxicology, and the increased public interest in the impact of chemicals on human health, there has been an increased availability of funds to investigate the impact of fluoride on public health. The number of papers identified in Chapter 8 attests to this fact. In today's climate of health awareness, and given the skepticism that often greets soothing medical pronouncements from the powers-that-be, the anti-fluoride charges of a health cover-up by the establishment have pretty much lost their zing.

It is not only government funding that raises anti-fluoridationist ire. The anti-fluoride camp is also wary of corporate funding of dental research. We have already learned in Chapter 6 of their suspicions of dark conspiracies between the aluminum industry and the fluoridation movement through the funding of scientific research at the Mellon Institute and the Kettering Laboratory in the 1940s and 1950s. However, as we also learned there, these charges are unlikely to be true, and in any case, they are a thing of the distant past. Brian Martin, in his assessment of this issue, concludes that the aluminum companies "have not played any substantial role in the promotion of fluoridation since the 1940s," and even then, he feels that the charges never had much basis in fact.[28]

Pharmaceutical companies, on the other hand, have provided considerable funding to universities for fluoride research over the years, primarily with the aim of developing and improving fluoridated toothpastes and fluoride supplements. The introduction of Crest toothpaste in 1955, for example, followed several years of research and development at the University of Indiana School of Dentistry under a grant from Proctor & Gamble.

The pharmaceutical giant Upjohn supported studies of childhood fluoride uptake in the hope that results would promote the need for its fluoride supplements.[29] However, once again, much of this funding took place in the early years of the fluoridation movement, and it was always done openly and aboveboard. Clearly, the funding was provided in support of self-interested motives, but in the private sector, that is how the world goes around. Like it or not, corporate funding of self-interested research is now a common feature of the town-and-gown relationship between universities and their host communities. It is a source of considerable research funding in most university departments of science and engineering. Dental schools have no qualms in accepting similar largesse, especially in view of their belief that they are helping to develop products that aid in the eradication of dental caries.

Perhaps the largest corporate supporter of pro-fluoride research over the years has been the sugar industry.[30] It is not difficult to discern the motive. Sugar is clearly implicated as the dietary cause of dental caries, and any scheme that promises to reduce decay without requiring a cutback in sugar intake is bound to attract the interest of the sugar companies. In the early years, funding was channeled to university dental schools and nutrition programs through the Sugar Research Foundation, an industry organization dedicated to two ends: the "scientific study of sugar's role in food," and the "communication of that role to the public." In 1968 the foundation was split into two separate entities, the Sugar Association, which continues the media mandate, and the World Sugar Research Association, which develops and supports scientific research.[31] The latter group is a "worldwide alliance of sugar producers, processors, marketers, users, and their associates." It has 76 member companies from 33 countries. It is "dedicated to the development of a better understanding of the role of sugar in health and nutrition, based on accredited scientific research." The nature of this understanding can be found in the statement on "the role of sugar" in their fact sheet *Sugar and Dental Caries*. It states that "the relationship between the amount of sugar consumed and the levels of decay in individuals is actually very weak. Caries prevalence is much more strongly related to age, social class, and level of oral hygiene. The most effective means of preventing caries is routine use of fluoride in conjunction with proper oral hygiene practices."[32] Research support from the sugar industry has gone primarily to studies that are likely to support this position.

Research funding from the soft drink industry has also been considerable. As recently as March 3, 2003, the American Academy of Pediatric Dentistry announced a "collaborative research and education partnership" between the AAPD Foundation and the Coca-Cola Foundation. Coca-Cola is providing a grant of $1 million to AAPD to "promote improved dental health for children." Mindful of the likely skeptical response to this partnership, the AAPD announcement is very clear that all research will be conducted by "independent investigators" and that Coke will not be able to dictate the kind of research undertaken or its outcome.[33] Critics of the pact are not mollified. "It is astonishing and outrageous that the AAPD would enter into a partnership with the world's biggest producer of soft drinks," says Michael Jacobson, executive director of the Center for Science in the Public Interest. "The Coca-Cola Company has effectively bought a health professionals' organization for a million bucks."[34]

Clearly, research support from both government funding agencies and the private sector has been strongly biased in favor of research that is likely to uphold the fluoridation paradigm. Opinions as to whether this bias is appropriate or inappropriate probably rest almost entirely on one's view of the anti-fluoride scientific community itself. Some see Waldbott, Yiamouyannis, Sutton, and others as reputable scientists persecuted by an unfair system. Others see them as unsophisticated purveyors of junk science acting in the cause of a fiercely held political goal. Perhaps there is some truth in both viewpoints.

FLUORIDATION IN THE COURTS: THE ANTI-FLUORIDATIONISTS' LAST STAND

The role of science in the courtroom has always been a touchy issue. Reputable scientists who are hired by lawyers as expert witnesses anticipate that the methods of science will be used to decide scientific questions in court. They are often not prepared for the adversarial nature of the enterprise, where the truth is reached through brutal conflict rather than reasoned scientific debate. Moreover, as described by Peter W. Huber in his book *Galileo's Revenge: Junk Science in the Courtroom*, they often find themselves in competition with fringe scientists who have sufficient credibility to be qualified as experts but who provide support for positions not accepted by mainstream science.[35] From the pro-fluoridation perspective, anti-fluoride litigation is the definitive example of junk science in the courtroom. In their eyes, clever lawyers parade the George Waldbotts and John Yiamouyiannises of the world past credulous judges and juries, subverting the scientific method with ill-informed rhetoric. Not surprisingly, anti-fluoridationists have a different take. They see the courts as the only establishment venue that gives them their say. And of course, they question which side it is that is producing the junk science.

Anti-fluoridationists have never been shy about taking their case against fluoridation into the courts. In city after city across the nation they have brought suit against city councils, health boards, and water supply agencies, seeking injunctions against the implementation (or the threat of implementation) of community water fluoridation programs. In a legal sense, they have been spectacularly unsuccessful. No court of last resort has ever determined fluoridation to be unlawful. However, some lower courts have afforded a sympathetic hearing, and in a few cases, anti-fluoridation judgments at this level gave the pro-fluoride camp a scare until they were overturned at the appellate level.

In a few of their unsuccessful cases, anti-fluoridation activists have appealed the negative judgments they received in state courts all the way to the U.S. Supreme Court. However, the Supreme Court has never deigned to hear one of these appeals. In the 13 cases that reached the highest court between 1954 and 1984, for example, seven were dismissed for lack of a "substantial federal question," and six were denied a writ of certiorari, which simply implies that the court does not feel that the case deserves its attention. In all such cases, the decisions reached in state appellate courts stand.[36]

The constitutional basis for fluoridation lies in the preamble to the U.S. Constitution, where it is stated that the purpose of government is "to promote the general welfare." More specifically, it lies in the 10th Amendment, which gives to the states all powers not specifically delegated to the federal government. These powers include control of public health legislation. The states have the further right to delegate some of this power to local jurisdictions or to administrative agencies such as health boards or water supply agencies.

Public health statutes and regulations come under the legal concept of *police power*, which is defined as "the power to enact and enforce laws to protect and promote the health, safety, morals, order, peace, comfort, and general welfare of the people." There are many examples of state police power that are virtually uncontested by the public, among them such long-standing policies as minimum wage laws or the need to take a blood test before getting a marriage license. The use of police power by the legislative or executive branches of state government is subject to the supervision of the judiciary. It is this constitutional promise of judicial protection that brings anti-fluoridationists to court.[37]

The development of public health law often highlights the conflict between the rights of the individual (or of an identifiable minority) and decisions that are made for the greater good of the greater number. Historically, the courts have always upheld "laws of overruling necessity," such as those necessary to prevent or control contagious diseases such as smallpox, diphtheria, polio, and tuberculosis. They have accepted the need for state-mandated programs of compulsory smallpox vaccination, for example, and the quarantining of patients with highly communicable diseases. More recently, public health bodies have recognized their broader responsibilities, turning their attention to the control of environmental factors that are related to chronic diseases and a general lack of well-being of the community. To this end, the courts have supported the need for regulations to exert control over such practices as industrial air emissions, toxic waste disposal, and timber harvesting. It is in this context that community water fluoridation has thus far received the support of the courts.

Legal challenges to fluoridation are based on the claim that adding fluoride to public drinking water is an arbitrary and unreasonable exercise of police power. Anti-fluoridationists have tried to get the courts to so rule by using one or the other of two broad arguments. The first claims that fluoridation is a violation of the personal liberties, freedom of religion, and due process guaranteed in the 1st, 9th, and 14th Amendments. The second focuses on the purported harmful effects of fluoride on the health of the populace. Most of the early cases tried the first tack; most of the more recent cases followed the second tack. The second strategy has been marginally more successful.

Among the "due process" arguments made in the early cases, we find claims that fluoridation constitutes a form of mass medication that is beyond the authority of the state; that it is an unacceptable form of "class legislation" because it benefits only children; that it is a violation of statutes forbidding the unauthorized practice of medicine; and that it is an illegal use of public funds because less intrusive alternative approaches are available to obtain the same end. When these arguments failed in the lower courts, many of the plaintiffs appealed to state appeals courts. Some of the rulings in these individual appellate cases make interesting reading.[38]

In *Krause v. City of Cleveland* in 1953, an anti-fluoride plaintiff claimed that fluoridation of the Cleveland water supply was a violation of his fundamental liberties "in the orderly pursuit of happiness by free people." Among the personal liberties he claimed had been violated were the right of parents to rear children and care for them as they deem best; the right of individuals to be free of medical experimentation; the right of individuals to control their own body; and the right of certain religious groups to be free of compulsory medication that is against their beliefs. He recognized the police power of the state but argued that individual rights are subordinate to police power only when there is an overriding public purpose. He argued that no such purpose exists to justify fluoridation. The seven-judge appeals court disagreed, stating that 1st Amendment rights do not prevent states from enacting reasonable laws to protect the public health. They quoted from earlier case law on individual rights: "Liberty implies the absence of arbitrary restraint, not immunity from reasonable regulation." As for the freedom-of-religion issue: "Two concepts are involved: freedom to believe, and freedom to act. The first is absolute. The second is subject to regulation for the protection of society." As would happen in many subsequent cases, the court also noted the similarity of water fluoridation to water chlorination, a measure that has been upheld in the courts many times. They were clearly nervous that an anti-fluoridation ruling could put chlorination in jeopardy.

In the case of *Dowell v. City of Tulsa* in 1954, a group of residents sought to prevent the implementation of a fluoridation program passed by the Tulsa Board of Commissioners. They argued that fluoridation was a form of compulsory medication designed to treat the chronic disease of dental caries, and that the state of Oklahoma had never before attempted to regulate or control any disease that was not "contagious, infectious, or dangerous." The court was not impressed with this argument and denied the injunction. The judge who wrote the opinion stated that the maintenance of a "healthy, normal, and socially sound populace" was a valid exercise in police power. He rejected the contention that fluoride was a form of medication, stating that fluoridation is "no more practicing medicine or dentistry . . . than a mother would be who furnishes her children a well balanced diet." He felt that trying to distinguish between contagious and chronic diseases was "immaterial, ridiculous, and of no consequence to the promotion of public health."

In the same year, in *Chapman* v. *City of Shreveport*, the plaintiffs tried to halt the fluoridation of Shreveport, Louisiana, by invoking the equal protection clause of the 14th Amendment. They argued that it is unreasonable to fluoridate public water supplies when such a step only benefits children, and that any such law represents "class legislation." The three-person judicial panel rejected the argument, noting that the exercise of police power need not extend to all classes of people to be valid. In any case it was their opinion that reduced tooth decay benefits parents as well as children and that the benefits to the children extend into adulthood. One judge apparently dissented, but he did not write a countervailing opinion.

In *Paduano* v. *City of New York* in 1965, the plaintiff sought an injunction against the fluoridation of New York City's public water system based on the privileges and immunities clause of the 14th Amendment, which protects against unequal freedoms from state to state. The court rejected the argument, finding the actions of the New York Board of Health valid and no citizen rights invaded. They also held that the existence of alternative methods for obtaining fluoride was irrelevant as long as the proposed method was lawful.

By 1965, almost all the arguments relating to personal liberties and due process had been rejected by the courts. However, in the *Paduano* judgment, anti-fluoridationists thought they saw a crack in the wall. In a section commenting on the role of the judiciary in fluoridation cases, the appellate court had written: "Until scientific evidence as to the harmful effects of fluoride exceeds the speculation now existing, the courts will not interfere and the controversy should remain with the legislative and executive branches of government." The opinion went on to state that while the judiciary does not have the power to impose fluoridation on anyone, it does have the power to overrule legislation authorizing acts that are not in the public interest if convincing proof of harm is offered.

This was music to anti-fluoride ears. "Convincing proof of harm" is what they thought they had in abundance. So began a series of assaults on the courts by experts and quasiexperts who were willing to testify to all the bad things that fluoride is doing to us: cancer, bone disease, genetic damage, allergic reactions, and more. The defendants countered with their own experts from the Public Health Service, the Centers for Disease Control, and the American Dental Association, who refuted the anti-fluoride claims. The courts were forced into a role for which they are not well suited: the judgment of competing scientific theories. Some courts questioned the entire process. One appeals court judge wrote that the "introduction of these studies as evidence at trial is technically irrelevant, because the court's purpose is to determine whether the regulation has no reasonable basis and is arbitrary as claimed by the plaintiffs. The true test of arbitrariness would depend upon what information was before the legislative body when it made the decision to fluoridate and not what evidence is before the court during the trial."[39]

The anti-fluoride camp persisted, but their initial forays into the courtroom were not encouraging. In *Rogowski* v. *the City of Detroit* the court held that it was "common knowledge" that fluoridation is beneficial to prevent dental caries and that the court did not require evidence to establish this fact. Furthermore, "the fact that a belief is not universal is not controlling, for there is scarcely any belief that is accepted by everyone." In the case *Minnesota State Board of Health* v. *City of Brainerd, Minnesota*, the court ruled that the Minnesota mandatory fluoridation law was constitutional, bowing to the "overwhelming weight of scientific opinion that fluoridation is a safe and effective means of reducing dental caries." They found that "in light of the substantial health benefit of fluoridation and its innocuous effect on the individual, fluoridation of the public drinking water is a justified intrusion into an individual's bodily integrity." In a case brought to the South Carolina Court of Appeals, *Charleston Committee for Safe Water* v. *Commissioners of Public Works* of that city, the three-person court noted that all the witnesses appearing for the committee were "ardent anti-fluoridationists, whose views, though sincerely held, were inconsistent with the medical and scientific opinion of the great majority of medical and scientific experts in this country."

However, by 1982, in three separate cases, anti-fluoridationists finally gained some small measures of success. In *Safe Water Foundation of Texas* v. *City of Houston*, the judge ruled in favor of the plaintiffs, concluding in his written opinion that "artificial fluoridation may cause or may contribute to the cause of cancer, genetic damage, intolerant reactions, and chronic toxicity ... in man." However, an appeals court quickly overturned the verdict, ruling that the plaintiffs would have to produce "overwhelming evidence" in support of their case before the courts could void a legally enacted fluoridation statute.

In *Illinois Pure Water Committee* v. *State of Illinois*, the judge took the opposite tack to that of the *Houston* case, ruling that it was not the plaintiffs who ought to be required to produce overwhelming evidence of the harm done by fluoridation, but rather, the state which ought to be required to produce overwhelming evidence of its safety. It was his opinion that they had not done so, and he ruled in favor of the plaintiffs. On appeal, the Illinois State Supreme Court reversed the verdict of the lower court, but anti-fluoridationists in Illinois felt that for the first time they had put their foot in the door.

In the most widely touted of the three cases, *Aitkenhead* v. *Borough of West View*, first filed in 1978, a group of citizens from West View, Pennsylvania, in the western suburbs of Pittsburgh, brought suit in the Allegheny Court of Common Pleas seeking an injunction against the fluoridation of their community. The case lasted five months, and both sides trotted out a long string of expert witnesses to debate the "sole issue before the court," which was whether or not fluoride is a carcinogen. The primary experts for the plaintiffs were John Yiamouyiannis and his colleague Dean Burk, who testified as to the results of their study showing an increased incidence of cancer in fluoridated communities. The defendants' experts, who refuted Dr. Y's claims, included Leo Kinlen from Britain, Donald Taves of the University of Rochester, and several scientists from the Public Health Service and the National Cancer Institute. The lawyer for the plaintiffs was John Remington Graham, who is now widely feted as the Perry Mason of the anti-fluoridation camp for his bravura performance in this and other fluoridation cases. He made effective use of his own experts' unwavering claims while cajoling the defendants' experts into acknowledging doubts about the absolute safety of fluoridation. The judge, John P. Flaherty, Jr., who has become a figure of heroic stature in the anti-fluoridation pantheon, ruled in favor of the plaintiffs. He was "compellingly convinced" by their evidence. He felt that "simple prudence indicates that the best evidence must be scrutinized now, not after tragedy has struck."

The Flaherty decision made big news in the nation's press. Several articles appeared that questioned the future of fluoridation. The American Dental Association treated the decision as apocalyptic. The alternative medicine fraternity was elated. However, as fate would have it, the anti-fluoridation victory was relatively short-lived. The borough of West View appealed the case to the Commonwealth Court of Pennsylvania, and in 1982 this court reversed the decision of the lower court. However, as the anti-fluoridation literature is quick to point out, the reversal was based solely on jurisdictional grounds, not on the judge's opinion as to the merits of the scientific question at hand. The decision of the common pleas court was reversed because decisions with respect to the State Water Supply Law under which the fluoridation program was mandated are not reviewable by a common pleas court. Anti-fluoridation literature still revels in the Flaherty decision and highlights the Pittsburgh case as if it were the only court battle ever fought.

The years since these semi-successes in the early 1980s have not brought any further legal solace to the anti-fluoride cause. Judge Flaherty moved on to the Pennsylvania Supreme Court. John Remington Graham moved to Canada. John Yiamouyiannis is dead. In *Safe Water Association* v. *City of*

Fond-Du-Lac, Wisconsin in 1994, the plaintiffs tried to cash in on the enlarged scope of the right-to-privacy clauses in the Constitution, which they felt had been opened up by the judicial opinions offered in the famous abortion case, *Roe* v. *Wade*. The court, however, could see no relation between the right to reproductive choice and the purported right to be free of fluoridation. The anti-fluoride camp also saw hope in the 1990 *Washington* v. *Harper* decision, in which the U.S. Supreme Court ruled that "the forcible injection of medication into a nonconsenting person's body represents a substantial interference with that person's liberty." It will undoubtedly be used as a basis for future fluoridation challenges, but has not been so to date.[40]

Perhaps it is best to end this section on a light note. In 1966, during a fluoridation referendum in Cudahy, Wisconsin, James Quirk, the leading light of the Greater Milwaukee Committee Against Fluoridation, wrote a brochure in which he challenged the Cudahy Junior Chamber of Commerce to prove that "a daily dose of four glasses of fluoridated water cannot cause dermatologic, gastrointestinal, and neurological disorders." He went on to write: "If the Jaycees should find that we have misrepresented matters, we will pay them the sum of $1000." After the referendum, the Jaycees brought suit to claim the $1000. A jury trial was held, and judgment was granted in favor of the Jaycees. Quirk appealed the decision to the Supreme Court of Wisconsin, which considered the case in 1969. The appeals court decided that what Quirk had offered the Jaycees was a wager. They then ruled that participants in a wager cannot use the courts to settle their dispute, because gambling debts cannot be established or collected in the courts. The judgment was reversed, and the case dismissed.[41]

THE CONGRESSIONAL PULPIT

The anti-fluoridation camp has been more successful with the legislative branch of government than with the judicial branch. Although Congress has never passed any overtly anti-fluoridation measures, they have often provided a forum for anti-fluoride views. Ever since the beginning of the fluoridation era, opponents of the practice have kept steady pressure on their Congress members to look into the safety of fluoridation and to hold hearings that give them a chance to voice their concerns. Given the more-or-less even split in public attitudes toward fluoridation, as indicated by the razor-thin results of so many referendums, perhaps it is not surprising to find that there are a goodly number of Congress members who lean toward opposition and are willing to accede to these requests. As a result, there has been a steady parade of congressional hearings over the years that addressed the fluoridation controversy.

The earliest such deliberations took place during the hearings of the Delaney Committee in 1952. Officially known as the House Select Committee to Investigate the Use of Chemicals in Food and Cosmetics, the committee took its informal name from the chairmanship of James J. Delaney, a young Democratic congressman from New York who eventually served 14 terms in Congress. He later became well known as the author of the *Delaney clause* in the Food, Drug and Cosmetic Act of 1958, which specifies that *any* additive that has shown *any* evidence of causing cancer in humans or animals at *any* dosage may not be used in *any* amount in *any* food, drug, or cosmetic. It is a simple position, perhaps simplistic, certainly extreme, and it has caused much handwringing in the food and drug industry.

During the course of the Delaney hearings, the seven-person congressional committee looked at the role of chemicals and additives in the production of a variety of foods and drugs, including bread, canned food, antibiotics, cosmetics, and pesticides. In the last seven sessions of the hearings, they addressed the fluoridation issue. The most active member of the committee in this regard was Representative A. L. Miller, a Republican from Nebraska, a medical doctor and former Nebraska State Health Officer, who had sponsored a bill in Congress the previous year to fluoridate the water supply of Washington, DC. As fate would have it, both he and Delaney changed their minds about fluoridation on the basis of the evidence they heard in the House Select Committee hearings. Both became lifelong, ardent, and outspoken foes of public water fluoridation. The report that was eventually issued by the committee, while acknowledging the views of the medical and dental establishment that fluoride is a safe and effective procedure for the control of dental caries, urged communities to "err on the side of caution" when considering the fluoridation of their domestic water supplies. The report did not recommend any federal legislation, but it put on record the opinion that there were enough unanswered questions concerning the safety of fluoridation to warrant the conservative recommendation.[42]

The dental research community had anticipated a friendly rubber stamp from Congress. They were flabbergasted by the tone of the Delaney report. They immediately fired an answering salvo in the form of a critical analysis of the report, published in the *Journal of the American Dental Association*, authored by J. Roy Doty, the secretary of the ADA Council on Dental Therapeutics and one of those who had testified in favor of fluoridation at the Delaney hearings. It accused the committee of paying too much attention to those with "inadequate backgrounds to warrant their testifying as experts in this matter," failing to adhere to the "proper standards of investigative procedure," and acting on "vague concerns which are contrary to the vast majority of scientific opinion."[43]

In actual fact, most of those who testified against fluoridation at the Delaney hearings were reputable scientists who were not opposed to fluoridation in principle as much as they were nervous that things were moving too fast. At the very least, they counseled, the Public Health Service ought to wait for the end of the Grand Rapids trial before encouraging widespread fluoridation of community water supplies.

If the pro-fluoridation camp was upset by this somewhat-muted opposition, imagine their shock and dismay at what happened next. In 1954, Representative Roy Weir, a Democrat from Minnesota, introduced a bill to "protect the public health from the dangers of fluorination." If passed, it would have prohibited any agency of the federal, state, or municipal government from introducing a fluoride compound into a water supply.[44] The proponents of fluoridation trotted out their usual slate of experts, including Trendley Dean and Pokey Arnold of the Public Health Service and other highly reputable representatives of the American Dental Association and the National Research Council. This time, however, the opposition did not rely on reputable scientists with minor caveats against fluoridation. This time, they brought out the likes of Leo Spira and C. T. Betts from the old anti-aluminum crusade and the head of the National Committee against Fluoridation, who for the first time made public the anti-fluoridation charges against Oscar Ewing and his sinister Alcoa connections, the possibility of a communist conspiracy, and the likelihood of a government plot to poison the populace. Frederick Exner, who later wrote an anti-fluoridation book coauthored with George Waldbott called *The American Fluoridation Experiment*,[45] testified that "we are now committed to a giant steamroller, fabricated by the Public Health Service, powered with unlimited federal funds, and directed from Washington. It is designed to put over the greatest hoax in history, and destroy once and for all, the constitutional protections of the citizens." Weir's bill died with the adjournment of the 83rd Congress, but the anti-fluoridation movement gained considerable credibility in the next few years by quoting their own witnesses from the *Congressional Record*, always identifying the source as "the congressional investigation of fluoridation."

In the ensuing years, anti-fluoridationists continued to pepper their Congress members with petitions, letter-writing campaigns, and demands to be heard by congressional committees. They continued to get their chances every time a federally sponsored fluoridation program came up for reauthorization, especially during the long-drawn-out deliberations over the appropriate value for a maximum contaminant level for fluoride in drinking water. In the latter context, in 1975, James Delaney made a point of reading into the *Congressional Record* the full text of the study by John Yiamouyiannis and Dean Burk that purported to show higher cancer rates in fluoridated than in nonfluoridated cities. This study, which was widely debunked by the medical establishment and which was accepted for publication only in the anti-fluoridation journal *Fluoride*, is now claimed by anti-fluoridation forces to have the imprimatur of the U.S. Congress.

In 1977, another round of congressional hearings on fluoridation was held, this time in the House Subcommittee on Intergovernmental Relations under the chairmanship of Representative L. H. Fountain. This was the session where Yiamouyiannis and Burk took on the PHS/ADA establishment over the cancer question. It was this face-off that led to the congressional recommendation for an examination of the issue under the auspices of the National Toxicology Program.

In 1985, Representative John F. Sieberling of Ohio tried to introduce an amendment to the Safe Drinking Water Act mandating that "no chemical substitute may be added artificially to the water of any public water system for any purpose other than to render it safe for human consumption, or to test the water for contamination, or to improve the taste or clarity of the water."[46] The amendment was not included in the act.

The most recent flurry of activity took place in 2000 in both houses of Congress. In the Senate it was the Subcommittee on Wildlife, Fisheries, and Drinking Water (of the Committee on Environment and Public Works), that heard William Hirzy's anti-fluoridation pitch on behalf of the union representing the environmental scientists at EPA headquarters. Meanwhile in the House, the Science Committee, under the chairmanship of James Sensenbrenner (through its Subcommittee on Energy and Environment, under the chairmanship of Ken Calvert), reacted to a strong letter writing campaign by the anti-fluoridation community and began yet another investigation of fluoridation. In obvious response to the issues raised by anti-fluoridationists, Sensenbrenner and Calvert sent letters to the Centers for Disease Control, the Food and Drug Administration, the National Academy of Sciences, and the Environmental Protection Agency, requesting answers to a series of questions.

Readers of this book will recognize the questions and may even by now know the answers. In their letter to CDC, they asked at what incidence and level of fluorosis the CDC would consider that the population as a whole is receiving too much fluoride. In their missive to NAS, they requested the most recent information on file on the dietary reference intake, acceptable fluoride dosage, and crippling skeletal fluorosis. They asked the EPA about the apparently slim margin of safety offered by the 4.0 ppm maximum contaminant level, and they requested information from the NSF on the possibility of heavy-metal contamination of fluoridation-grade hydrofluosilicic acid.

Perhaps the most barbed question went to the FDA. They were asked whether any *New Drug Applications* for fluoride supplements have recently been accepted, rejected, or even tested; or whether they are still all classified as *Unapproved New Drugs*. At the same time, a New Jersey assemblyman, John V. Kelly, petitioned FDA to take action on this front. He pointed out that fluoride supplements were first marketed in 1946. As he put it: "The manufacturers of fluoride supplements have had fifty years to conduct clinical trials and toxicological studies to demonstrate the safety and effectiveness [of the supplements] and submit them for FDA approval. They have not done so. Fifty years is a long time, even for the FDA."[47]

Fair or unfair, proper watchdog activity or misuse of the public purse, congressional hearings and the publicity they spawn have probably done more to keep the fluoridation controversy alive than any other single set of activities by either side. We suspect that the great majority of the public at large are now ready to accept fluoridation as a done deal and let sleeping dogs lie, but just when they get comfortable, up pops another congressional hearing to give the anti-fluoridationists another day in court. Maybe this is the way that democracy is supposed to work, and maybe it isn't. Your opinion probably depends on which side of the fence you sit.

In any case, to bring us back to the role of science in all this, it should be clear that neither the courts nor the Congress are set up to illuminate scientific truth. Science works best within its own social milieu, through the testing of hypotheses by experiment, the development of consistent theories that explain experimental results, the use of accepted statistical interpretations, and the publication of results in reputable journals, where they become subject to experimental replication and peer review. For the public (including judges and Congress members), it is often difficult to tell the difference between establishment science, maverick science, and junk science. For many social decisions that need to be made, fluoridation perhaps among the least important of them, this is a serious societal failing. On the other hand, scientists often fail to appreciate the social, cultural, and psychological impacts of their findings on the common man. C. P. Snow's *Two Cultures* continue to keep their distance from one another as we move into the twenty-first century.

REFERENCES

1. C. Sagan, *The Demon-Haunted World: Science as a Candle in the Dark*, Ballantine Books, Des Maines, IA, 1996.

2. W. Broad and N. Wade, *Betrayers of the Truth: Fraud and Deceit in the Halls of Science*, Touchstone Books, Simon & Schuster, New York, 1982.

3. P. W. Huber, *Galileo's Revenge: Junk Science in the Courtroom*, Basic Books, New York, 1991.

4. Ibid.

5. Sagan, 1996, op. cit.

6. Broad and Wade, 1982, op. cit.

7. References to studies mentioned in this section may be found in Chapter 8.

8. *Fluoride* does have a section that reproduces abstracts of fluoride articles from other journals, including those from the establishment press, but few if any of the authors of these articles ever appear on the byline of an original research submission to the journal.

9. http://www.fluoride-journal.com.

10. G. L. Waldbott, A. W. Burgstahler, and H. L. McKinney, *Fluoridation: The Great Dilemma*, Coronado Press, Lawrence, KS, 1978.

11. S. P. S. Teotia and M. Teotia, Dental caries: a disorder of high fluoride and low dietary calcium interactions, *Fluoride*, 27(2), 59–66, 1994.

12. S. L. Manocha, H. Warner, and Z. Olkowski, Cytochemical response of kidney, liver, and nervous system to fluoride ions in drinking water, *Histochem. J.*, 7, 343–355, 1975. A description of their publishing experience is included in B. Martin, *Scientific Knowledge in Controversy: The Social Dynamics of the Fluoridation Debate*, State University of New York Press, Albany, NY, 1991.

13. G. E. Smith, A surfeit of fluoride? *Sci. Prog. Oxford*, 69, 429–442, 1985.

14. As posted on the anti-fluoride website of the Health Action Network, http://www.fluoridation.com.

15. P. R. N. Sutton, Letter to the editor, *Chem. Eng. News*, 67(4), 3, January 23, 1989.

16. Martin, 1991, op. cit. The other two are pesticides and nuclear power.

17. American Dental Asociation, Comments on opponents of fluoridation, *J. Am. Dent. Assoc.*, 65, 694–710, 1962; and 71, 1155–1183, 1965.

18. Waldbott et al., 1978, op. cit.; Martin, 1991, op. cit.

19. The quotes from Mullenix are taken from her "Statement on central nervous system damage from fluoride" of September 14, 1998, posted at http://www.rvi.net; and from her letter of May 5, 1999, to BSA Environmental Services about the possible fluoridation of Fort Detrick Army Base, Maryland, posted at http://www.nofluoride.com.

20. P. J. Mullenix, P. J. Denbesten, P. K. Schunior, and W. J. Kernan, Neurotoxicity of sodium fluoride in rats, *Neurotoxicol. Teratol.*, 17, 169–177, 1995.

21. http://www.fluoridation.com.

22. Mullenix letter to BSA Environmental Services, op. cit.

23. J. Griffiths and C. Bryson, Fluoride, teeth, and the atomic bomb, *Waste Not*, No. 414, September 1997.

24. For a summary of Groth's views on fluoridation, see E. Groth III. The fluoridation controversy: Which side is science on? Appendix to Martin, 1991, op. cit.

25. J. Colquhoun, Why I changed my mind about water fluoridation, *Perspect. Biol. Med.*, 41(1), 1997.

26. K. Foss, Are we getting too much fluoride? *Toronto Globe and Mail*, May 4, 1999.

27. B. Forbes, Prominent researcher apologizes for pushing fluoride, *The Tribune*, Mesa, AZ, December 5, 1999.

28. Martin, 1991, op. cit.

29. Waldbott et al., 1978, op.cit.

30. Martin, 1991, op. cit.; W. Varney, *Fluoride in Australia: A Case to Answer*, Hale and Iremonger, Marickville, NSW, Australia, 1986.

31. http://www.sugar.org.

32. http://www.wsro.org.

33. http://www.aapd.org.

34. L. Tanner, Coke's dental grant flawed: critics, Associated Press release, March 4, 2003.

35. Huber, 1991, op. cit.

36. L. E. Block, Antifluoridationists persist: the constitutional basis for fluoridation, *J. Publ. Health Dent.*, 46, 188–198, 1986; P. Bergen, Legal status of fluoridation, *J. Am. Med. Assoc.*, 211, 555–556, 1970.

37. P. J. Frazier and E. Newbrun, Legal, social and economic aspects of fluoridation, Chapter 5 of *Fluorides and Dental Caries: Contemporary Concepts for Practitioners and Students*, edited by E. Newbrun, Charles C Thomas, Springfield, IL, 1986, pp. 115–154.

38. Copies of the judicial opinions for the cases under discussion in the following paragraphs can be found on the website of the Pennsylvania Fluoride Leadership Team, http://www.penweb.org/fluoride/lawandcourts. A pro-fluoridation discussion of some of these cases can be found in G. A. Strong, Liberty, religion, and fluoridation, *J. Am. Dent. Assoc.*, 76, 1398–1409, 1968; and in M. W. Easley, C. A. Wulf, K. S. Brayton, and D. F. Striffler, eds., *Proc. Workshop on Fluoridation, Litigation, and Changing Public Policy*, University of Michigan, Ann Arbor, MI, 1984. An anti-fluoridation discussion of some of these cases can be found in D. A. Balog, Fluoridation of public water systems: Valid exercise of State police power or Constitutional violation? *Pace Environ. Law Rev.*, 14(2), 1997; and in J. R. Graham and P. J. Morin, Highlights in North American litigation during the Twentieth Century in artificial fluoridation of public water supplies, *J. Land Use Environ. Law*, 1999.

39. Block, 1986, op. cit.

40. Balog, 1997. op. cit.

41. See http://www.penweb.org/fluoride/lawandcourts.

42. D. R. McNeil, *The Fight for Fluoridation*, Oxford University Press, New York, 1957.

43. J. R. Doty, An analysis of the Delaney committee report on the fluoridation of drinking water, *J. Am. Dent. Assoc.*, 45, 351–356, 1952.

44. McNeil, 1957, op. cit.

45. F. B. Exner, G. L. Waldbott, and J. Rorty, *The American Fluoridation Experiment*, Devin-Adair Co., New York, NY, 1975.

46. Block, 1986, op. cit.

47. Citizens for Health; http://www.citizens.org.

CHAPTER 12

MONEY, MOTIVE, AND RISK

Up to this point in our story we have learned many things about fluoride: that it reduces the prevalence of dental caries in young people; that this reduction is accompanied by an increase in cosmetically unattractive dental fluorosis; that there is some risk of more serious health impacts at higher dosages; and that the dosage that is delivered by current fluoridation systems, although within the range that is usually considered "safe," is probably higher than is needed to attain optimal levels of caries reduction. What we have not attempted yet is an overall assessment of the fluoridation enterprise to see whether the benefits that accrue to society clearly outweigh the costs and risks that are generated by the undertaking.

THE UNEASY SCIENCE OF RISK–COST–BENEFIT ANALYSIS

Public-sector policymakers often have to decide on which course of action to recommend given a suite of alternative possibilities. Or, there may be only one course of action under consideration and the policymaker must decide whether to proceed down that road or not. For decisions of either type that do not involve any risk to life or limb, the standard economic tool is a *cost–benefit* analysis. For decisions that involve risk, it is a *risk–cost–benefit* analysis.[1]

The unit of measurement in these types of analyses is usually *dollars*, and we shall go down this road as far as we can. The *costs* in our case relate to the expenses associated with the installation and operation of fluoridation systems for municipal water supplies, and they can usually be quantified in a fairly straightforward manner. The economic valuation of *benefits* and *risks* is a far trickier business. The *benefits* in our analysis come in the form of reduced dental caries, but there are also *disbenefits* in the form of increased dental fluorosis. We need to estimate the savings in dental costs

The Fluoride Wars: How a Modest Public Health Measure Became America's Longest-Running Political Melodrama   By R. Allan Freeze and Jay H. Lehr
Copyright © 2009 John Wiley & Sons, Inc.

that accrue from reduced caries as well as the additional expenses that arise from increased fluorosis.

The pro- and anti-fluoridation camps differ on whether there is any *risk* associated with the fluoridation process. Anti-fluoridation activists are vociferous in their claims of danger, and they pander to the fears of the populace on this front in every referendum. They see risk on two fronts: first in the form of *chronic* health risk from a lifetime ingestion of fluoridated water, and second in the form of *acute* health risk due to fluoride poisoning from possible overfeeds caused by engineering failures of fluoridation equipment. We have reviewed the evidence for and against the chronic risks to health in Chapter 8. We review the potential for engineering failure later in this chapter. We believe that a reasonable reader will conclude that such risks are small, but they are probably not zero, and as such they deserve some measure of our attention.

Like the benefits and costs, we would like to measure the risk in dollars. But unlike the benefits and costs, which are firm, the risk is probabilistic. Risk costs are borne only if our fears are realized. In the case of a potential engineering failure of a fluoridation system, for example, no additional costs accrue to society unless a failure actually occurs. *Risk* is therefore defined as the cost associated with failure multiplied by the probability of such a failure (which puts the risk into a form that is measured in dollars). It must be recognized that even where the probabilities are thought to be quite low, the consequences in some instances could be very great. In any case, the available estimates of both the probabilities of failure and the potential costs associated with such a failure are extremely uncertain. Clearly, it is much easier to estimate the annual operating costs of a fluoridation system than it is to place a dollar value on some small but finite increase in the risk of bone disease.

Because the valuation of the risks is so subjective, some risk analysts argue that the risk component, especially when it involves threats to health or potential loss of life, should be kept in a separate account, with no attempt made to place a dollar value on it. There is something seamy, they argue, in trying to place a dollar value on life, health, or happiness. As E. F. Schumacher put it in his wise and influential book *Small Is Beautiful*, "To undertake to measure the unmeasurable is absurd. The higher is reduced to the level of the lower and the priceless is given a price."[2]

In truth, it probably doesn't matter how the risks are calculated. The parties are not likely to agree. There are many players in the fluoridation game, and each sees the risks from his or her own perspective. Some, like those in the traditional health care community, are so solidly pro-fluoridation that it is unlikely that any analysis would sway their opinion. Their perception of the benefits is very high, and they see the risks as unproven, remote, and miniscule. Others, such as those in the alternative and holistic health care community, are viscerally anti-fluoridation. Their perceptions of the benefits and risks are the mirror image of those of their opponents, and equally unassailable. It is well known in risk-analysis circles that politically prominent risks often provoke a disproportionate level of outrage, and such outrage is certainly evident for the issue at hand.

Even within these various groups, individuals differ greatly in attitude and motive. Some people operate from a position of altruistic love for their fellow beings. Others operate with naked self-interest. Each assessment of risks, costs, and benefits is likely to reflect one or other (or both) of these proclivities. How should we judge the pro-fluoridation stance of the members of the American Dental Association, for example? Should we see their position as that of public benefactors or as that of a self-interested trade organization? What about the Public Health Service? The environmental movement? What are the motives of the health food industry, the bottled water industry, the sugar industry, and the toothpaste manufacturers? Are the fluoride producers from the aluminum and fertilizer industries evil polluters, as the antis have them pegged, or just good businesspeople?

In other words, perspective is everything. The discussions that follow are carried out from a *societal* perspective. We take the position of a rational public-policy analyst who is asked whether the benefits of fluoridation to society as a whole truly outweigh the costs and risks. It should come as no surprise that it is difficult to reach a simple, clear, and concise answer to this question that will satisfy everyone. The quantification of benefits, costs, and risks is a difficult exercise, and no two people are ever likely to agree. A cavity-free mouth is of great value to some people; others could not care less. A one-in-a-million risk of a hemodialysis failure is a trifle to the optimist but an unacceptably fearful outcome to the pessimist. Everyone has his or her own *perception* of the degree of risk involved in the fluoridation process, and his or her own attitude to the *aversion* of such risk. The best that we can do is to lay out the template for such an analysis and try to present some more-or-less value-free numbers. Each reader has every right to finagle these vital statistics to fit his or her own biases.

THE COST OF FLUORIDATION

The cost of a municipal water fluoridation system has two components: the initial capital expense for equipment, and an annual operating expense for chemicals, labor, and maintenance. Using dollar figures appropriate to the year 2002, the capital cost for a system that serves a major metropolitan area runs on the order of $200,000 to $1.5 million, depending on the population served. Operating costs for such a system are reported to be in the range $100,000 to $1 million per year.[3] To put these numbers into perspective, the annual operating cost of $220,000 for the city of Cleveland in the year 2000 represented roughly one-tenth of 1% of the total city budget of $200 million.[4]

By annualizing and discounting the capital costs, adding them to the operating costs, and dividing by the population served, one can produce a statistic that places costs in terms of dollars per person per year. Both the American Dental Association and the National Institute of Dental Research (of the Public Health Service) have carried out such a calculation.[5] The ADA results are representative. They state that the average cost of water fluoridation across the nation is about 50 cents per person per year. However, the range of reported values from the various municipalities across the land is quite large, running from $0.12 to $5.41. The primary control on this per capita cost is the population served by the reporting system, with smaller systems being the most expensive and larger systems the most cost-effective. A study carried out in 1992 in 44 communities of varying sizes in Florida is widely quoted in this regard.[6] This study reported a cost of $2.12 per person per year in towns with a population less than 10,000 and $0.31 per person per year in cities with a population greater than 50,000.

If one accepts the ADA average cost of 50 cents per person per year, the total nationwide cost of providing fluoridated water to the 151 million Americans who get it (see Table 2.3) is $75.5 million.

To most of us, 50 cents a year seems like a very small price to pay to avoid the pain and suffering of tooth decay. However, anti-fluoridationists have an argument that brings the effectiveness of even this small outlay into question. They point out that public water supplies are used for a wide variety of purposes that do not involve ingestion by humans. Water is used for industrial processes, fire protection, lawn sprinkling, toilet flushing, car washing, and so on. In fact, less than one-tenth of 1% of public water supplies is actually ingested by children in their tooth-forming years. In this argument, 99.9% of all the fluoride that is added to public water supplies is wasted. Dan Montgomery, an anti-fluoridation activist from Oakland, California has calculated (using 1977 data) that the total fluoride requirement for all the children who live in the area serviced by the East Bay Municipal Utility District (EBMUD) is about 7 ounces (at 1 mg/day per child, as recommended by the American Dental Association), whereas the total fluoride added to the system each day (to bring it to the optimal concentration of 1.0 ppm) amounts to 7636 pounds. "The EBMUD," he says, "is using 7636 pounds a day to do a 7-ounce job!"[7]

Whether you view this argument as important or a bit of a red herring, the facts seem pretty clear that fluoridation costs are low, certainly much lower than lots of other widely accepted preventive health care costs.

THE WRANGLE OVER BENEFITS

Anti-fluoridation forces have never argued very strenuously with the cost estimates. It is on the benefits side of the equation that they wish to start the economic battle. Looking at the pro-fluoridation position first, spokesmen for this community list a great number of benefits that they see coming from the fluoridation of public water supplies. Direct dental benefits include reduced numbers of childhood cavities, fewer missing teeth, fewer teeth requiring root canal procedures, and a reduced need for dentures and bridges in later years. All these things, they claim, should lead to significantly reduced family dental costs. In addition, they draw attention to the indirect benefits that arise from the decrease in time lost from work and school, the reduction of pain and discomfort, and the more positive self-image that comes from good dental health.[8]

When trying to put a dollar value on these benefits, the dental establishment has generally zeroed in on the value of cavities prevented. The American Dental Association estimates the average cost of a two-surface silver amalgam restoration in a permanent tooth to be about $102 (in 2005). This leads to their claim that the lifetime cost of fluoridation, taken as $40 per person (50 cents per person per year over 80 years), is less than the cost of one dental filling.[9] The Centers for Disease Control estimate the dental savings produced by fluoridation to be $53 per person per year in larger communities (although it is admitted to be significantly less in smaller communities).[10]

Looking at the larger picture, Michael Easley of the National Center for Fluoridation Policy and Research has suggested that each $100,000 investment in community water fluoridation prevents 500,000 cavities.[11] Even if we conservatively cut this figure in half to account for inflation and over-optimism, at $102 per cavity, this still converts to a saving of $25 million for each $100,000 invested. This seems to imply that the $75.5 million invested in fluoridation each year prevents as many as 188 million cavities per year (about one and a quarter cavities per person) and buys $14.3 billion worth of benefits. This value would strike most of us as incredibly high, and indeed, other estimates of the annual benefits of fluoridation, although still large, are significantly lower. In a 1985 textbook entitled *Understanding Dental Caries*, Gordon Nikiforuk stated his belief that the nationwide savings produced by community water fluoridation are on the order of $1 billion per year,[12] while the Centers for Disease Control cites a study that claims savings of $3.9 billion per year (in 1990 dollars) over the 10-year period 1979–1989.[13] Updating the latter figure for inflation suggests benefits on the order of $5 to 6 billion per year in 2008 dollars.

These pro-fluoridation economic arguments drive anti-fluoridationists wild. Forget all this arm-waving about reduced cavities and the purported dental savings, they argue. These savings are calculated, not observed. They are *theoretical* savings that bear no resemblance to reality. It makes infinitely more sense, they say, to look at figures for *actual* family dental costs, *actual* numbers of dentists practicing, and *actual* dentist incomes. They recommend comparison of these reality-based economic statistics between fluoridated and nonfluoridated communities (and in fluoridated communities, between pre- and post-fluoridation conditions).

Such studies have been carried out both inside and outside the dental community, and although they are not widely quoted by the dental establishment, they do seem to provide fodder for anti-fluoridationist arguments. One representative study of 30 U.S. cities, the results of which were featured in a 1976 segment of *CBS Reports*, found that there were more dentists per capita in fluoridated than in nonfluoridated cities (76.7 dentists per 100,000 population versus 59.2). Another documented an increase in the nationwide cost of dental services from $13.6 billion to $27.1 billion per year during the period 1979–1985.[14] This rate of increase exceeds the inflation rate during a period of steady growth in fluoride exposure. A more detailed study carried out in Illinois in 1972, some 20 years after the widespread adoption of fluoridation in that state and reported in the *Journal of the American Dental Association*, compared conditions in five fluoridated communities against those in five nonfluoridated communities. The authors found that whereas there were slightly fewer dentists per capita in the fluoridated cities than in the unfluoridated cities, those in the fluoridated cities tended to have higher incomes. Moreover, the average number of visits to the dentist in a year was higher in the fluoridated than the nonfluoridated cities, and the cost of dental care (in terms of cost per patient per year) was also higher in those cities. None of the differences were large, and the authors concluded their study by stating that the onset of fluoridation "did not affect dentists' incomes or fees to any significant degree."[15] A report of a similar study carried out much more recently and reported in the journal *Medical Care* in 1997 asked "Does Fluoridation Reduce the Use of Dental Services Among Adults?" The authors' answer in a nutshell was yes, but not much.[16]

The tenor of these articles makes it clear that they were written not as critiques of fluoridation effectiveness but to assuage the fears of rank-and-file dentists that this crusade on the part of the dental research community was not going to put them out of business. In her anti-fluoridation book *Fluoridation and Truth Decay*, Gladys Caldwell gleefully recounts the story of J. C. Muhler, the scientist who developed the formula for Crest toothpaste, addressing a technical session on preventive dentistry in Charleston, South Carolina in 1963. Caldwell claims that Muhler hailed fluoridation as "a revolution in dentistry that will eliminate cavities and enable dentists to do the type of work they prefer, and make more money doing it." He promised that dentists who are freed from having to fill cavities will "have longer vacations, will be able to afford to take trips to Europe, will own bigger houses, and will be able to buy their wives fur coats."[17]

All of this evidence leads the anti-fluoridation camp to believe that dentists have benefited from fluoridation legislation. They decry the dentists' claim that they supported fluoridation on purely humanitarian grounds, regardless of the harm that might be done to the dental profession. The more conspiracy oriented among them feel that the dental fraternity knew all along that fluoridation would be good for business and acted not on their Hippocratic oath but as a self-interested trade group with predictable motivations. Specifically, they charge that the dental community knew that increased fluoride in the environment would lead to increased dental fluorosis and that the restoration of fluorosed teeth would be a more lucrative business than the restoration of decayed teeth. They see the economic data, with its clear-cut message that dental costs have not decreased nor dentist incomes fallen, as unequivocal proof that fluoridation simply traded one disease for another, with no net benefit to society.

The dental community argues strenuously against this interpretation. They claim that problems related to dental fluorosis represent only a small part of modern-day practice. Rather, they point to the transformation of dentistry over the years from an extractive to a restorative technology, from a curative to a preventive philosophy, and from a medical to a cosmetic emphasis. In particular, they cite the tremendous growth in orthodontics and other services driven by cosmetic concerns. They argue that this growth has been driven by public demand, not by undue promotion on the part of dentists. In this view, the current preoccupation of the dental profession with cosmetic dentistry is a part of the contemporary social climate that strives for perfection in appearance. This emergence of the "me" generation, together with the general prosperity of the middle class, has created a massive new leisure market in the form of fitness clubs and weight-loss clinics, and a significant medical market for tummy tucks, breast implants, and liposuction. It has also allowed for a continuation of traditional dental budgets, but with a new emphasis on the perfect smile. Dentists join with their cosmetic cousins in touting the inestimable value of improved self-image.

This interpretation begs an important question. How should we now view the dental profession? Is our friendly family dentist still a part of the Hippocratic community? Should we view his or her advice as medical advice, similar to that provided by the heart specialist or oncologist, or should we be wary, as we would, say, to the advice of the stock promoter? Are his or her orthodontic recommendations for our children driven by concern for their health, or concern for his or her pocketbook? An article that appeared in *Reader's Digest* in 1997 under the title "How Honest Are Dentists?" does not provide solace. The author reports the results of a study in which 50 dentists in 28 states were asked to examine the same set of x-rays. They recommended a widely differing set of treatments, with costs that ranged from $500 to $30,000. In an understated conclusion, the author remarked: "I got 50 opinions, and I am not comforted."[18]

In his previously quoted study of the social dynamics of the fluoridation debate,[19] Brian Martin rejects the arguments of both extremes in favor of a more pragmatic interpretation of the motives of the dental community. Taking a historical perspective, he argues that the motives of dentists in the early years of the fluoridation controversy were complex, and like the rest of us, sometimes in conflict. There seems little doubt that the profession had a sincere desire to improve the dental health of the populace, but they also wished to avoid conflict with powerful groups in society and to protect the interests of their profession and their own economic well-being. Among the alternative courses of action available to them at that time were the espousal of community fluoridation, emphasis on improved oral hygiene, and the promotion of less-sugary foods. Climbing on the fluoridation bandwagon was in many ways the path of least resistance. It accomplished the primary health-based goal; it gave the appearance of self-sacrifice; it pleased the medical establishment in the Public Health Service; and it avoided conflict with the sugar lobby.

With respect to the uninterrupted stability of dentist incomes, Martin draws attention to the closed-shop nature of the dental profession. Dental incomes are maintained in part by professional control of the number of dentists in practice, which is carried out through limitations on university entrance and through professional licensing requirements. The dental profession has exerted more control in this area then have most other professions, such as engineering and law. He also accepts the argument that the continuity of dentist incomes reflects the transition of the profession from restorative to cosmetic dentistry. Nor does he flay the profession for their role in promoting their new cosmetic services. All the players in the fluoridation game are motivated to some degree by self-interest, and the dental community is no exception. In short, like most of us, he concludes that dentists are neither angels nor charlatans, just plain folks.

Burt and Eklund in their 1999 textbook on *Dentistry, Dental Practice, and the Community* put the blame at least partly on the dental community for the continued high cost of dental care. "If dentists continue to see children twice a year," they lament, "and apply the full battery of diagnostic and preventive services each time, the substantive savings that can be realized in the cost of restorative treatment will be drastically reduced."[20]

So what is a defensible bottom line on the question of the benefits of fluoridation? On the one hand it is hard not to accept at least part of the pro-fluoridation argument. If one grants the case made in Chapter 7 that increased fluoride in the environment is responsible for the observed decline in dental caries, it seems that one must also grant the fact that fluoridation proponents delivered on their promises. They promised to reduce caries. They did so. They deserve to claim the benefits of their actions. The fact that society chose to increase its use of dental services for cosmetic purposes, or that dentists have successfully convinced parents to buy into more preventive care, represent interesting cultural developments but they are not really relevant to the calculation of the benefits of fluoridation.

Working on this credo, and ignoring any potential risk costs, dental economists have tried to integrate the cost data and the benefit data through the calculation of a benefit–cost ratio. If we accept the ADA estimate of an annual nationwide cost of $75.5 million and the CDC estimate of annual nationwide benefits of $5 to 6 billion, the benefit–cost ratio of community water fluoridation comes out to be almost 7.0. This is within the values range 2.5 to 11.5 reported by a team of dental economists who reviewed eight independent benefit–cost studies from the dental literature.[21]

The higher end of this range represents a spectacularly high ratio of benefit to cost, far higher than is claimed for any other public health measure. Readers who are skeptical have every right to be so. Benefit–cost ratios for most public policies lie in the range 1.0–2.0. A respected dental researcher, Brian Burt, in his role as convenor of a 1989 international symposium on cost-effectiveness of caries prevention programs, presumably recognized this when he stated that fluoridation is "one of the few public health procedures that actually saves more money than it costs."[22] This statement does not claim a benefit–cost ratio of 7.0, only a value greater than 1.0.

Although all these calculations are interesting, the fact is that benefit–cost calculations do not tell the entire story. First and foremost, these calculations do not take into account the *disbenefits* that are brought on line by fluoridation. A disbenefit is defined as an undesired cost that is created by a policy decision or chosen course of action. The dental services that are needed to address increased levels of dental fluorosis brought on by increased fluoride levels are such a cost. Chapter 7 makes it clear that increased levels of dental fluorosis have indeed occurred under fluoridation and that the costs associated with their treatment ought to be included in a cost–benefit analyses.

Unfortunately, the dental community has not been as resolute in publishing economic data on this issue as they have been in proclaiming the value of the benefits. Not one of the economic analyses quoted above mentioned dental fluorosis (although one of them did admit to not including "social costs").[23] If we take the figure of $27 billion quoted above for the annual nationwide cost of dental services in 1989, round it up to $36 million for inflation, and assume that only 10% of these services deal with fluorosis, the resulting disbenefit of $3.6 billion wipes out a goodly portion of the benefits claimed by fluoridation proponents.

Furthermore, the cost–benefit ratios quoted above seem to give community water fluoridation the credit for *all* the cavities prevented by the increased level of fluoride intake by the public. Chapter 7 makes it clear that researchers are still unsure of the relative roles played by community water fluoridation, topical fluoride applications in a dental office, and the use of fluoridated toothpastes. It is felt that the latter two are less effective than the former, but they are certainly not totally ineffective. If the dental economists are going to take credit for all the benefits, their analysis ought to include all the costs, including the very significant annual costs laid out for topical fluoride applications and fluoridated toothpaste (or at least the added cost of a *fluoridated* toothpaste relative to an *unfluoridated* one, if such a difference exists).

The lack of published economic data on some of the factors identified in the discussion above makes a defensible final value for the benefit–cost ratio of community water fluoridation unattainable. Certainly, the value of 7.0 implied by pro-fluoridation data is far too high. However, we are inclined to agree with Brian Burt in his assessment that it is well above 1.0. The weight of the evidence suggests that the benefits of fluoridation outweigh the costs by a significant margin. But, of course, even this statement does not tell the entire story. We still have the risks to worry about, and it is over these subjective probabilistic costs that arguments forever swirl.

THE ULTIMATE BATTLEGROUND

There is no topic that can be raised on which there is so little common ground as the question of chronic health risks and whether such risks are (or are not) engendered by a lifetime of drinking fluoridated water. It is the ultimate battleground of the fluoride wars. Most anti-fluoridationists are convinced that increased fluoride intake is responsible for an increased prevalence of hip fractures, heart disease, and cancer. It is only a matter of time, they feel, before crippling skeletal fluorosis becomes a serious problem in the United States, just as it is in many third-world nations where the natural fluoride content of water is high. They are further worried by the emerging evidence that fluoride, like lead, may be sapping the intelligence of our children. They feel that the costs, and potential costs, of these various health risks are so great that they easily overwhelm the modest benefits that may accrue to society from a reduction in dental caries. Their perception of these risks is very high, and their aversion to them greater yet.

Anti-fluoridationists have tried to put some dollar figures on their fears. In one of the several fluoridation battles that have been waged in Calgary, Alberta, David Hill, an emeritus professor from the University of Calgary and one of the leaders of the anti-fluoridation movement there, made a formal presentation at a public forum convened by the Chemical Institute of Canada, in which he estimated the annual cost of hip fractures in the United States at $7 billion per year. He admitted that it was difficult to estimate the percentage of these hip fractures that had been precipitated by fluoride in the water supply, but he noted that even a 10 to 15% reduction in their number would save millions of dollars per year, perhaps as much as $1 billion.[24]

A more holistic estimate of health risk costs has been made by H. Lewis McKinney, a professor of the history of biology and medicine at the University of Kansas, and a coauthor of George Waldbott's early anti-fluoridation book *Fluoridation: The Great Dilemma*. McKinney estimated that at least 1% of the population, and perhaps as many as 10 to 20%, are subjected to the "misery, suffering, missed days of work, deaths, and medical costs" that are caused by fluoridation. In 1988 he calculated that if even 1% of the 130 million people then receiving fluoridated water experienced health problems, and if their average medical costs were on the order of $5000 per year, the total cost to society would be $6.5 billion per year.[25]

The pro-fluoride community finds these kinds of calculations ludicrous. Review the evidence, they say (which we have done in Chapter 8). The weight of evidence strongly suggests that none of these health fears are justified, certainly not for heart disease or cancer, and probably not even for hip fractures. They acknowledge the worldwide significance of crippling skeletal fluorosis, but they point to the EPA's maximum contaminant level for fluoride, which they say is suitably protective against this disease, and they claim that there have only been almost no documented cases in the United States. Get real, they are saying. We have enough genuine health threats to worry about; we should not be distracted by fanciful ones.

Furthermore, they argue, if fluoridation were truly harmful to our health, surely there would be some indication of that fact in national health statistics. At first glance there would seem to be solid evidence to the contrary. Average life expectancy in the United States has been steadily rising ever since records were first kept in the mid-nineteenth century. The average life lasted about 50 years or a little less in 1900, 60 or more in the 1940s, and 75 in the 1980s. If these trends continue, it will soon hit 80. Between 1920 and 1985, average life expectancy increased at the rate of about four months per year.[26]

It is also possible to look at the situation on a disease-by-disease basis. It turns out that the age-adjusted mortality rates for almost all diseases, including heart disease and most cancers, have been decreasing in recent years. The only notable exceptions are certain types of cancers, such as lung cancer and melanoma, whose causes are apparently related to twentieth-century lifestyles (too much smoke, too much sun). In the most comprehensive treatise available on the causes of cancer, up to 40% of all cancers are ascribed to tobacco use and no more than 2% to environmental factors. The possible impact of fluoridation is not even mentioned.[27]

Of course, the improvement in overall national health has many facets. The increase observed in human resistance to disease has been brought about in part by advances in medical treatment and by improvements in nutrition, maternal care, health education, and fitness. Nevertheless, there is simply no statistical evidence that fluoridation has brought about any significant decline in societal health. On the contrary, the very period in which fluoride exposure has been increasing has been a period of steady health improvement in the nation. As summarized in Chapters 7 and 8, apart from the documented increase in dental fluorosis and the unproven but potential influence on bone health, the evidence for health risk from community water fluoridation is essentially absent.

ENGINEERED SYSTEMS AND HUMAN ERROR

There is another type of risk that deserves our attention. Ever since the first fluoride was introduced into the water supply at Grand Rapids, the antifluoridation camp has questioned the ability of water treatment engineers to design and operate fluoridation equipment that can function without accident. In particular, they fear a breakdown in fluoridation equipment, or a breakdown in management control, such that a toxic overdose of fluoride is allowed to flow to community taps, leading to acute fluoride poisoning, illness, and perhaps even death.

Here at least, we should be on firmer ground than in our discussions of chronic health risk. In the case of chronic-health-risk assessments, it is difficult not to sink into the quagmire of mushy data and value-laden interpretations, whereas here we should be able to carry out a more objective perusal of the historical record. With 50 years of community water fluoridation now on the books, it should be possible to assess the safety performance of the engineered systems (and their keepers) in a more-or-less straightforward fashion.

Viewed in the abstract, it seems that anti-fluoridation concerns could well have some merit. When engineers design a mechanical system to meet some objective, they do so in full knowledge that no design (or at least no affordable design) can ever be considered *perfectly* reliable. They recognize that there may well be some unanticipated combination of loads or stresses or flow rates that could potentially lead to a failure of their design. The most widely used engineering-design process utilizes the concept of a safety factor, which is set in such a way that it reduces the probability of failure to some extremely low level. The system of pipes, pumps, valves, basins, and hoppers that make up a fluoride delivery system at a water treatment plant are undoubtedly designed with a very high factor of safety and a very low probability of failure. However, *absolute* safety can never be guaranteed.

To add to the concern, there is the ever-present possibility of human error. Human beings are not perfect. Some are lazy, some are stupid, and some are impaired or hung over as they work. Some are just clumsy now and then. There are taps that can be left open, meters that can be misread, and warning signals that can be missed. Most water treatment plants have strict protocols designed to prevent all these mistakes and safety programs to try to cut down the number of accidents. These programs certainly reduce the proclivity for human error, but it is unlikely that they can eliminate it totally. The combination of very low probabilities of equipment failure, and perhaps somewhat higher (but hopefully still quite low) probabilities of human error, implies that accidents at water treatment plants should be rare, but it is not possible to discount them entirely.

If we look at the process in more detail, we find that there are three different fluoride compounds that are used in water fluoridation systems: sodium fluoride, sodium silicofluoride, and fluosilicic acid. The first two come in the form of white crystalline powder, the third as a liquid. All three are considered hazardous substances, and all three are toxic to humans in their concentrated form. The first two are fed into the water supply through the use of a dry feeder, while the third uses a solution feeder. The result is a fluoride concentration of about 1.0 ppm in the water flow that is distributed to municipal households. Water treatment engineers argue that these feeder systems are extremely simple to use and very reliable. Operators receive comprehensive training on the installation and operation of the equipment.

Managers can choose from training manuals put out by the American Water Works Association, the Environmental Protection Agency, or the Centers for Disease Control, all of which contain detailed engineering and administrative recommendations.[28]

Furthermore, they point out, there are a large number of checks and balances to ensure safety. For example, protocols require that the holding tanks for the feeders hold only one or two days' supply of fluoride (on the order of a few tens to a few hundred pounds of sodium fluoride, depending on the size of the population served), thus limiting the amount of fluoride that could be released accidentally into the water distribution system in a single event. Monitoring of flow rates and feed rates is carried out routinely. There is regular sampling of the water, and analysis for fluoride concentrations at the source and at representative outlet points of the distribution system. The California mandate, for example, requires that fluoridation systems have continuous 24-hour monitoring, a warning system that is triggered by any overfeed, and an emergency response protocol that comes into play when a warning is triggered.

Despite these several layers of protection, it appears that many fluoridation systems are often out of compliance. The usual operational goal is to stay within 10% of the target concentration (which is usually 1.0 ppm). A study of 249 systems in Illinois during the period 1977–1981 found that even the best run systems were out of compliance about 20% of the time. Sometimes fluoride concentrations were too low and sometimes too high. Apparently, many of the flagged events were only slightly out of compliance, and there is no mention in the article of any toxic-level overfeeds. The most successful systems were those in the larger population centers with better trained operators and lower operator turnover. The least successful systems were those in smaller communities.[29] More recent data are available from the state of New Hampshire for the period 2000–2002. Fluoride concentrations delivered were in the optimal range 0.7 to 1.2 ppm only 50% of the time. Of the rest, 42% were underfeeds and only 1% were overfeeds (the missing 7% were unmeasured).[30] There are undoubtedly ongoing improvements in the equipment and in the hazard response systems as time goes by, so one might expect a steadily improving level of performance over the years. On the other hand, there are ever more systems in place with time, and the uncertainty of future terrorist targets hangs in the air. It seems likely that some overfeed situations are still likely to arise somewhere in the nation each year.

The impact of some of the worst of these overfeeds is well documented. In a letter to the editor on Bette Hileman's article in *Chemical and Engineering News* in 1988, Evelyn Hannan, chairman of the environmental committee for the town of Merrick, New York, claimed that there have been "dozens of documented accidents, overfeeds, spills, leaks, and mishaps, which have caused illness, hospitalization, and even fatality."[31] Philip Heggen, in his chronology of *How We Got Fluoridated*, states that "dozens of verified fluoride overfeeds have occurred in cities across the country" and that "fatalities have occurred when fluoride saturation levels ran too high due to faulty flow control systems."[32] In his book *Fluoridation: the Great Dilemma*, George Waldbott cites two cases of "mass poisoning" from mechanical difficulties with fluoridation equipment.[33] Among the U.S. communities that are identified by these and other anti-fluoridation authors as having suffered from fluoridation accidents are Annapolis, Maryland; Harbor Springs, Michigan; Hooper Bay, Alaska; Los Lunas, New Mexico; New Haven, Connecticut; Marin County, California; Poplarville, Mississippi; Portage, Michigan; Potsdam, New York; Rice Lake, Wisconsin; Saratoga Springs, New York; Stanley County, North Carolina; Wakefield, Massachusetts, Westby, Wisconsin; and even the first city of fluoridation, Grand Rapids, Michigan.[34]

The cases for Poplarville, Mississippi, Annapolis, Maryland, and Hooper Bay, Alaska, are particularly well documented, not only in the anti-fluoridation literature but also in the medical literature. In Poplarville, a small rural community in Mississippi, a faulty feed pump at the town treatment plant allowed saturated fluoride solution to be pumped accidentally directly into the town system. Concentrations up to 200 ppm were documented in tap water near the treatment plant. Ice samples made from contaminated water in a nearby restaurant ran to 40 ppm. There was widespread gastrointestinal illness throughout the small community.[35]

The event in Annapolis, Maryland, occurred on November 13, 1979, when a technician at the Annapolis water treatment plant failed to close a valve. A feed container overflowed and 1000 gallons of fluonosilicic acid was funneled into the city water supply. The accident was not reported to the proper authorities until one week later. Studies carried out at that time by the Maryland State Department of Health and Mental Hygeine found that soda bottled on the day after the event had fluoride concentrations of 30 ppm. A check of the admission records at a local hospital and at a nearby pediatric clinic failed to uncover any anomalous occurrence of illnesses resembling fluoride poisoning. However, eight chronic renal-failure patients who were undergoing kidney dialysis at that time became ill, and one died. An autopsy on the deceased patient showed elevated fluoride levels throughout the body.[36] In the weeks following the event, the *Annapolis Evening Capitol* invited John Yiamouyiannis and George Waldbott to carry out an epidemiological survey in the community. They claim to have identified 10,000 people who suffered acute symptoms of fluoride poisoning, 62% musculoskeletal, 65% neurological, 59% urological, and 13% dermatological.[37] In a later publication, Yiamouyiannis further claimed that there were five times the normal number of heart failure deaths in Annapolis in the week following the overfeed.[38]

Hooper Bay, Alaska, is a Yup'ik Eskimo settlement on the coast of the Bering Sea with an aboriginal population of 950. In May 1992 the community water supply was provided by two water wells. The fluoridation system on one of the wells malfunctioned, delivering fluoride to some of the residents in the community at a concentration of 150 ppm. A retrospective study showed that 292 people served by the malfunctioning system suffered symptoms of fluoride poisoning, including gastrointestinal problems, headaches, numbness, and fatigue. One 41-year-old man died. The cause of death was listed on his death certificate as an acute overdose of sodium fluoride.[39]

THE CONCEPT OF ACCEPTABLE RISK

The way that one views the fluoridation safety record of the water treatment industry probably depends on one's predilections with respect to fluoridation. It is clear from the record that many of the smaller systems are quite often slightly out of compliance, and that serious overfeed events with identifiable health impact, occasionally even death, occur somewhere in the country, perhaps on the order of once per year. Anti-fluoridationists see each event as a disaster, proof positive that fluoridation is not worth it. Even a single event is seen as totally unacceptable. Ergo, fluoridation must go.

Pro-fluoridationists are more likely to take a broader view, trying to place the risks associated with fluoridation into context with the broad suite of technological risks that are already shouldered by society. Given the nearly 60 years of fluoridation history, with systems now operative in thousands of U.S. communities, it appears that the probability of failure of a given fluoridation system in a given year is probably on the order of 1 in 10,000. That is, for every 10,000 fluoridation systems put in place, one might expect an overfeed event leading to some identifiable level of health impact in one of them each year. This probability of failure is similar to that for many other technological systems that are widely accepted by the public.[40] The risk of dam failure, for example, falls in the same range.

Not only that but the consequences of fluoridation failures are quite small relative to those from other technological accidents. The number of potential deaths from a fluoride-poisoning event would be much less than that for a dam failure, for example. While each individual death is undoubtedly a tragic event to those close to the victim, policymakers must view the situation from a societal perspective. In this light, the risk of death from a fluoridation overfeed is slight, perhaps on the order of 1 in a million. In a widely quoted treatise entitled *Analyzing the Daily Risks of Life*, risk analyst Richard Wilson identifies many actions that increase the risk of death by one in 1 million. They include smoking 1.4 cigarettes, drinking 0.5 liter of wine, traveling 30 miles by car, and flying 1000 miles by commercial plane.[41] In other words, the probability of getting cancer from smoking or from dying in an automobile accident on our nation's highways is orders of magnitude higher than the chances of dying from a fluoridation over-feed. It is clear that the public accepts some risks much more readily than others.

Many studies have been designed to address the reasons that some people exhibit such pessimistic risk perceptions and such strong aversion to certain types of risks. It seems that many people are particularly averse to risks that are involuntary rather than voluntary, human-made rather than natural, difficult-to-detect rather than readily observable, and unfamiliar rather than familiar.[42] Fluoride poisoning fits into this risk-averse profile.

If we wish to carry our risk–cost–benefit analysis to fruition, it would be necessary to put a monetary value on the chronic health risks associated with daily use of fluoridated drinking water and the acute health risks associated with potential accidents at water treatment plants. However, trying to place a dollar value on risks that involve sickness and death is notably difficult. One can try to estimate the cost of the health response, but it is clear from the discussions and case histories presented above that total national costs on this front are not very large. They would be on the order of millions per year at most, rather than billions, and are therefore much smaller than either the direct costs or the apparent benefits of fluoridation. If the risk term is to have any significant impact on risk–cost–benefit calculations, it can only be because the *perceived* risks are much greater than these health costs alone. It would be necessary to assign a dollar value to the feelings of *dread* that are felt by those who are receptive to the anti-fluoridation message. It is probably better to accept E. F. Schumacher's advice and keep the risk in a separate account from the costs and benefits, recognizing the appropriateness of an assessment that is more subjective than it is purely quantitative.

Ultimately, we reach the question of what constitutes an *acceptable risk*. This is not a technical question; it is a social one. For each person, it depends on risk perception, risk aversion, economic status, values, and beliefs.[43] For the body politic, it is some type of integrated sum of these individual acceptable risks. It is not a fixed or known quantity. It is determined by the democratic process through elections, referendums, and public hearings, and under the influence of adversarial lobbies. As one pundit put it, "it is the level at which the political pressure dies down or the budget runs out."[44] It is determined by common consent, not by any sophisticated analysis. It may sound like a tautology, but acceptable risk is the risk associated with the most politically acceptable decision.

The number of Americans who have access to fluoridated water supplies has been increasing steadily over the years and now constitutes about 67% of the population. To the extent that this statistic reflects the public will, it can be argued that the public now considers the risks associated with community water fluoridation as acceptable. However, it must be remembered that referendums are still fiercely fought, often lost, and when won, are usually won by a narrow margin. There is still much uncertainty in the public mind about the acceptability of fluoridation risks. Or more likely, the public reticence reflects continuing doubts about whether the small but undeniable benefits associated with improved teeth are worth the apparently miniscule but still-uncertain risks that may arise from the daily use of fluoridated water and from the possibility of engineering accidents such as those that occurred in Annapolis, Poplarville, and Hooper Bay.

THE PRECURSORS

To some degree, the battle that is being fought over fluoridation today has been fought twice before: first when the *chlorination* of public water supplies was introduced, and again when some quixotic moves were made toward the *iodization* of water supplies. Chlorination has become a staple of the water treatment business, almost universally used, and subject to almost no dissent. Iodization was a short-lived experiment that never caught on.

As public health efforts, chlorination, fluoridation, and iodization have much in common. In the first place, chlorine, fluorine, and iodine all belong to the same chemical family (the halogens), and have similar properties. Second, all three efforts proposed to use the public water supply as the delivery vehicle to distribute an apparently beneficial supplement to the populace. And third, all three faced opposition, with opposing arguments that were very similar in the three cases. The question arises as to why one has become standard practice, one a source of ongoing conflict, and one a historical footnote. The answer probably lies in their respective costs, benefits, and risks.

The practice of water chlorination took root in this country early in the twentieth century. The first U.S. patent on chlorination was granted to a professor of chemistry at the Stevens Institute of Technology in Hoboken, New Jersey, in 1888. The first American application, in 1908, was at the Boonton Reservoir waterworks, which serves Jersey City, New Jersey. In 1909, Philadelphia became the first major city to fully chlorinate its public water supply.[45] The success of these early programs in reducing the prevalence of acute waterborne diseases such as cholera and typhoid fever spurred the proliferation of chlorination plants across the country. The practice is now used as standard disinfection methodology in over 98% of the public water supply systems in the United States. *Life* magazine has called chlorination "the most significant public health advance of the millennium."[46]

The value of chlorination lies in its ability to kill the bacterial and viral microorganisms that are capable of transmitting such diseases as typhoid fever, cholera, hepatitis, salmonellosis, and legionellosis to human beings. Early in the twentieth century there were upward of 25,000 deaths each year from typhoid fever in the United States, a death rate that is similar to that now ascribed to automobile accidents. By 1960, there were fewer than 20 such deaths per year. Between 1920 and 1936, there were 470 outbreaks of typhoid fever in the United States and Canada; between 1971 and 1985, there were five.[47] The role of water chlorination in these reductions is unquestioned.

Furthermore, proponents of chlorination pointed out that it does more than just provide disinfection control to water distribution systems. It also provides biological control by preventing the growth of algae, molds, and bacterial slimes in water reservoirs. It also provides odor control by oxidizing many of the foul-smelling gases that are released during the water treatment process, such as hydrogen sulfide and ammonium.

Despite all this, early chlorination programs were not without opposition. Many prominent water engineers were opposed to the chlorination of public water supplies because they felt that any water source that was not potable ought to be abandoned. They felt that it was better to search out a pure water supply than to add a powerful disinfectant to public drinking water. The public at-large may or may not have agreed, but they certainly objected to the chlorinous taste, which was common in early chlorination practice. And foreshadowing the claims against fluoridation some 50 years later, there were charges of enforced medication, and there was exploitation of health fears related to the public knowledge that chlorine, in its pure gaseous form, is toxic to humans.[48]

Regardless of the appeal of these arguments to a small minority, the anti-chlorination movement never attracted the public fancy in the way that the anti-fluoridation movement did later. The great majority of the populace viewed chlorination as hugely cost-effective: an incredibly small price to pay for the benefits received. The public satisfaction associated with the near-eradication of cholera and typhoid fever far exceeded any fears associated with the small health risks that were then thought to be associated with chlorination.

In recent years it has been recognized that the health risks associated with chlorination may be somewhat higher than originally thought. It turns out that chlorine can react with natural organic matter in water to form *disinfection by-products* in the form of trihalomethanes, the most common of which is chloroform. A number of epidemiological studies have indicated an association between trihalomethanes and increased cancer mortality. To date, the results are suggestive but not definitive, and risk analysts are quick to point out that the health risks from these by-products are extremely small in comparison with the risks associated with inadequate disinfection.[49]

Additionally, it has been recognized that whereas chlorination kills bacteria and viruses effectively, it does not eradicate protozoans such as *Giardia* and *Cryptosporidium*. In recent years, outbreaks of disease carried by these parasitic microorganisms have been on the increase in the United States. Alternative methods of disinfection which are effective against all microorganisms, such as ultraviolet radiation treatment, are under consideration in many cities. However, treatment costs with these alternative approaches are significantly higher.

Even with these modern fears added to the mix, there has been little public outcry against water chlorination. Certainly, no anti-chlorination movement has arisen to mirror the strength of the anti-fluoridation movement. The costs for the two practices are of similar magnitude, as are the apparent health risks from chronic use or acute exposure. It is the benefits that differ: a few less cavities in one case; eradication of several deadly diseases in the other. In those areas of the third world where water chlorination is still not available, waterborne diseases may be responsible for as many as 3.4 million deaths per year.[50] This is a powerful reminder of the value of chlorination. Fluoridation cannot call on benefits that even remotely rival those of chlorination. A cost–benefit analysis of fluoridation still leaves the protagonists something to fight about, whereas that for chlorination is a slam dunk.

Let us turn now to the almost-forgotten proposals to add iodine to drinking water, which first surfaced in the United States in the early 1920s. It was recognized by that time that the widespread prevalence of goiter, especially in young girls and in certain specific areas of the nation, was due to an iodine deficiency that adversely affects the production of growth hormones in the thyroid gland. Worse yet, it was known from evidence from other countries that *severe* iodine deficiency can lead to endemic cretinism, a sad disease whose victims are not only deaf and mute but also suffer from mental and physical retardation.[51]

Under normal circumstances, iodine is taken into our body from the fruits and vegetables we eat, which in turn pick it up from the soils in which the fruits and vegetables are grown. In areas where soils are deficient in iodine, usually in inland regions far removed from the sea, dietary iodine deficiency can arise. This was the case in the Great Lakes states in the early years of the twentieth century. As with fluoridation, proposals to add iodine to drinking water were given a huge boost by a famous experiment in which 5000 schoolgirls in Akron, Ohio were given iodine supplementation in their water over a three-year period. As with the Grand Rapids data on tooth decay, the Akron results indicated a huge positive impact of supplemental iodine on the prevalence of goiter.[52]

Iodization of water supplies was proposed in many U.S. cities, but it actually came into place in only three of them: Rochester, New York; Sault Ste. Marie, Michigan, and Anaconda, Montana, and even in these three, it lasted only a few years.[53] In most cities there was strong opposition by Christian Scientists and by the American Medical Liberty League. Fears of the toxic effects of over-iodization (which, like fluoride, are not entirely fanciful) came to the fore. Even the American Water Works Association at their annual conference in 1923 concluded that "the practice of using the public water supply as a medium of medication is undesirable." Proponents argued that it was "no more medication than the addition of chlorine, lime, soda, or alum to our water supplies, and the day has passed since we objected to these." As would fluoridation proponents years later, they argued that "as a preventive method against an important disease, iodization is comparable to chlorination."[54]

As fate would have it, the iodization movement was overtaken by events. Several European countries had already turned to the use of iodized salt to treat iodine deficiency. In 1924, iodized salt was introduced in the state of Michigan, and by 1929 the prevalence of goiter in that state had been reduced from 38.6% to 9.0%. By 1955, over 75% of all U.S. households used iodized salt on their table. By 1972, a multistate survey in the Great Lakes region indicated that there was no remaining indication of widespread goiter in these states.[55]

There is no reason that salt could not be used as a delivery vehicle for fluoride as well as iodide, and indeed this has been tried with some success in Switzerland. In the United States, however, for the reasons outlined in Chapter 10, fluoridation proponents pushed for the public water supply as the preferred path of distribution. Perhaps they wanted the public to accept the contention that the prevention of tooth decay is a cause more akin to the prevention of typhoid than the prevention of goiter.

PUBLIC HEALTH OR HOME REMEDY?

Although the absolute value of the benefit–cost ratio for fluoridation remains elusive, the use of a benefit–cost methodology can still prove useful in a comparative sense to assess the relative cost-effectiveness of alternative delivery systems. As long as the method of calculation remains consistent across the various alternatives investigated, the results should be informative. One such exercise was carried out for the international symposium on the cost-effectiveness of fluoride therapy held in 1989. It included a benefit–cost analysis for community water fluoridation and comparative analyses for home-based fluoride supplementation in the form of fluoride tablets and fluoride mouthwashes. Results showed that the community water fluoridation program was significantly more cost-effective than home-based programs.[56]

Once again, this study did not include consideration of the health risks associated with the various alternatives. As we will see, when the risks are added to the mix, comparative analyses tip even further in favor of a public health approach rather than private supplementation. The risks associated with fluoride tablets and mouthwash lie in the possibility of accidental overdoses by children. A study of the records of the Rocky Mountain Poison Center for the year 1986 identified 87 cases of toxic fluoride ingestion by children.[57] There was one fatality due to ingestion of a sodium fluoride insecticide (which we judge to lie outside our frame of reference). All the rest of the cases were limited to relatively short-lived gastrointestinal distress. Two of these arose after fluoride treatment in a dental office, while the remaining 84 involved the accidental ingestion of fluoride tablets, drops, or rinses in the home.

An even larger study of 73 poison control centers (serving 250 million Americans) reported 10,596 calls about suspected cases of overingestion of fluoride in 1994 (0.5% of all calls). Of these, 33% involved dietary supplements, 32% toothpaste, and 12% mouthwashes. No fatalities were reported; a few hundred required treatment in health care facilities; most of the cases were not serious.[58]

Anti-fluoridation websites highlight several tragic stories of childhood fatalities from fluoride ingestion, and some of them have received detailed coverage in the medical literature as well. In their textbook *Fluorides in Caries Prevention*, Murray, Rugg-Gunn, and Jenkins describe three such cases of fatal ingestion of fluoride tablets by small children.[59] The acute fatal dose for a child may be as low as 1.0 gram or less, so a bottle of one hundred 10-mg tablets, if left within a child's reach, represents a similar threat to their safety as do other toxic household products, such as garden pesticides and cleaning solvents. Most poison control centers now include fluoride supplements on their list of dangerous household items. There is also one well-documented case of a 3-year-old child who died after swallowing fluoride mouthwash containing 435 mg of fluoride in a dentist's office in a New York City dental clinic in 1974. In 1979, a jury awarded the parents of the victim compensatory damages of $750,000.[60]

As first noted in Chapter 10, even fluoride toothpastes present some danger to small children. A large tube of fluoride toothpaste contains an amount of fluoride that is greater than the acute lethal dose for a small child. Although we have not located any documented reports of death, it is certainly not outside the bounds of anticipated behavior that a child could consume a full tube of toothpaste. To address this eventuality, the Food and Drug Administration decided in 1997 to strengthen the "do not swallow" warnings that appear on any fluoride toothpaste endorsed by the American Dental Association. In addition to the ADA warning, fluoride toothpastes must now add the FDA caution: "If you accidentally swallow more than used for brushing, seek professional help or contact a poison control center immediately." Toothpaste manufacturers (and the American Dental Association) oppose this added warning. They feel that it fails to take into account the excellent safety record of fluoride toothpastes, and that mention of poison control centers unnecessarily frightens parents and children. It is their contention that a child cannot absorb enough fluoride from swallowing toothpaste to cause a serious problem.[61]

Consideration of all this anecdotal data leads us to believe that the probability of getting an unhealthy acute dose of fluoride is probably greater from home supplements, rinses, and dentifrices than it is from the mechanical breakdown of fluoridation systems. If that is the case, an argument can be made from the societal perspective that lower costs and lower risks both favor community water fluoridation over home-based alternative delivery systems. The only argument left in favor of any of the latter approaches is that of freedom of choice.

THE BOTTOM LINE ON THE ECONOMICS OF FLUORIDATION

So what have we accomplished in attempting this societal economic assessment of the fluoridation game? It seems that the direct costs of fluoridation are well established and not contentious. If we consider the value of the cavities prevented by fluoridation as our measure of the benefits, as most dental economists do, it is apparent that the benefits of fluoridation outweigh the costs by a significant margin. Economic studies carried out on this basis calculate a benefit–cost ratio on the order of 7.0, and perhaps as high as 11.5. In our opinion, these values are demonstrably optimistic, because they fail to take into account either the disbenefits or the health risks that may be associated with fluoridation. Assessment of the data available suggests that the disbenefits of dental fluorosis are societally significant. The

economic costs of the chronic health risks associated with a lifetime ingestion of fluoridated water, on the other hand, are small. Acute health risks
associated with overfeeds caused by engineering failures, while distressing
and occasionally even fatal, are also small compared with other technological risks that are accepted by society. When the disbenefits and risk costs are
factored into the analysis, a defensible quantitative value is hard to come
by, but it seems clear that the benefits of fluoridation still outweigh the costs
and risks by a healthy margin. It is apparent that when viewed through an
economic prism, fluoridation is one of the most cost-effective of all public
health measures.

The anti-fluoridationist argument that points to the stability of dentist
incomes as proof that fluoridation provides no net benefit to society does not
stand up to rational scrutiny. The fluoridation movement promised to reduce
cavities and they deserve credit for doing so. The fact that society has chosen
to continue its use of dental services for preventive and cosmetic purposes is
not relevant to the calculation of the benefits of fluoridation.

The argument that it is inappropriate to try to place a dollar value
on risks to health and life has greater merit. If risks are kept in a separate
account, the societal acceptance of fluoridation rests on the subjective bal-
ancing of the quantifiable benefits and costs against the unquantifiable risks.
This approach allows for greater weight to be placed on pessimistic societal
risk perceptions and the public aversion to such risks. It is in this latter arena
that anti-fluoridationists must make their case.

Perhaps it is best to close this chapter with a shrug. Some people like
cost–benefit ideas; some people hate them. "Benefit–cost analysis," write the
authors of a well-known treatise on the subject, "can be viewed as anything
from an infallible means of reaching a new Utopia to a waste of resources in
attempting to measure the immeasurable."[62] One hopes that "the application of this technique to dental programs lies somewhere between these two
extremes."[63]

REFERENCES

1. For a clear and concise introduction to the principles and methodology of risk–
   cost–benefit analysis, see D. V. Lindley, *Making Decisions*, Wiley-Interscience,
   New York, 1971; or E. A. C. Crouch and R. Wilson, *Risk/Benefit Analysis*, Ballinger
   Publishing, Cambridge, MA, 1982.
2. E. F. Schumacher, *Small Is Beautiful*, Harper & Row, New York, 1973.
3. These figures are taken from E. Newbrun, Water fluoridation and fluoridation
   supplements in caries reduction, *J. Calif. Dent. Assoc.*, 8(1), 1980.; and from A. L.
   Garcia, Caries incidence and costs of preventive programs, *J. Publ. Health Dent.*,

49(5)(Special Issue), 259–271, 1989. The dollar values from both sources have been corrected for inflation.

4. F. Henry, The invisible fear, *Cleveland Plain Dealer*, Sunday Supplement, March 26, 2000.

5. American Dental Association, *Fluoridation Facts*, http://www.ada.org; National Institute of Dental and Craniofacial Research, http://www.nidcr.nih.gov.

6. M. L. Ringelberg, S. J. Allen, and L. J. Brown, Cost of fluoridation: 44 Florida communities, *J. Publ. Health Dent.*, 52, 75–80, 1992.

7. D. Montgomery, On the economics of the "recommended amount" of fluoride, http://www.sonic.net/~kryptox/fluoride.htm.

8. ADA, *Fluoridation Facts*, op. cit.

9. ADA, *Fluoridation Facts*, op. cit.

10. U.S. Public Health Service, Centers for Disease Control and Prevention, Achievements in public health, 1900–1999: fluoridation of drinking water to prevent dental caries, *MMWR* 48(41), 933–940, 1999.

11. M. W. Easley, Fluoridation: a triumph of science over propaganda, *Priorities*, 8(4), 1996.

12. G. Nikiforuk, *Understanding Dental Caries*, Vol. 2, *Prevention: Basic and Clinical Aspects*, Karger, Basel, Switzerland, 1985, pp. 13–44.

13. USPHS, CDC, 1999, op. cit.

14. P. Heggen, *How We Got Fluoridated*, Stop Fluoridation USA, http://www.rvi.net/~fluoride/, 1999.

15. B. L. Douglas, D. A. Wallace, M. Lerner, and S. B. Coopersmith, Impact of water fluoridation on dental practice and dental manpower, *J. Am. Dent. Assoc.*, 84, 355–367, 1972.

16. D. Grembowski, L. Fiset, and P. Milgrom, Does fluoridation reduce the use of dental services among adults? *Med. Care*, 35, 454–471, 1997.

17. G. Caldwell and P. E. Zanfagna, *Fluoridation and Truth Decay*, Top Ecology Press, Reseda, CA, 1974.

18. W. Ecenbarger, How honest are dentists? *Reader's Digest*, February 1997.

19. B. Martin, *Scientific Knowledge In Controversy: The Social Dynamics of the Fluoridation Debate*, State University of New York Press, Albany, NY, 1991.

20. B. A. Burt and S. A. Eklund, *Dentistry, Dental Practice, and the Community*, W.B. Saunders, Philadelphia, 1999.

21. B. A. White, A. A. Antczak-Bouckoms, and M. C. Weinstein, Issues in the economic evaluation of community water fluoridation, *J. Dent. Educ.*, 53, 646–657, 1989.

22. B. A. Burt, ed., Proceedings of workshop on cost effectiveness of caries prevention in dental public health, *J. Publ. Health Dent.*, 49(5)(Special Issue), 251–344, 1989.

23. Garcia, 1989, op. cit.

24. D. R. Hill, Fluoride: risks and benefits? Disinformation in the service of big industry, presented to Chemical Institute of Canada public forum on fluoridation, Calgary, Alberta, Canada, September 29, 1992; available from Health Action Network, http://www.fluoridation.com.

25. H. L. McKinney, Letter to the editor regarding article by B. Hileman entitled "Fluoridation: Contention Won't Go Away", *Chem. Eng. News*, October 31, 1988.

26. L. A. Sagan, *The Health of Nations*, Basic Books, New York, 1987.

27. R. Doll and R. Peto, *The Causes of Cancer*, Oxford University Press, New York, 1981.

28. American Water Works Association, *Water Fluoridation: Principles and Practices*, 2nd ed., AWWA, Denver, CO, 1996; E. Belleck, *Fluoridation Engineering Manual*, U.S. Environmental Protection Agency, Washington, DC, 1980; U.S. Public Health Service, Centers for Disease Control, *Water Fluoridation: A Manual for Engineers and Technicians*, U.S. PHS, Washington, DC, 1986.

29. R. A. Kuthy, C. Naleway, and J. Durkes, Factors associated with maintenance of proper water fluoride levels, *J. Am. Dent Assoc.*, 110, 511–513, 1985.

30. A. R. Pelletier, Maintenance of optimal fluoride levels in public water systems, *J. Publ. Health Dent.*, 64(4), 237–239, 2004.

31. *Chem. Eng. News*, October 17, 1988.

32. P. Heggen, *How We Got Fluoridated*, Stop Fluoridation USA, http://www.rvi.net/~fluoride/, 1999.

33. G. L. Waldbott, A. W. Burgstahler, and H. L. McKinney, *Fluoridation: The Great Dilemma*, Coronado Press, Lawrence, KS, 1978.

34. The website of the Pennsylvania Fluoride Leadership team, http://www.penweb.org, features a list of 75 accidents involving fluoride releases. Eleven of them involve releases into drinking water distribution systems.

35. A. D. Penman, B. T. Brackin, and R. Embrey, Outbreak of acute fluoride poisoning caused by fluoride overfeed, Mississippi, 1993, *Publ. Health Rep.*, 12(5), September 1997.

36. See the news item under the heading "Noted, Quoted, and Exerpted" in *J. Publ. Health Dent.*, 40, 360–362, 1980; also the news item in *MMWR*, March 28, 1980, pp. 134–136.

37. G. L. Waldbott, Mass intoxication from accidental overfluoridation of drinking water, *Clin. Toxicol.*, 18, 531–541, 1981.

38. J. Yiamouyiannis, *Fluoride, The Aging Factor: How to Recognize the Devastating Effects of Fluoride*, Health Action Press, Delaware, OH, 1983.

39. B. D. Gessner, M. Beller, J. P. Middaugh, and G. M. Whitford, Acute fluoride poisoning from a public water system, *N. Engl. J. Med.*, 330(2), 95–99, 1994.

40. H. W. Lewis, *Technological Risk*, W.W. Norton, New York, 1990.

41. R. Wilson, Analysing the daily risks of life, *Technol. Rev.*, Feb. 1979.

42. C. R. Cothern, ed., *Handbook for Environmental Risk Decision Making: Values, Perceptions, and Ethics*, CRC Press, Boca Raton, FL, 1996.

43. B. Fischoff, S. Lichtenstein, P. Slovic, S. L. Derby, and R. L Keeney, *Acceptable Risk*, Cambridge University Press, New York, 1981.

44. Lewis, 1990, op. cit.

45. M. N. Baker, *The Quest for Pure Water: The History of Water Purification from the Earliest Records to the Twentieth Century*, American Water Works Association, Denver, Co, 1949.

46. Based on information from the Chlorine Chemistry Council, http:/c3.org/chlorine_knowledge_center.

47. G. C. White, *Handbook of Chlorination and Alternative Disinfectants*, Wiley, New York, 1999; American Water Works Association, *Water Quality and Treatment: A Handbook of Community Water Supplies*, 4th ed., AWWA, Denver, CO, 1990.

48. Baker, 1949, op. cit.; White, 1999, op. cit.

49. Chlorine Chemistry Council, op. cit.; American Water Works Association, 1990, op. cit.

50. Chlorine Chemistry Council, op. cit.

51. J. B. Stanbury and B. S. Hetzel, eds., *Endemic Goiter and Endemic Cretinism: Iodine Nutrition in Health and Disease*, Wiley, New York, 1980; R. I. S Bayliss, and W. M. G Tunbridge, *Thyroid Disease: The Facts*, Oxford University Press, New York, 1998.

52. Stanbury and Hetzel, 1980, op. cit.

53. Baker, 1949, op. cit.

54. Quotes are from Baker, 1949, op. cit.

55. Stanbury and Hetzel, 1980, op. cit.

56. Garcia, 1989, op. cit.; see also L. C. Niessen and C. W. Douglass, Theoretical considerations in applying benefit–cost and cost-effectiveness analyses to preventive dental programs, *J. Publ. Health Dent.*, 44, 156–168, 1984.

57. W. L. Augenstein, D. G. Spoerke, and K. W. Kulig, Fluoride ingestion in children: a review of 87 cases, *Pediatrics*, 88, 907–912, 1991.

58. J. D. Shulman and L. M. Wells, Acute fluoride toxicity from ingesting home-use dental products in children, birth to 6 years of age, *J. Publ. Health Dent.*, 57, 150–158, 1997.

59. J. J. Murray, A. J. Rugg-Gunn, and G. N. Jenkins, *Fluorides in Caries Prevention*, 3rd ed., Butterworth-Heinemann Publishers, Boston, MA, 1991.

60. J. R. Mellberg and L. W. Ripa, *Fluoride in Preventive Dentistry*, Quintessence Publishing, Hanover Park, IL, 1983; see also *Am. Dent. Assoc. News*, February 5, 1979.

61. See the American Dental Association, http://www.ada.org.

62. A. R. Prest and R. Turvey, Cost–benefit analysis: a survey, *Econ. J.*, 75, 683–735, 1965.

63. Niessen and Douglass, 1984, op. cit.

CHAPTER 13

THE LIGHT AT THE END OF THE TUNNEL

If there is light at the end of the tunnel, perhaps it can serve us best through the illumination it throws on the undeniable facts and the shadows it leaves over the undeniable uncertainties. If this book has done nothing else, we hope it has clarified the facts without obscuring the uncertainties.

As promised in the introduction, some of the facts support the views of the pro-fluoridation movement, while others support those of the anti-fluoridation movement. On balance, I suspect that most readers will feel that the known facts favor the fluoridation paradigm. There seems little doubt, based on current scientific and medical understanding, that fluoridation does more good than harm. In that sense, this book provides affirmation for 60 years of public policy with respect to the fluoridation of public water supplies. However, we hope that readers will also come away with a greater sympathy and respect for the remaining uncertainties and the societal risks that these uncertainties engender. The final stance for each of us on the fluoride question rests squarely on our assessment of the degree of risk that remains and our level of aversion to it. In the following short sections we summarize the essential findings of our ramble through the complexities of the fluoridation issue, with respect to both the facts and the uncertainties.

TEETH

When all is said and done, fluoridation is about teeth. It is fitting, then, that the conclusions about teeth are among the strongest and most solidly based that we can set down.

- There has been a precipitous decline in the incidence of tooth decay among children in the years since World War II. Reductions in the incidence of this disease have been so significant that dental caries is no longer considered a major public health problem in the developed countries of the world.

- The evidence is indisputable that the decline in caries over this period is due primarily to increased fluoride intake. Better dental care, better nutrition, and improvements in dental hygiene have played an important but subsidiary role. The two main vehicles for fluoride delivery are the ingestion of fluoridated drinking water and the use of fluoridated toothpaste.

- The mechanism of fluoride action on tooth enamel is now understood to be primarily topical and post-eruptive, rather than systemic and pre-eruptive, as originally thought by the dental research community. The ingestion of fluoridated drinking water plays an important role under either mechanism.

- Reductions in tooth decay have been observed in more-or-less equal measure in fluoridated and nonfluoridated communities in the United States. These observations do not represent a disproof of the value of fluoride, as the anti-fluoridation camp claims. They can be explained by the widespread use of fluoridated toothpaste and by the "halo effect" caused by the regional distribution of processed food and beverages prepared with fluoridated water.

- Increased fluoride intake has caused a significant increase in the occurrence of dental fluorosis. Most of the increase has been in the form of very mild to mild mottling of the teeth. Pro- and anti-fluoridationists differ as to whether such levels of dental fluorosis are a minor cosmetic problem or a harbinger of more serious health problems.

Most objective observers feel that the positive social impact associated with the near-eradication of dental caries far exceeds the negative impact associated with the observed increase in dental fluorosis. Viewed from this perspective, fluoridation must be judged as an effective public health measure.

HEALTH RISK

Effective as fluoride may be in its primary goal, the real battleground of the fluoridation debate lies not with teeth but with health. The battles are fought over whether there is, or is not, chronic health risk associated with the long-term intake of fluoridated drinking water. The hostilities follow a predictable path: The anti-fluoridation camp raises health concerns; the pro-fluoridation camp tries to lay them to rest. Medical researchers contribute to the fray by means of epidemiological studies of human populations or by laboratory studies on experimental animals. Both approaches are fraught with problems. Epidemiological studies are statistical in nature, and are open to misinterpretation when the appropriate confounding factors are not carefully evaluated. Laboratory studies require questionable extrapolation from animal to human populations. The findings of both types of study are often uncertain and always controversial. As consensus slowly emerges, it has become apparent that most of the health concerns are baseless, a few remain uncertain, and a very few have merit.

- Fluorine is the most exclusive bone-seeking element known to medical science. Roughly 50% of the fluoride ingested is taken up by the mineral crystals of the body's hard tissues, the bones, and the teeth. Given this physiological response, the nexus of legitimate concern with respect to the health impact of fluoride revolves around diseases of the bone. It has long been known that excessive intake of fluoride can lead to osteosclerosis, a hardening of the bone. The severest form of osteosclerosis is a tragic disease known as crippling skeletal fluorosis, which is endemic in several third-world countries, including India and China. It arises from long-term ingestion of naturally fluoridated drinking water at concentrations exceeding 10 ppm fluoride. The disease is extremely rare in the United States, with only five documented cases in the past 35 years. People who live in North American communities that are artificially fluoridated at the usual concentration of 1 ppm are not at risk of developing crippling skeletal fluorosis.

- Results of epidemiological studies are almost evenly divided on the question of whether those who live in fluoridated communities are at greater risk of suffering hip fractures in later life than those who live in nonfluoridated communities. Recent reviewers of this body of work are unconvinced that any association between fluoridation status and the incidence of hip fractures has been identified, but the issue remains on the table.

- There is no evidence to suggest that fluoride intake is in any way responsible for loss of kidney function in otherwise healthy people. However, fluoride intake is implicated in the accelerated development of skeletal fluorosis in those who already suffer from kidney dysfunction, especially those undergoing hemodialysis. It is now recognized that dialysis treatment requires the use of deionized water to avoid the danger of fluoride poisoning.

- Long-standing claims of adverse allergic reactions from drinking fluoridated water are no longer given much credence by the medical establishment, who note the difficulties in distinguishing purported fluoride allergy from other more established allergies, the absence of a convincing immunological mechanism, and the likely role of psychological distress in most of the claims.
- There is no credible evidence to support any relationship between fluoride intake and heart disease.
- Early experimental and epidemiological evidence that linked fluoride intake with such genetic disorders as Down's syndrome and other chromosomal abnormalities has now been thoroughly repudiated.
- There have been many epidemiological studies designed to investigate a possible relationship between fluoride and cancer. All recent reviews of this body of work have concluded that there is no credible evidence that water fluoridation increases the risk of any type of cancer. The only possible exception is some equivocal evidence that fluoride intake could be implicated in the occurrence of osteosarcoma, a rare form of bone cancer, in young males. The medical establishment is extremely skeptical, and ongoing studies should clarify the situation in coming years.
- A recent epidemiological study has led to the claim that some of the chemicals used in water fluoridation could cause diminished brain development and behavioral dysfunction in children. Neurological deficits have also been observed in experimental animal studies under high dosage. The initial response of the medical research establishment to the possibility of neurotoxic effects at low fluoride intake has been skeptical. Further studies can be expected.
- Acute fluoride poisoning can result from industrial accidents that release fluoride chemicals in liquid or gaseous form from aluminum smelters (and perhaps other industrial processes) into the human environment. Fatal toxic events have been recorded. These accidents are in no way related to the fluoridation of water supplies.
- Fluoridation systems are often marginally out of compliance with regulatory requirements. More seriously, there have been several instances of fluoride releases from malfunctioning fluoridation equipment at water treatment plants over the years. Such events are rare, and the impacts societally small, but the possibility of their occurrence creates a small additional health risk in fluoridated communities.

- The acute toxic dose for fluoride can be exceeded by overingestion of home fluoride products such as fluoridated toothpastes, supplements, or mouthwashes. A large tube of fluouride toothpaste contains an amount of fluoride greater than the acute lethal dose for a small child. Care should be taken in the use and storage of such products.

In summary, it is apparent that harm can arise in special circumstances from ingesting very high doses of fluoride. The harm is most likely to appear in the form of diseases of the bone. However, there is little credible evidence of adverse health impact from long-term ingestion of drinking water that is fluoridated at the usual concentration of 1.0 ppm. Risk analyses suggest that the chronic health risk associated with a lifetime ingestion of fluoridated water is inconsequential compared with many other risks that are widely accepted by society.

DOSAGE

Fluoride is both savior and devil: A little bit of it is good for us; a lot of it can do us harm. Choosing an optinum fluoride intake involves an unavoidable trade-off between the reduced incidence of dental caries and the increased incidence of dental fluorosis. Moreover, the jury is still out on some of the bone-related health impacts. Under these circumstances, it is reasonable to ask whether the current total fluoride load in society is acceptable or whether it has reached a level where unacceptable harm could be done to some members of society.

- Fluoride is ingested into the human body from many sources. There are traces of fluoride in the air we breathe, the water we drink, and the food we eat. Some of it is natural, and some of it is placed there by humans. The anthropogenic contribution comes from fluoridated drinking water, fluoride content in foods that are processed with fluoridated water, inadvertent ingestion of fluoridated toothpastes, and fluoride supplements and mouthwashes.
- There has been a significant and continuing increase in total fluoride intake in the United States over the past 50 years due to the fluoridation of public water supplies. Under current fluoridation policy and practice, such intakes are likely to increase even more in the future.
- Total fluoride intake in fluoridated communities exceeds that in nonfluoridated communities by a factor of 2 or 3 to 1.

- An average adult (who lives in a fluoridated community, drinks a liter of water a day, uses fluoridated toothpaste, but doesn't take fluoride supplements or mouthwash) will receive a total fluoride intake in the range 2 to 5 mg/day. This is considerably less than the tolerable upper intake level set by the Food and Nutrition Board of 10 mg/day.
- There are upward of 2 million Americans who drink more than 5 liters of water a day. Representatives of this group who live in fluoridated communities, use fluoridated toothpaste, and/or take fluoride supplements, could have a daily intake that approaches or exceeds the tolerable upper intake level.
- There is considerable controversy surrounding the maximum contaminant level (MCL) for fluoride in drinking water, as set by the Environmental Protection Agency. Many critics see the value of the MCL (4 ppm) as perilously close to the concentrations that are known to cause harm (10 ppm) and consider the margin that exists between the usual concentration of fluoridated water (1 ppm) and the MCL as alarmingly thin.

Given widespread concerns about possible overdosage, there is growing agreement in the dental research establishment that a recalibration of the "optimum" fluoride concentration for drinking water may be in order. An appropriate value for the new reality may lie closer to 0.5 ppm than the traditional 1.0 ppm. It seems likely that lower fluoride concentrations, coupled with widespread use of fluoride toothpastes, would be sufficient to ensure the continued caries miracle while protecting against the unwelcome increase in dental fluorosis. There is growing recognition that fluoridation strategy should promote the lowest fluoride levels capable of producing the desired therapeutic effect.

CREDIBILITY

None of us can expect to be expert in all the issues that arise in the fluoridation debate. We are beholden to some degree to the opinions of those who ought to know. To this end, an assessment of the credibility of the various available sources of information is in order.

- The historical leadership of the pro-fluoridation movement in the United States has come from the Public Health Service. Although the PHS may at times have bowed to political expediency in downplaying the problems of dental fluorosis and even the possibility of bone-related health problems, the best available evidence suggests that their unwavering support for fluoridation is based on a sincere and well-founded belief in the societal value of reduced dental caries.

- The American Dental Association has also given steadfast support to the fluoridation movement since its inception. It has done so in the interests of improved dental health. Anti-fluoridation charges of hidden agendas and self-interested motivations on the part of the dental profession are unfounded.

- Support for fluoridation from establishment medical organizations is rock solid. Among the national and international health agencies that have specifically stated their unqualified approval are the American Cancer Society, the National Cancer Institute, the American Public Health Association, the American College of Physicians, the World Health Organization, the American Heart Association, and the American Academy of Allergy, Asthma, and Immunology.

- The great majority of individual doctors, dentists, and dental researchers favor fluoridation, but there have been a small number who have publicly declared their conversion to the anti-fluoride cause in recent years.

- Every Surgeon General and every sitting President since Kennedy has publicly endorsed fluoridation.

- Historical leadership of the anti-fluoridation movement has come primarily from the alternative and holistic medical health community, as represented by such organizations as the National Health Federation and the National Nutritional Foods Association and from a small number of zealously committed research scientists who have been willing to give up their standing in the medical establishment to fight on behalf of their anti-fluoride convictions.

- Opposition to fluoridation has also come from some quarters of the environmental movement, especially the more activist organizations such as the Natural Resources Defense Council. Perhaps the most credible of all fluoridation opponents is the union that represents the scientists and professional staff at the headquarters location of the Environmental Protection Agency. Their initial concern arose over political machinations associated with the setting of the MCL for fluoride.

- Anti-fluoridationists have not been successful in taking their case against fluoridation into the courts. No court of last resort has ever determined fluoridation to be unlawful. However, some lower courts have afforded a sympathetic hearing, and in a few cases, anti-fluoridation judgments at this level have given the pro-fluoride camp a scare until they were overturned at the appellate level.

- The anti-fluoridation camp has been more successful with the legislative branch of government than with the judicial branch. Although Congress has never passed any overtly anti-fluoridation measures, congressional hearings of one kind or another have often provided a sympathetic forum for anti-fluoride views.

- Anti-fluoridation conspiracy theories involving dark motives and secret plots on the part of government agencies, the aluminum industry, university-based industrial research laboratories, and the Manhattan Project are unconvincing and seem to be based on an overly suspicious interpretation of innocuous historical events.

- Credibility with respect to the possible health impacts of fluoridation falls more favorably on the pro-fluoride camp. They can usually point to replicated scientific studies published in leading peer-reviewed journals. The anti-fluoride camp often has to turn to maverick scientists for support, and to unpublished, unreplicated, or repudiated work. In particular, the two influential epidemiological studies of John Yiamouyiannis, the first purporting to prove the ineffectiveness of fluoride in fighting dental caries, and the second claiming a relationship between fluoridation and cancer incidence, are less credible than the establishment studies that attempt to prove the opposite.

- The most likely explanation of the often negative outcomes of fluoride referendums is risk aversion on the part of individual voters. Many citizens who vote against fluoridation probably do so because they choose to avoid the high-consequence risks (such as cancer and skeletal fluorosis), even though they judge these risks to be of low probability, rather than accept the almost certain but fairly small benefits (fewer cavities for their children).

Overall, the pro-fluoridation movement is the clear winner on the credibility front. Those to whom we usually turn for expertise on scientific, medical, and technical matters speak pretty much with one voice in favor of the fluoridation paradigm. Unfortunately, they have not always worn the victor's mantle with grace. There are many documented cases of the suppression of anti-fluoridation articles in establishment journals and the shunning of reputable scientists who developed an anti-fluoride viewpoint. These actions represent an embarrassing stain on the record of the dental research establishment.

THE NEED FOR CIVIL DISCOURSE

The greatest obstacle to progress lies in the polarity of views of the major players on both sides of the chasm. Their entrenched positions and adversarial mentality mitigate against any type of civil discourse. Their unwillingness to take into account new evidence as it comes online leads to a stagnation in viewpoint and a failure to reach available compromises. The two sides seldom talk to one another. Their research communities hold separate symposia and publish in separate journals. Their political leaders refuse to appear together on the same stage. Both sides engage almost exclusively in a spirited battle to gain the attention and support of a largely disinterested public.

If these hard positions could be softened, and this spirit harnessed for the greater good, perhaps some societal benefit could be salvaged from all these years of adversarial wrangling. If the anti-fluoridation camp could accept that fluoride is indeed responsible for stemming the tide of childhood tooth decay; if the pro-fluoridation camp could bring itself to examine the dosage problem; or if both sides could just sit down and study the health issues together with reason and respect, then perhaps this long-standing and somewhat silly dispute could finally be laid to rest.

It is even possible at some future date that good diet, good hygiene, and carefully controlled use of fluoridated toothpaste could become sufficiently universal that a rational argument could be made for the cessation of public water fluoridation. However, at this point in time, no other delivery vehicle provides the safety, efficacy, cost-effectiveness, and social equity of public water fluoridation. The entire community benefits regardless of age, educational attainment, or socioeconomic status. The benefits are derived without any direct action on the part of each citizen and without dependence on professional dental services or the ability to afford them.

The true challenge facing society is to rationally assess the huge storehouse of currently available information on fluoride and to put such an assessment to use to determine just how much fluoride is enough, how much is too much, which therapeutic strategies are best, and what combination of fluoride-delivery vehicles gets the fluoride most effectively to those who need it most.

INDEX

365